Nordic Social Polic

Nordic Social Policy
Changing welfare states

**Edited by Mikko Kautto,
Matti Heikkilä, Bjørn Hvinden,
Staffan Marklund and
Niels Ploug**

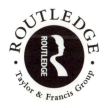

London and New York

First published 1999
by Routledge
11 New Fetter Lane, London EC4P 4EE

Simultaneously published in the USA and Canada
by Routledge
29 West 35th Street, New York, NY 10001

Routledge is an imprint of the Taylor & Francis Group

Typeset in Times by
J&L Composition Ltd, Filey, North Yorkshire
Printed and bound in Great Britain by
Biddles Ltd, Guildford and King's Lynn

British Library Cataloguing in Publication Data
A catalogue record for this book is available
from the British Library

Library of Congress Cataloguing in Publication Data
Nordic social policy: changing welfare states/
edited by Mikko Kautto *et al.*
    p.   cm.
Includes bibliographical references and index.
1. Social service—Scandinavia.   2. Scandinavia—Social policy.
3. Welfare state.   I. Kautto, Mikko, 1965–   .
HV318.N57   1999
361.948—dc21   98-49961
                                                        CIP

ISBN 0 415 20875 0 (hbk)
ISBN 0 415 20876 9 (pbk)

Contents

vi *Contents*

Figures

Tables

Contributors

Rolf Aaberge is Senior Research Fellow in the Research Department of Statistics Norway. He has worked on labour supply and taxation, unemployment, local government economics, poverty, income distribution and social welfare.

Ådne Cappelen is Director of Research at the Division for Macroeconomics and Statistics Norway. His interests are in macroeconomics, econometric modelling and defence economics.

Jon Anders Drøpping is Research Fellow and Doctoral Student in the Department of Sociology and Political Science at the Norwegian University of Science and Technology (NTNU) and affiliated with the Institute for Applied Social Science (FAFO), Oslo. His research interests are comparative social policy, active labour market policy, disability policy, policy rationale and implementation.

Johan Fritzell is Associate Professor of Sociology at the Swedish Institute for Social Research, Stockholm University. He has for several years been operative director of the Swedish level of living project and his main research interests are social inequality, income distribution research and comparative social policy.

Jørgen Goul Andersen is Professor of Political Sociology in the Department of Economics, Politics and Public Administration, University of Aalborg. He is Director of the Centre for Comparative Welfare State Studies and Co-director of the Danish Election Programme. His research fields include the welfare state, political behaviour, democracy and political power.

Björn Gustafsson is an economist and holds a position as Associate Professor of Social Work at the University of Göteborg, Sweden.

He is also a Senior Researcher in Social Policy at the Swedish Social Research Council (SFR).

Björn Halleröd is Reader in the Department of Sociology, Umeå University (Sweden). His principal research interests are distribution of economic resources, standard of living, and poverty. He has written about different theoretical definitions of poverty and explored how choices of definition influence the outcomes of empirical analysis. He is currently engaged in longitudinal research on the distribution of economic well-being and on intra-household distribution of resources.

Matti Heikkilä is Research Professor at the National Research and Development Centre for Welfare and Health (STAKES) in Helsinki, Finland. He is also Associate Professor at the University of Turku, Finland. His principal research interests are the issues of poverty, deprivation and the welfare state. He worked as a Detached National Expert in the European Foundation for the Improvement of Living and Working Conditions, Dublin, Ireland in 1997–98.

Bjørn Hvinden is Professor of Sociology in the Department of Sociology and Political Science at the Norwegian University of Science and Technology (NTNU). He has carried out research on employment policies, especially for people with disabilities, the administration of social security, and self-organisation among disadvantaged groups. He is currently co-directing a cross-national study of disability policies in a number of European countries. He is also co-ordinating a research programme on policies aimed at Travellers and their counter-strategies.

Mikko Kautto is Researcher at the National Research and Development Centre for Welfare and Health (STAKES) in Helsinki, Finland and Coordinator of the 'Nordic welfare states in the 1990s' researcher network. His research interest is in comparative welfare state research and welfare state development. He has published on European social services, social protection for the elderly and partnerships in Finland.

Juhani Lehto is Professor of Social and Health Policy at Tampere University, Finland. He has worked at the National Board of Social Welfare, at the National Research and Development Centre for Welfare and Health (STAKES) and at the WHO's Regional Office for Europe. He has published on alcohol and drug treatment systems, alcohol and drug control policies, financing and management of social and health care, reforms in social and health care and urban social policy.

Staffan Marklund was Professor of Sociology at the University of Umeå, Sweden (1990–98). Marklund has mainly been working with comparative social policy and studies of poverty and labour market exit in Sweden. At present he is Professor at the National Institute for Working Life, Sweden, working on long-term sickness, inequalities in work and health and sustainable work ability.

Nina Moss is Researcher at the Danish Institute of Clinical Epidemiology (DIKE).

Anders Nordlund is a Doctoral Student in the Department of Sociology, University of Umeå. He is currently working on a doctoral thesis on Nordic social policy development.

Peder J. Pedersen is Professor in the Department of Economics at the University of Aarhus and Research Director at the Centre for Labour Market and Social Research at Aarhus, Denmark. His current research interests are labour economics, income distribution and low income problems.

Per Arnt Pettersen is Professor of Political Science in the Department of Sociology and Political Science at the Norwegian University of Science and Technology (NTNU). He has produced several books on the development of the Norwegian welfare state and published internationally on legitimacy of welfare state arrangements, local democracy and political behaviour.

Niels Ploug graduated from the University of Copenhagen in 1985 and has since then been employed at the Danish National Institute of Social Research (SFI) in various positions, currently as Research Director. He has also worked for the Danish Government's Social Commission and for the Rockwool foundation research unit.

Tine Rostgaard, is a PhD student at the Danish National Institute of Social Research (SFI). She received her Masters Degree in European Social Policy Analysis at the University of Bath, England in 1995. Her present research project concerns social care services and cash benefits for the elderly and children in Europe.

Nina Smith is Professor of Economics at Aarhus School of Business, and Research Director at the Centre for Labour and Social

Research, CLS Aarhus University, Denmark. Her research and publications concentrate on labour supply, income distribution and poverty, gender wage gap and applied welfare analyses.

Stefan Svallfors is Senior Lecturer in the Department of Sociology at the University of Umeå, Sweden. His main research interests concern attitudes and values in the population and their links to social structure and institutions. He is currently heading the Swedish part of the International Social Survey Program, a comparative project on attitudes and values in industrialised nations. He has been a visiting scholar in London, Sydney and Oxford.

Hannu Uusitalo is Professor and Deputy Director General at the National Research and Development Centre for Welfare and Health (STAKES). He has done research since the 1970s on the level of living and income inequality in particular in the Nordic countries, on Finland in a broader comparative perspective and causes and outcomes of the welfare state in terms of living conditions. In the 1990s his research has been oriented to more politically relevant issues in Finland.

Kirsten Vik is a graduate of the cand.polit. degree in Sociology at the Department of Sociology and Political Science at the Norwegian University of Science and Technology (NTNU). Her thesis is a comparative investigation of public disability policies to influence employers in Denmark, Norway and Sweden in the period 1990 to mid-1998.

Acknowledgements

This book results from the joint efforts of a number of scholars from four Nordic countries. Our aim has been to produce a comparative study which is international both at the design level and in the analysis of data and its interpretation. The approach has necessitated deep collaboration that was made possible with financial help from Nordic bodies.

The grant from the Joint Committee of the Nordic Social Science Research Councils (NOS-S) helped to launch the study in 1996–7. The Nordic Academy for Advanced Study (NORFA) provided funding to establish the 'Nordic welfare states in the 1990s' researcher network, starting 1997. The research work was carried out with a grant from the Nordic Council of Ministers and its 'Norden och Europa' programme. We have benefited from the willingness of these Nordic bodies to promote inter-Nordic co-operation and comparative research and wish to express our warm thanks to all of them.

We also thank Laura Keeler and Sheryl Hinkkanen for improving our written English.

The editors

1 Introduction

The Nordic welfare states in the 1990s

Mikko Kautto, Matti Heikkilä, Bjørn Hvinden, Staffan Marklund and Niels Ploug

Are the Nordic welfare states facing a new era?

In international settings it has become customary to speak of the Nordic, or Scandinavian,[1] countries as a distinct unit of nations that share a variety of common features, be they in terms of geography, religion, language, history, politics or economics. A closer look reveals substantial differences in most areas, pointing to country-specific traits. Similarly, in welfare state research, by speaking of a 'Nordic (or Scandinavian) model' one can transmit a multitude of information about public policy, social policy arrangements, labour markets, etc. shown to be common to Denmark, Finland, Norway and Sweden. For those interested in a closer examination of the Nordic model, the similarities between the countries may sometimes prove arbitrary and be subjected to criticism.

Much of the literature about and around the Nordic model has been produced with data from the 'Golden era'; in the 1980s all Nordic countries were among the most prosperous industrialized countries, with good records of economic development. In all countries economic prosperity was combined with policies aiming at high levels of equality and low levels of poverty. Comparative evidence pointed to the success of the Nordic model; it was possible to combine good economic performance and social justice. The treatment of the Nordic countries as an entity already had its critics, but keeping in mind the differences in development in various spheres during the early and mid-1990s could make one even more dubious about the common practice of looking at the four countries as an homogeneous group.

The Nordic countries' political and macroeconomic development shows a picture of diverging paths since the beginning of the 1990s. Politically, the deepening of European integration has meant new questions for the welfare states in the northern corner of Europe. Finland and Sweden revised their policy in the early 1990s, applied for membership and, after a negotiation process and referendums that followed, became new members of the European Union in 1995. Norway negotiated with the European Commission about membership simultaneously with Finland and Sweden, but after referendum it opted to remain out of the Union. As Denmark has been a member since the mid-1970s, three of the Nordic countries now are EU member states, while Norway, co-operating under different rules laid out by the EEA (European Economic Area) agreement, is also affected by integration although in a slightly different manner.

The countries' domestic policy development in the 1990s has seen a period of power changes between the conservative and social-democratic parties that has perhaps not ended, but has at least challenged, the ruling position of social democrats in the governments. At least in the early 1990s, the social democrats had a weaker position in the national parliaments than in the middle of the 1980s in Sweden, Finland and Norway. In 1993 in Denmark, in 1994 in Sweden and in 1995 in Finland, social democrats were able to win back their position in the government. On the other hand, in Norway the social democrats found themselves in opposition after the elections in fall 1997.

Economically, the Nordic countries have also followed different paths. At the beginning of the decade, Sweden and Finland faced a severe recession, which ended a long period of steady economic growth. Denmark had already experienced economic difficulties from the 1970s, and for the Danes the economic developments of the 1990s have not been dramatically different compared to those of the late 1980s. Denmark's foreign debt is falling and it has achieved economic growth in the 1990s. Thanks to oil revenues Norway has been able to recover from its bank crisis and recession quickly, although from a level that never reached the depths experienced in Finland and Sweden.

From a social point of view, the unemployment trends suggest further differing paths. In Finland and Sweden unemployment has risen very sharply from the times of full employment that lasted until 1990. Denmark has had its ups and downs, leaving the country today with roughly the same unemployment rates that it had in the early 1980s. Norway has experienced some fluctuations, but overall a slowly increasing unemployment trend may be traced, although an unemployment rate of less than 5 per cent can hardly be deemed a problem in the same way as the unemployment rates in other industrialized countries.

Giving an intermediate summary of Nordic macroeconomic and political developments, one would have to draw attention to how the paths of Sweden and Finland differ from those of Denmark and Norway. Yet, there are also common elements when it comes to assessing the developments from a welfare state perspective. Noteworthy is the fact that, despite differences in economic performance, the countries seem to share a common preoccupation with the state of public finance. Growing public debt and deficit are, at least in political speeches, named as key problems. Fast-growing budget deficits have been a major preoccupation especially in Finland and Sweden during this decade, with consequences for public expenditure and the preservation of welfare states. But cuts, or at least cost-containment in public spending, are suggested not only in Finland and Sweden, but to some degree also in Denmark and, perhaps surprisingly, in Norway, although their economic situations are far better than those of their neighbours.

For some reason, during the first half of the 1990s discussion has revolved mainly around 'economic necessities' or 'constraints', and here the Nordic countries seem to share something in common. But it is not only a question of changing external conditions that have affected the four countries, but there are also internal developments that have forced politicians and administrators to rethink some aspects of the welfare state. Ageing of populations, changes in family stability and gender relations and changes in the organization of work are the most important internal factors that power the push for reforms. It is possible that these internal factors may better explain welfare state development, although their importance seems to vanish in rhetorics that stress external pressures.

In most political speeches the state of the public economy and dependency ratios have become the most crucial question for the future of the welfare state. Increased dependency ratios are mainly due to unemployment and ageing, but also other forms of 'passivity' (e.g. early retirement, disability pensions) have to be taken into account in order to form a coherent picture of dependency ratios. The fact that a considerable part of the population does not participate in gainful employment creates needs (and consequent expenditures) while it simultaneously undermines the economic sustainability of welfare state programmes by decreasing revenues. In contrast to the situation in Finland, Sweden and Denmark, where the equation is already seen as alarming, in Norway the warnings about unsustainability are dressed more in the form of future problems that nevertheless have to be solved today. So, policy-wise the preoccupations in this respect seem to have been the same. At first glance at least, there does not seem to be a uniform Nordic response to the changed circumstances. The governments in Finland and Sweden have curbed public spending by introducing cuts in the social security system starting from 1992. Reforms have been justified by citing mainly economic reasons. On the other hand, Denmark and Norway have adapted to new circumstances by changing their social security legislation in some sectors in ways that can be assessed to be a further expansion of the welfare state, questioning claims that this era is a period of retrenchment.

In sum, there are many grounds on which to claim that in the 1990s the Nordic welfare states have been under pressure to make changes in their welfare state systems. It is also true that all Nordic countries have introduced reforms, but what has remained unclear so far is *the character and direction of changes*. Have the Nordic countries entered a new era or not? Have they developed similarly?

The framework of the book

From a research point of view the differences in the preconditions for welfare state development pose an interesting starting point. According to theories of welfare state development one should expect differences also in the routes followed by the four welfare states since the beginning of the 1990s. Thus the Nordic welfare states in the 1990s provide a most stimulating research setting and research questions because external factors have affected the national economies differently and some societal development patterns seem to vary. This book aims first and foremost to give an empirically based account of the recent developments in different welfare state aspects of the Nordic countries. The empirical examination provides answers to the character of changes, but should also give material to rethink theories of welfare state development.

The framework adopted for this book is one that tries to look at the Nordic countries from a comparative, intra-Nordic perspective. This strategy may highlight the differences between the countries and challenge the prevailing view in comparative welfare state research about the uniformity of the Nordic countries. Yet again, it can bring stronger evidence in support of some particularly Nordic characteristics.

The effort arises from a combination of interests in welfare state development and in the Nordic model. First, as to welfare state development, there is a wide collection of contributions assessing the current period as one of welfare state curtailment. The common view holds that the 1990s are a different period in the long-term history of the welfare states because the period of expansion is definitely over. This assumption now prevails in the Nordic countries, too. However, despite often-heard claims about the withering of welfare states, their decline is not at all evident. Whether the Nordic welfare states have already entered a period of retrenchment and cutbacks is the main question this book tries to answer. Are there structural changes in the premises of the Nordic model? How have the Nordic welfare states reacted to pressures? Is there any proof of major curtailment? Do the Nordic countries follow a similar path of development and if not, where do they diverge and why?

Second, the existence of a Nordic model has been acknowledged in the scientific community without sharp criticism. In fact, in the modelling branch of research, it is the least controversial example and, for instance, in a relatively recently published comparative study, it is the Scandinavian group of nations which after analysis features most conspicuously as a distinctive group (Castles 1993: xxi). There are therefore good reasons to take the existence of a Nordic model as the starting point of our scrutiny, to 'revisit' the Nordic model. A diverging pattern of adjustments could cast a shadow on the existence of a special Nordic model. However, it should be emphasized that this is not a book about the Nordic model. The research interest is rather in changes over time in welfare state development of individual Nordic countries and in intra-Nordic comparison of policies and their outcomes. In the following, we consider these two interest areas which have served as the starting points for this book.

How should we interpret the recent phase of welfare state development in the Nordic countries?

In all industrialized countries the main question concerning the welfare state has become its affordability (see George and Miller 1996) or sustainability (see Koslowski and Føllesdal 1997). Balancing between available resources and expenditure-creating needs is not a new issue, of course, but it could be argued that it has entered the day-to-day politics of the Nordic countries only during this decade. In a recent book *Restructuring the Welfare State* it has been stated that we have moved from a stage of modifications to a period of restructuring

(Koslowski 1997). Other terms used that are characteristic of these times of welfare state development are 'retrenchment' or 'dismantling' (e.g. Pierson 1994, 1996); even the old term 'crisis' seems to have reared its head.

But what exactly do we mean by these notions describing the current period of welfare state development? Retrenchment points more to straightforward cutting of budgets that is based on mainly economic logic. Admittedly, retrenchment has a political connotation, too, when it is used to advocate a smaller public sector. Restructuring in turn does not mean just economic adjustments to balance the budget. It also entails questions of legitimacy and questions about the outcomes of the welfare state apparatus (Koslowski 1997), in other words the efficiency of the welfare state both in economic and social terms. Thus, to make a social reform that benefits some groups of society may well be classified under the notion of restructuring but not under the notion of retrenchment, and in this way restructuring seems to be close to the notion of adjustment.

In many ways the present discussion about the sustainability of the welfare states echoes earlier debates. At different times the discussion about welfare states has revolved around different issues. If in earlier decades the questions have touched upon issues like state involvement or equality, the prevailing debate, which started in the 1980s and has gained impetus in the 1990s, is more concerned with the relation between economy and social policy.

One can track debates about the unsustainability of welfare state arrangements to their roots in early Bismarckian social security schemes. Criticism is often both economic and political. There is a 25-year-old tradition in welfare state research on the notion of welfare state 'crisis', that in a way has combined all variants of criticism. The start has been traced to the mid-1970s' oil crisis, which gave rise to such books as *Fiscal Crisis of the Welfare State* by James O'Connor (1973), *The Political Economy of the Welfare State* by Ian Gough (1979), *Legitimation Crisis* by Jürgen Habermas (1975) and *The Contradictions of the Welfare State* by Claus Offe (1984 in English). Basically the argument put forward in these books was an analysis of the welfare state that concentrated on the state's role to both legitimize the capitalist economy and constrain its outcomes. The welfare state's crisis was seen in the light of a deeper crisis in capitalist economies. This leftist critique was complemented by criticism from the right. The 'overload' thesis argued that government functions kept on expanding, while their capacity to fulfil promises became weaker (Brittan 1977). Both Marxist and right-wing critiques agreed that a crisis existed; the disagreement was on its causes and consequences.

However, a central message from all empirical research trying to verify the existence of a welfare state crisis is that despite beliefs, assumptions and forecasts of radical changes in welfare states, empirically oriented research has shown the opposite to be true. Jens Alber could conclude in his article 'Is There a Crisis of the Welfare State?' (1988) that there were neither signs of a general welfare backlash nor of a legitimation crisis caused by the curtailments. Staffan Marklund's (1988) analysis of the developments in the Nordic welfare states from the oil crisis to the mid-1980s confirmed that the crisis debate consisted of little actual proof in the everyday practice of the Nordic welfare states. The Nordic welfare states proved to be stable. They were economically efficient, strongly work oriented, with high labour market participation also involving women and were widely publicly supported (Esping-Andersen 1985; Marklund 1988). In trying to evaluate welfare state research in an article titled 'O'Goffe's Tale', Rudolf Klein (1993) wanted to remind researchers that as there were no empirical signs of crisis, emphasis should rather be directed at analysing the welfare states' capacity to adapt to changed circumstances.

If anything, crisis debate in one form or another has proven its sustainability for a century. For a research-oriented person this should not mean that there cannot be a crisis of the welfare state. In fact, discussion about the effects of globalization on the welfare state, which has prevailed in the 1990s, seems to raise the 'crisis of the welfare states' issue again, but in a revised form. In the 1990s one is constantly confronted with views about the uncompetitiveness of European welfare states in the global market, about their high costs and consequent failures in terms of social integration. There is not much positive said for the welfare states these days.

In the rhetorics at least, it is held that in a globalized economy enterprises are forced into increased competition in world markets. Competitiveness has become the key word both for companies and national economies as well. Companies are forced to adjust their costs and states have to take side costs and social wage into account when formulating policies. Moreover, it is argued that owing to international pressures, states have less room to manoeuvre their economic policies, which in turn affects social policy (Kosonen 1994a). As Pfaller *et al.* (1991: 1) put the issue, the principles of the welfare state are at stake as: '[A]bstractly speaking, social and non-economic objectives in general might be sacrificed to the overriding priority of efficient production for highly contested markets.'

Subject to research, the often heard argument about the welfare state as a burden to the economy has remained controversial. Alfred Pfaller and Ian Gough (1991: 15–43) tried to characterize this linkage by looking at various growth indicators together with welfare state indicators in a number of nations over time, but saw no stable negative or positive relationship. Other research on the subject has not supplied definite answers about the relationship either. In the Nordic context the question is especially interesting due to high taxes and high welfare spending. Walter Korpi (1985) found no evidence to support the argument that the Nordic welfare states are economically inefficient. He later espoused the same view in replying to strong criticism especially in Sweden, where the economists have tried to dub Sweden the worst example of 'eurosclerosis' (see *The Economic Journal*, 106, for discussion about the controversy with articles by Korpi 1996, Henrekson 1996 and Agell 1996, but also Lindbeck *et al.* 1995).

Economically based criticism against the welfare state has another variant, too, expressed in the discussion on incentives. The argument holds that welfare states create disincentives to work and further undermine the work ethic and morals of the society. Evidence from studies concentrating on incentives is as controversial as that on uncompetitiveness. Here again research cannot give simple answers. In the Nordic countries it has been claimed that generous social insurances contribute to labour force participation because of the tight link of benefits to work participation (Esping-Andersen 1985). Besides, there can be efficient work enforcement rules despite high standards, i.e. high benefit levels (Marklund and Svallfors 1987; Lindqvist and Marklund 1995). On the other hand, comparative studies about compensation levels indicate that the Nordic countries might experience more incentive problems than other OECD countries, at least when measured by effective marginal tax rates (Eardley *et al.* 1996 on social assistance) or net replacement rates (*Unemployment Benefits and Social Assistance in Seven European Countries* 1995).

So, both variants of economic critique remain controversial as no final truth about the pernicious effects of the welfare state on the economy has appeared. In any case, this kind of criticism has affected policy.[2] What has research been able to say about the reaction of governments to economic criticism? Martin Rhodes (1996) recently presented two points that are relatively uncontroversial in the existing literature on welfare state adjustment. First, the welfare states have borne the cost of increasing unemployment and industrial adjustment, although the opposite, retrenchment, has probably been a more expected reaction. Rhodes refers to Garrett (1995) and Garrett and Mitchell (1995) who speak about an 'expansionary compensation effect'. Second, 'governments have failed to scale back welfare spending, even when they set out explicitly to do so' (Rhodes 1996: 307). Here Rhodes referred to Paul Pierson's analysis in his book *Dismantling the Welfare State* (1994), where Pierson suggests that the support of electorates and vested interests make the politics of retrenchment difficult to carry out, resulting in no or just minor changes in welfare state arrangements. If these two findings hold true, we seem to end up at the same conclusion as empirically oriented researchers did a decade ago: there is a lot of talk about deep problems but no incontestable evidence to support such claims.

Keeping in mind this lesson, one starting point for the book is that we will not speak about crisis, retrenchment, curtailment or any other notion that has a connotation suggesting a decline in the welfare state. We prefer to start looking at the changes using more value-neutral terms, such as restructuring, reorientation or adjustment. This is not to say that there could not be major structural adjustments. In fact, evidence from the development in the Nordic welfare states suggests that Rhodes' second point, that of governments failing to scale back welfare spending, is not true in the Nordic context. There have been major savings in some areas of social policy, especially in Finland and Sweden, that have been carried out surprisingly easily. Our stand at this point is that we are not desperately looking for signs of curtailment, but rather are trying to take account of positive restructuring as well. We thus first aim to give an assessment of the changes in the development of the four Nordic welfare states, and only then try to evaluate the nature of this much debated era in the light of the empirical evidence presented in the book.

In addition to economically oriented criticism, there are doubts about how successful the welfare state is. Many observers hold that something in the functioning logic of the Nordic welfare states has changed. First, it has often been mentioned that the questions welfare states are supposed to answer are not the same as 50 years ago. Demographic changes (mostly ageing but also new family structures), changes in the gender balance and changes in the labour market have altered the needs of people, and welfare states have had to (or soon will have to) take these into account when reforming their programmes. Although this is an obvious remark, there is not much research that has concentrated on examining changes in risks and needs with regard to welfare state development. Second, there is criticism about welfare state failures. Despite the highest social spending in GNP per head in history, the welfare states have a hard time guaranteeing security for the individual. Increasingly, this has led to questions about the efficiency and legitimacy of the welfare state. If these are more important factors for change than economic pressures, there should be no reason to talk about crisis or retrenchment whenever reforms are made. Solving problems related to needs created by dependency, addressing the issue of gender equality and working towards better social inclusion are something the welfare states have tried to solve throughout their history, and the efforts to do so should rather be looked at as positive restructuring of the welfare states. One of our tasks in this book is to assess how well the Nordic welfare states have been able to address these questions. How has the well-being of the population evolved? Is inequality rising? Are there new risk groups? Do the four countries experience problems of poverty and exclusion?

What is the Nordic model?

Typologies of welfare states can be traced from Richard Titmuss in the 1950s, but it is in the 1990s that comparative welfare state research has increasingly been occupied with typologies. Gösta Esping-Andersen's work *The Three Worlds of Welfare Capitalism* (1990) is a landmark in this respect. Esping-Andersen's interest lay in the relation of state and economy in different 'welfare-state regimes', a concept he used as the organizing concept of the book. The work builds on earlier research, where he has defined regimes to be 'the specific institutional arrangements adopted by societies in the pursuit of work and welfare' (Esping-Andersen 1987: 6). More precisely, '[R]egimes are defined in terms of the relation between politics and markets, or perhaps more appropriately, between state and economy' (Esping-Andersen 1987: 7). Francis Castles *et al.* prefer to speak of 'families of nations, defined in terms of shared geographical, linguistic, cultural and/or historical attributes and leading to distinctive patterns of public policy outcomes' (Castles 1993: xiii).

Typologists claim there exist models that differ from each other in their policy practices and outcomes. To speak about a Nordic model is not new, of course. For instance, already before Esping-Andersen's typology, there existed sketches of the 'Scandinavian model' (e.g. Erikson *et al.* 1987) laying out some typically Scandinavian characteristics. And even earlier, the works of Titmuss (1974) and of Korpi and Palme (see their forthcoming article in *American Sociological Review* for English version) referred to certain different ways of arranging social security, pointing to similarities among the Nordic countries.

So what exactly is the Nordic model? In an earlier contribution to defining the Scandinavian model the cornerstone in social policy was stated to be universalism (Erikson *et al.* 1987: vii). 'The goal [of Scandinavian welfare states] is a set of egalitarian institutions which not only give the poor access to a minimum standard of income and social services but also bring those who would otherwise have been poor closer to the general standard of their society, decrease the need of the well-to-do to develop exclusive services, and bring about some overall redistribution of income and other resources' (Erikson *et al.* 1987: viii). Esping-Andersen and Korpi (1987) named three important features: the comprehensiveness of social security systems, institutionalized social rights and solidarity accompanied by universalism. The principle of universalism has been stated to be an important reason for the high equality in the Nordic countries. The importance to the Nordic model of even income distribution accomplished through redistributive policies has also been shown (Ringen and Uusitalo 1992).

The preconditions for the Nordic model have often been addressed. Importantly, one of them is an organized and mobilized working class. Strong trade unions have in turn been in co-operation with social-democratic parties (e.g. Stephens 1979; Korpi 1988). Some stress the importance of social democracy by naming the model 'social democratic' (Esping-Andersen 1990). A high level of public support, due to the fact that the systems created were attractive also to the middle classes, has been mentioned as an important factor in the development of welfare policies (Esping-Andersen 1990). Moreover, the public service sector created jobs for women. When private employment declined in all the Nordic countries in the 1970s, public employment in the education, health and social sectors increased (Alestalo *et al.* 1991). This contributed to full employment, as a number of articles in books edited by Jon Eivind Kolberg (1991, 1992a, 1992b) stress, and to more resources for social policies.

Despite these and other numerous attempts to outline characteristics of 'Nordicness', we do not have at our disposal an undisputable list of characteristics, or one agreed set of criteria of what constitutes the Nordic model. Why is this? There has been a lot of interest in defining the important features of the Nordic model, giving a wide collection of traits but leaving uncertainty as to what these important features exactly are. The criticism of Esping-Andersen, for instance, has been targeted at the number of regimes (e.g. Leibfried 1992), their composition (e.g. Castles and Mitchell 1990), their blindness to gender differences (e.g. Orloff 1993), their neglect of services (e.g. Anttonen and Sipilä 1996) and so on. The characteristics that count depend on the perspective chosen. From a social care perspective (Sipilä 1997) the Nordic model looks different than from a health care perspective (e.g. Alban and Christiansen 1995). While Sipilä (1997) argues that social care services are a specific feature of the 'Scandinavian model' with similarities that distinguish them from other parts of the world, Alban and Christiansen (1995) realize there is no such thing as one 'Nordic approach' in the organization and financing of health care, although admittedly there is the dominance of public funding. Besides, there are of course marked differences in the development of the Nordic countries that should be taken into account while formulating general arguments about the Nordic welfare states as a unit (e.g. Flora 1986). Furthermore, as Olli Kangas has shown (1994) by analysing longitudinal patterns in social policy formation, belonging to a model is contingent upon a specific point in time as well as upon the dimension of welfare state development.

It is not our ambition to embark on the route of finding the right definition for the Nordic model. For our purposes it is enough, as Castles (1993) argues, that there are groupings of nations that to varying degrees share common historical and cultural experiences, and that these nations defined in this sense do, in some areas, appear to manifest rather similar policy outcomes. The Nordic countries do form such a group. We are interested in development trends, and for the purpose of trying to indicate the direction of change of the four countries as a group, it is helpful to have a reference point on the characteristics of the Nordic model as it existed in the 'Golden era' of the 1980s, at least as an ideal-typical construct.

It is clear that the welfare state can be approached both narrowly and broadly, and in this sense our approach adopts the narrower route of scrutinizing the welfare state mainly from the point of view of social policy, as it is understood in the Nordic context. A narrower definition is justified by our focus, which is on both welfare state inputs, meaning social security schemes, services and activation measures, and on outcomes, meaning income distribution, poverty and level of living.

This definition delimits the list of characteristics of 'Nordicness'. For the purposes of this book, we are concerned with the criteria that have been mentioned concerning our focus. Here the characteristics of the welfare state's inputs (paragraphs 1–5) and outcomes (paragraphs 6–7) are listed in an order relevant to our object of study.

1   *The scope of public social policy is large.* It encompasses social security, services, education, housing, employment, etc. with an aim to meet most basic needs.

2   The State's involvement has been strong in all policy areas. The political commitment to full employment has been based on both macroeconomic and social policies. There is of course historical variation and variation between the Nordic countries, but *an emphasis on full employment* nevertheless could be regarded as one trait. It is often *accompanied by active labour market measures* and tripartite wage-bargaining negotiations that sometimes have resulted in sociopolitical legislation as well.

3   The Nordic welfare system is based on *a high degree of universalism*, meaning that all citizens/residents are entitled to basic social security benefits and services, regardless of their position in the labour markets. There are also targeted measures, but they are applied only as a last resort safety net. It is argued that universalism has contributed to wide public support for welfare policies.

4   Income security is based on two elements. In most schemes, there is *a flat-rate basic security and an earnings-related part* for those with a work history. The strength of the central organizations of employers and employees in administering earnings-related parts of social insurances varies in the Nordic countries. Compared to other industrialized countries, the Nordic countries can be characterized as transfer-heavy states. Thus *the share of social expenditure of GNP has been high.* As public financing of transfers has been considerable, the Nordic countries also have had *high taxation.*

5   The Nordic countries have also been characterized as *service states*. The role of local democracy is strong. Social and health services are financed through taxation without high user fees, and are targeted at all residents in need. They are provided by the local authorities and, also, mostly produced by them.

6   *Income distribution* is relatively even. Both in terms of wage dispersion and disposable income, the Nordic countries have low income inequality compared to other countries. There are no big cleavages between different income groups. Partly for this

reason *poverty* rates and differences in *levels of living* have been relatively low.

7   *Gender equality* has been stated as one of the guiding principles of the Nordic welfare states. The Nordic countries have the broadest participation of women in wage labour and in most families there are two breadwinners. Social policy measures are based on *individual rights*, so women are not economically dependent on their husbands.

Focus of the book and research questions

Esping-Andersen's definition of regimes looks at the welfare state from a broad view, which often frames its questions in terms of political economy, and its interests focus on the state's larger role in managing and organizing the economy (see Esping-Andersen 1990: 1–2). On the other hand, the 'families of nations' (Castles 1993) conceptual approach is more linked to a large set of attributes affecting the welfare state. The chapters in this book have been written from a different starting point. By 'welfare state' in this book we mean state measures that via both cash benefits and services aim to redistribute resources between its members. These functions, cash benefits and services, make up the largest part of welfare expenditure and the biggest share of all public spending; this is the reason why they are often characterized as the essence of the welfare state (e.g. Wilensky 1975).

The book aims to give answers to two series of questions. The first set of questions relates to development in the welfare state system itself. How have the Nordic welfare states survived political changes, periods of economic difficulties, demographic changes and consequent pressures on financing? What has happened to welfare state measures in the Nordic countries? Are there signs of curtailment? What changes have been made? Should we speak of restructuring, curtailment or crisis? How do the Nordic countries compare in terms of adjustment patterns? Do the development trends follow a similar path? What are the similarities and differences experienced in the four Nordic countries? The second set of questions asks how the welfare and well-being of the citizens have developed during the changes in the welfare state. How have the Nordic welfare states been able to fulfil their tasks during a period of economic and political changes? Do we see widening income differences? Is there increasing poverty or social exclusion? What groups have suffered in the 1990s? The time period under study covers the years from 1980 to 1995, the 1980s being a period of 'Golden years' to start from, but the study concentrates on changes in the 1990s.

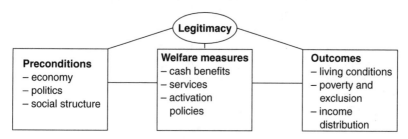

Figure 1.1 Conceptual model for the book's approach

The conceptual model behind our approach is presented in Figure 1.1. A common aim for the individual chapters is to look at actual changes and to give a concise analysis, based on comparative empirical data, of the trends during the last 10 to 15 years. In the concluding part of the book, we give a synthesis of the findings and concentrate on the relations and eventual causalities in the connections between the different dimensions of the welfare state.

As the welfare state's essence is subject to changes, the main body of the book starts with an analysis of the factors behind those changes, most importantly those of economy and politics (Chapter 2 by Staffan Marklund and Anders Nordlund). Nordic economic development is contrasted with the development of the OECD countries. In addition the chapter gives an account of shifts in political power. Besides problems in economic growth and labour market performance, the Nordic welfare states also face changes in their social structure. Recent population and family developments are examined to assess the pressures they create for the welfare states (Chapter 3 by Mikko Kautto).

The way welfare state arrangements have been adjusted to meet the changes in preconditions is examined first by looking at the social security system (Chapter 4 by Niels Ploug). Ploug's analysis puts emphasis on the institutional structure of cash benefit systems. The chapter presents the developments for different cash benefit schemes by investigating both resources and recipients. On the basis of this information major trends in developments are outlined and discussed.

These chapters are followed by an analysis of trends in the service system (Chapter 5 by Juhani Lehto, Tine Rostgaard and Nina Moss). The aim in this chapter is to study whether the characteristics attributed to the service side of the Nordic welfare states were actual characteristics of the four Nordic countries in the 1980s. Earlier studies argue that the Nordic welfare states are public service states and that they are based on the principle of universalism to guarantee services to everyone in need. A third argument has been that the services aim at equality in access and use of services and equity in health and welfare. Fourth, there is the link between female employment and services. In addition there has been discussion of the nature of the welfare state as employer and criticism of the paternalism related to the Nordic model of service provision. After an assessment of developments relating to these characteristics, the chapter will investigate whether and to what extent there is a tendency towards weakening of these characteristics in the 1990s.

We also look at how the Nordic governments have tried to shift their policies towards a stronger emphasis on 'active' measures over the period in question (Chapter 6 by Jon Anders Drøpping, Bjørn Hvinden and Kirsten Vik). A common concern in the Nordic countries has been the increasing number of people of working age living on 'passive' forms of public financial support. The chapter seeks to clarify what is meant by activation and examines the reasoning behind a turn towards activation. Furthermore, the chapter asks to what extent we can see attempts to prevent further increase in expenditure through activation measures in the Nordic countries. Are such measures adopted to the same extent or are there striking differences between the Nordic countries? To what extent have the activation measures been associated with tightening of rules for receiving cash benefits?

Besides our aim to capture in which direction and how the welfare state arrangements have altered, we intend to examine how their overall target, people's well-being, has changed during this period. Individual welfare can be seen as the outcome of individual actions in relation to at least three societal institutions, such as the welfare state, the labour market and the family. The link between changes in welfare state measures and the well-being of the population is of course not straightforward, but knowledge about their developments is imperative if one is interested in the effects of policies. The outcome side of welfare state measures is addressed in three subsequent chapters (Chapters 7, 8 and 9).

An analysis of changes in living conditions will provide a picture of the well-being of the population (Chapter 7 by Johan Fritzell). What changes in overall welfare in the Nordic countries have occurred during the last decade? Do we find the distribution of welfare to be similar in the Nordic countries? Do we find similar changes in inequality in living conditions in the Nordic countries during the last decade? Besides trying to answer these questions, the aim is to try to answer to what extent recent changes in living conditions are the outcome of changes in the systems of the welfare state and/or of other factors, such as changes more directly related to the labour market.

A look at poverty and social exclusion (Chapter 8 by Björn Halleröd and Matti Heikkilä) adds another dimension to the examination of developments in well-being. In this chapter the authors honour the Nordic tradition of utilizing level of living surveys when it comes to empirical analysis of these much discussed concepts. Poverty and social exclusion are treated as two independent but interrelated concepts. Poverty is defined as dealing with problems directly related to economic resources, while social exclusion deals with a broader range of questions concerning individuals' integration in the society. Thus social exclusion is seen as an effect of accumulation of welfare deprivation that occurs in a broad range of areas. Does the relationship between different areas of deprivation differ between countries? Does it change over time? Does it change differently in different countries? To what degree are 'classical' sociological background variables like class, gender, education and age connected with poverty and social exclusion? Answering these questions will clarify speculation about an increase or decrease in social exclusion in the Nordic welfare states.

These two analyses based on level of living surveys are complemented by documentation and analysis of changes in income distribution (Chapter 9 by Björn Gustafsson, Rolf Aaberge, Ådne Cappelen, Peder J. Pedersen, Nina Smith and Hannu Uusitalo). The idea in this chapter is first to describe the development of equivalent income in the four countries, based on national data. The chapter then moves on to an analysis of the causes of the changes. The focus is on the impact of unemployment, social policies and taxation.

Ultimately, the welfare state – as well as its reforms – depends on its legitimacy. There is a rich literature concerning the opinions and attitudes of the general public towards the welfare state, but comparative analyses are still rare because of the obvious reason that comparable data are largely lacking. Therefore we devote a part of our interest to the question of welfare state support in the Nordic countries (Chapter 10 by Jørgen Goul Andersen, Per Arnt Pettersen, Stefan Svallfors and Hannu Uusitalo). Some welfare state analysts have claimed that public support for the welfare state is declining, and this chapter examines whether a similar trend can be observed in the Nordic countries. It also asks what kind of commonalities and variations there are in the support for different welfare programmes and other state policies. Finally, the chapter examines the degrees of similarity and variation in the opinions of various population groups.

Are the structural cleavages of opinions similar or different between, say, social classes, between men and women or between the young and old in the Nordic countries? The underlying theme of this chapter is to try to find out the degree of stability in the support for the Nordic welfare states during the period under scrutiny.

The book's final chapter offers a synthesis of the findings. It concentrates on the relations between the different categories in our conceptual model and offers the editors' conclusions about welfare state developments in the 1990s in the Nordic countries.

Notes

1   The choice between using 'Scandinavian' or 'Nordic countries' is blurred in the literature. In this book we have preferred to speak about the Nordic countries, Nordic welfare states and the Nordic model. The use of 'Scandinavia' may be arbitrary and it sometimes refers only to Denmark, Norway and Sweden, whereas there is no such ambiguity with the Nordic countries. The Nordic countries are Denmark, Norway, Sweden, Finland and Iceland. To make things a little complicated, however, this study has had to leave Iceland out of the analysis. In what follows, by referring to the Nordic countries we therefore always speak of Denmark, Finland, Norway and Sweden.

2   For instance, in Finland, Prime Minister Paavo Lipponen's government programme named elimination of incentive traps as one main goal for the government, implying reforms in social policy.

2 Economic problems, welfare convergence and political instability

Staffan Marklund and Anders Nordlund

Introduction[1]

As was pointed out in the previous chapter, there is a sizeable literature arguing that the Nordic countries have devised a welfare state model distinct from the models applied in other industrialized countries. Characteristics such as a large state sector, extensive welfare provisions, high social welfare costs, high taxes, generous benefits and active labour market policies have been used by various writers to describe the degree of 'Nordicness'.

Theoretically as well as empirically, these characteristics refer to four different aspects of the welfare state: its economic foundation; its legal and administrative form; its coverage and compensation of needs among the population; and its ability to redistribute resources. The basic argument is that the Nordic countries have been able to construct a welfare state profile different from that of other nations but relatively similar to one another. Whether this was historically correct or is correct today can be analysed in different ways. This chapter provides information on the similarities and differences between the four Nordic countries with respect to some basic welfare state characteristics.

In addition to discussion of the situation in the mid-1990s, attention is also given to how the Nordic countries have changed in recent years owing to globalization of their economies and European integration (Kosonen 1994b). To what extent have the Nordic countries become more similar to other industrialized nations at large, or to other European nations in particular? Thus, this section aims to give an overview of basic economic and labour market conditions in the Nordic countries over the last 15 years. This together with a description of political structures will serve as a general background to the discussion of restructuring the welfare state in the Nordic countries.

As was described in the previous chapter, there is still some support for the argument that the Nordic countries constitute a relatively homogeneous group with respect to economic and political structures as well as with respect to welfare state institutions, welfare performance and living conditions. On the other hand, differences in historic developments and differences in vulnerability to recent external economic forces also support the idea that the four nations have become increasingly different.

A set of basic macro-level economic, political and labour market indicators can be used to examine such differences and similarities between the four countries. Information on similar indicators for the OECD nations can be used to relate the Nordic countries to other countries. The main reason for examining macro-level indicators is the need to obtain an overview without too much detail. However, it should also be pointed out that macro-level indicators, particularly those concerning economic performance and labour market conditions, have played an important role in political debate within these nations. Most political systems have become increasingly dependent on how the national economies fare in terms of public spending, growth rates and unemployment figures, as this information is presented by national or international sources. It may even be argued that politicians are becoming increasingly sensitive to market indicators and changes in interest rates in the international banking system.

The chapter is divided into two parts. The first part presents general economic indicators, indicators pertaining to the costs of social welfare and indicators pertaining to labour market conditions and unemployment. A large number of possible indicators are available and are more or less appropriate, depending on the specific question. The general idea here is to choose indicators dealing with how conditions in the different Nordic countries have changed in relation to each other and in relation to other industrialized countries. To avoid some of the problems of comparability of data, the sources are international or Nordic bodies.[2] The second part of this chapter deals with indicators of political structures. The indicators include data on national elections and Government composition during the last 15 years.

Economic crisis and economic growth

It goes without saying that the size and structure of the welfare state have at least partly been dependent on the economic situation. In general, all four Nordic countries have historically been relatively prosperous despite their relative smallness. They are rich even regarding the large differences between them in terms of their industrial level and structures, trading structures and international dependency. It is also a well-known fact that economic developments in the Nordic countries have been rather different during the last 15 years. Sweden and Finland have suffered severely from the recession of the early 1990s, whereas Denmark and Norway were affected to a much lesser degree. On the other hand, Denmark already had higher levels of unemployment than the other Nordic countries in the 1980s, and had started its restructuring of the welfare state a decade before the recession. In many respects, Norway has been spared the effects of the recession because of the large revenue from its oil resources. However, even Norway is experiencing some structural economic problems similar to those of the other Nordic nations.

One of the most used and important indicators of economic change is the annual change in the GDP per capita. However, the amount of change in the GDP is influenced by the size of the economy as well as by the relative level of the GDP, and should therefore be used with caution. The four Nordic countries are similar enough to limit the problems of comparability in this respect, and the GDP may serve as a crude measurement of their economic position (Figure 2.1).

There seems to be reason to conclude that the economy in the Nordic countries has gone through cycles during the last 15 years. In the first three years of the 1980s, Denmark, Norway and Sweden all had experience of individual years of negative or zero growth in

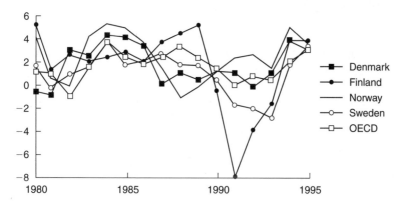

Figure 2.1 Annual percentage change in real GDP per capita in the Nordic countries and OECD average
Source: OECD 1997.

the GDP per capita. Thereafter the economies of all Nordic nations grew, and at a rate faster than that of other OECD nations for most years. In the second half of the 1980s, the Finnish economy was doing particularly well, but even the Swedish economy was prospering. After 1991, Finland and Sweden suffered severely from the effects of the international recession, while Denmark and especially Norway have continued to grow every year in terms of the GDP per capita. Finland and Sweden have both shown positive growth figures for 1994 and 1995, and are projected to have positive growth during the coming three years (OECD 1996b; Nordisk Ministerråd 1997).

Another aspect of the macroeconomy is the level of economic development. Economic prosperity, or the level of a nation's economic development, can be estimated in various ways. One problem in comparing nations is again the fact that the relative level of the economy will affect figures of change. Thus, there is a need for an indicator that takes the purchasing power of national currencies into account. Such a measure is the GDP per capita transformed into US dollars in purchasing power parities (OECD 1997). When compared to all OECD nations, the Nordic countries are close to or above the OECD average in terms of GDP per capita for most of the period after 1980. The exceptions are Finland after 1991 and Sweden after 1992. Thus, as a bloc, the Nordic countries have been, and still are, reasonably rich nations. Not surprisingly, these figures also show that Norway has been the most prosperous Nordic country in most of the period after 1980. Denmark has replaced Sweden as the second richest Nordic country, while throughout the period Finland has remained the poorest of the four nations.

Another important aspect of a national economy is how well its industry is doing in terms of external trade. A crude indicator of national industrial performance is the trade balance. Figure 2.2 shows the trade balance of the four nations.

Partly due to their relative smallness, all four Nordic countries are export-oriented over the whole period from 1980 to 1995. With the exception of Denmark in the early 1980s and individual years for the other three nations, the balance has generally been positive. In the period after 1990, all four nations made a trade surplus ranging between US$ 5 and 10 billion.

It is particularly worth noting that the 1980s were more problematic with respect to trade balances than the recession years of the 1990s. This indicates that the problems of the public economies were not fully shared by industry as indicated by its ability to generate

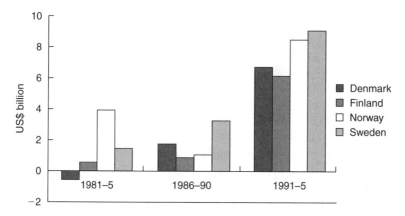

Figure 2.2 Trade balances, averages for five-year periods in the Nordic
countries (US$ billion)
Source: OECD 1997.

exports. On the other hand, the recession in the 1990s also meant that
the value of imported goods declined, owing to falls in domestic
consumption.

Big state, poor state

As pointed out in the previous chapter, one of the most visible
characters of the Nordic economies is the high level of public spending. When compared to other industrialized countries, all four
nations have high levels of public spending, but there are marked
differences between the four individual countries. The difference
between the Nordic countries and other nations has changed over
time. Figure 2.3 shows purchasing power parities of general government consumption per capita in relation to other OECD countries.
This index can be said to be a crude measure of the size of the state,
but it does not reveal anything about the 'social' character of the
state.

Denmark shows a stable relationship in government spending, at a
level some 60–70 per cent more than the average for OECD nations
over the entire period. For Finland, the relationship has a weak
tendency in the shape of an inverted u. During the first years of the
1980s, Finland was close to other industrial nations, but then
increased its public spending to a level some 20–30 per cent above
the average, the maximum being reached in 1991. In the last few

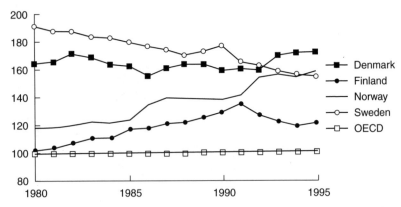

Figure 2.3 Government final consumption per capita in the Nordic countries, indices PPP OECD 100, 1980–95
Source: OECD 1997.
Note
PPP = Purchasing Power Parity.

years, Finland has reduced its relative public spending, but not very dramatically. In Norway, public consumption has grown rapidly throughout the entire period. While in the early 1980s Norway was lagging behind Denmark and Sweden in this respect, it reached the same level in the early 1990s. The trend for Sweden is opposite to that for Norway in the sense that its government consumption has been decreasing steadily since 1980. In this way Norway and Sweden have thus become rather similar, and Denmark stands out among the four nations as having the most costly state.

In the process of adjustment to external economic pressure and to the international recession, all four nations have striven to reduce spending by the public sector (Nordisk Ministerråd 1997; Benner 1997). Three interlinked dilemmas have surfaced during this process. One is how to cut public spending without increasing unemployment. The second dilemma is that unemployment itself gives rise to public costs. The third dilemma is the generation problem. The ageing of the population means increased expenditure for services, income transfers to the elderly and a decrease in resources available to meet the needs of young unemployed people and of families with children. The social policy solution to these dilemmas has usually meant that cash transfers have been more liable to cuts than services and that traditional measures of active labour market policies are preferred to cash payments. In general, the generation dilemma has been solved in favour of older citizens.

The relative lack of success in reducing public spending varies between the four countries, partly because of demographic changes and the different extent to which the individual countries were affected by the recession in the early 1990s. Differences between the countries also stem from the fact that Denmark started to take action to curb the growth in public spending in the 1980s, and from the fact that Norway is in a more favourable economic position owing to its oil resources. Thus, a visible decline in overall government spending occurred in Denmark in the 1980s, but Denmark has since been less active in this respect. Finland's government sector on the whole grew throughout the period after 1980, reaching its peak in 1993. This development is largely explained by the continuous process of reforms in welfare transfers and welfare services during the 1980s. Since 1993, a weak decline in government expenditure has occurred in Finland. In Norway, government expenditure has generally increased during the period, with a slight decline visible only for 1995. This decline, however, reflects the nation's increased prosperity more than cuts in welfare expenditure in real terms. Sweden had a rising trend of government spending in the early 1980s and a falling trend in the latter part of the decade. In the 1990s, Sweden's government expenditure again began to increase, peaking in 1993, after which there has been a moderate decline. However, Sweden has generally had higher figures of government spending than those of the other three countries, and this distinction persisted until 1993.

The level of public spending is closely related to the financial balance of the public economy, since the budget balance and international loans have usually been used to even out variations over time. Other factors that affect government financial stability include the costs for international loans, variations in national tax levels and variations in international trade.

As shown in Figure 2.4, the general government financial balance has been negative for all OECD nations every year since 1980. The deficit, which has usually been between 2 and 3 per cent of the GDP, can be seen as a crude measure of the level of unfinanced public spending. All of the Nordic countries have followed this pattern of public lending, but with some wide variations between the countries and over time.

In the first half of the 1980s, Denmark and Sweden had public deficits well over 5 per cent of their GDPs. Finland and Norway both

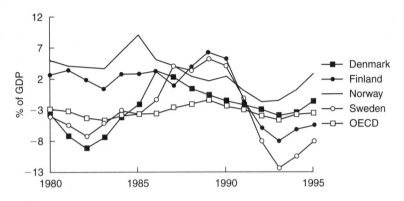

Figure 2.4 General government financial balances in the Nordic countries
        and OECD average, 1980–95
Source: OECD 1997.

had a surplus during this period. In the latter part of the 1980s, all
four nations except Denmark had, on average, a reasonable surplus.
Denmark had a small positive average during this period. During the
first half of the 1990s, Finland and Sweden had rapidly growing
public deficits and Denmark also showed negative figures. In Norway,
there were public deficits in the early 1990s but a surplus in 1994 and
1995.

Finland and Sweden, in particular, had large net lending figures
after 1992, amounting in 1993 to 8 per cent of the GDP in Finland
and 12 per cent in Sweden. Denmark began its public borrowing in
the 1980s and was also a net borrower in the late 1980s, but Denmark
did not reach the same level as Finland and Sweden in the 1990s.
Norway's financial balances were positive during the 1980s, but the
country was a net borrower in 1992 and 1993. The situation changed
again after 1994, when the balance showed a surplus.

In sum, the economic position of the Nordic countries has changed
over time. The problems encountered in the early 1980s were overcome, and the latter part of the decade was a general growth period.
This situation was again reversed by the recession of the early 1990s.
There are some differences between the four countries. Norway has
been least affected by economic fluctuations. Denmark experienced
problems earlier and was not as severely hit by the crisis of the 1990s
as were Finland and Sweden. In all four countries, the trade surplus
has been growing in the 1990s; this is a major sign that the economies

of the Nordic countries are still very strong when compared to those of competing countries. Denmark has overtaken Sweden in terms of public spending; Norway has rapidly approached these two and is now in a position very close to them. Finland, in contrast, is lagging behind despite the growth that has taken place since 1980.

High social welfare expenditure, high tax levels and shared finances

One of the major traits of the Nordic states has been devotion to social welfare. General government expenditures include all public activities and are thus not specifically related to social welfare alone. Unfortunately, strictly comparable data on social welfare expenditure in other nations are not available. In most respects, however, figures for the Nordic countries' social welfare expenditure as the share of their gross domestic product have a trend similar to that for general public spending (*Social Security in the Nordic Countries* 1996). Between 33 and 40 per cent of the gross domestic product is defined as social welfare expenditure. Table 2.1 presents some basic indicators of welfare structures, giving the situation in the mid-1990s and the change from the early 1980s. Data for the OECD are included when available.

Compared to other industrialized nations, the Nordic countries were spending a larger share of GDP on social welfare in the 1980s and 1990s. No dramatic development in this respect occurred

Table 2.1 Social spending, taxes and financial shares in ca. 1980 and ca. 1995 in the Nordic countries and OECD average

	Denmark	*Finland*	*Norway*	*Sweden*	*OECD*
Social spending as % of GDP in 1994 (change from 1983)	34(+4)	35(+14)	28(+6)	38(+4)	25(+5)
Payroll taxes and social security contributions 1994 as % of GDP (change from 1980)	34(+2)	30(+7)	30(+1)	35(+0)	14(+2)
General tax share of total social welfare spending 1994 (change from 1981)	80(−8)	49(+6)	64(+22)	55(+5)	n.a.

Sources: OECD 1996c; *Social Security in the Nordic Countries* 1996; Lazar and Stoyko 1997.

between 1980 and the mid-1990s. The four Nordic countries constitute a group where about one-third of the GDP is used for social welfare, compared to about 25 per cent in other OECD nations. The strong tendency for growth in social spending in Finland stems from the country's somewhat later introduction of costly social welfare programmes. For both Finland and Sweden, the development of social expenditures after 1991 is linked to higher costs arising from the much higher levels of unemployment in later years and with the decline in their GDP.

An important aspect of social welfare is its costs and the distribution of the cost burden. Table 2.1 presented information about tax levels. When payroll taxes, such as income taxes and social security contributions from employers and individuals, are included, the result is a picture similar to that of social spending. All four Nordic countries had tax levels close to one-third of their GDP, whereas the OECD average was around 15 per cent. There have been very minor changes in this respect over time, partly because of the general shift in most countries towards indirect taxes, such as consumer taxes.

Another notable character of the Nordic welfare states is the fact that, to a high degree, their welfare systems are publicly financed. The extent to which this was true during the 1980s and early 1990s varies between the four countries, and there have also been changes over time. The distribution of the financial burden between general taxes, employers' charges and designated contributions from citizens has changed only slightly during the last decade.

The major financial responsibility for social welfare has been borne by the state in all of the Nordic countries. General tax revenues have been used to cover between 50 per cent and over 80 per cent of the costs. Denmark has had a more clearly tax-based system than the other three nations. In Finland, the share of individual contributions has increased from 8 per cent in 1981 to 15 per cent in 1994. The same development has taken place in Denmark, where the increase in relative terms is very significant, although the share of tax revenues has remained dominant even in the early 1990s. In Norway, the trend has gone in the opposite direction, with the share of general tax revenues increasing and that of contributions from employers and individuals decreasing.

Another useful indicator of social spending is related to income transfers. These figures include the costs of cash benefits paid to individuals and households, but not the costs of welfare services. Annual OECD figures for spending on income transfers to households are not yet available for Norway after 1991 (Figure 2.5).

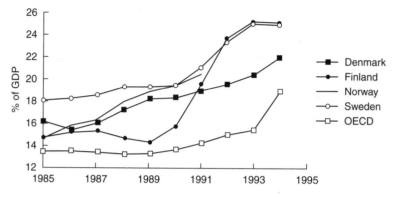

Figure 2.5 Income transfers in the Nordic countries and OECD average, 1985–94
Source: OECD 1997.

For the period 1985 to 1991, income transfers in the Nordic countries generally exceeded the OECD average for income transfers as the share of GDP by more than 5 per cent. During that period, the Nordic countries spent about 20 per cent of GDP for income transfers. Only very modest changes have occurred in the share of income transfers over time; income transfers in Finland and Sweden have shown a slight increase in the 1990s, largely owing to the costs of cash benefits paid to the unemployed. These figures provide no support for the idea that there has been a convergence of expenditure for income transfers between the Nordic countries and other industrialized countries, although the average OECD figures did rise in the 1990s. As already mentioned, the increased expenditure for income transfers that has occurred in recent years has been dependent both on ageing of the population and on increasing pressure stemming from unemployment.

The service-heavy and transfer-heavy welfare states

One of the basic ideas behind social welfare in the Nordic countries is its general and generous character. Social security provides protection for citizens in a large number of defined situations of income loss. Individuals and families are also covered by free or subsidised services related to old age, sickness, parenthood and various other situations. In addition, a number of cash transfers are distributed without regard to specific needs in the individual case. Child

Table 2.2 Transfers and services in Denmark, Finland, Norway and Sweden in 1994 as percentage of total social spending (and change from 1984)

	Denmark	*Finland*	*Norway*	*Sweden*
Services	33(−2)	32(−1)	31(−4)	35(−1)
Income transfers[a]	61(+3)	61(+0)	60(+4)	54(−2)
Cash transfers[b]	6(−1)	7(+1)	8(+0)	11(+3)
Total % (million FIM/SEK 1994)	100 (279.787)	100 (170.107)	100 (221.242)	100 (571.655)

Source: *Social Security in the Nordic Countries*, 1986, 1996.

Notes
a   Social insurance benefits: sickness and disability, old age pensions, unemployment insurance and parental leave.
b   Child allowances, child maintenance payments, housing allowances, social assistance and miscellaneous.

allowances, child maintenance payments and housing allowances are such benefits. Unfortunately, there is no available international information that would enable analysis of the qualitative aspects pertaining to the distribution of social welfare. In general, however, a number of studies indicate that the Nordic countries have been spending relatively less on means-tested benefits and more on general transfers and services. Thus, larger shares of the populations of the Nordic countries have been covered by public welfare than is the case in other nations. Table 2.2 gives information about the distribution of social spending in the Nordic countries in 1994 and changes in the last decade.

Between half and two-thirds of the national social welfare expenditure was allocated to income transfers such as pensions, sickness insurance and unemployment insurance. About one-third was used for free or subsidized services, of which health care, child care and old-age care constitute the major forms. There have been only minor changes over time with respect to the distribution between services and transfers.

The structure of social welfare expenditure and the allocation of resources to various areas and population groups are to a high degree based on the idea of a fair distribution of living conditions. A number of dimensions of equality and equity as well as of the effects on distribution and redistribution of various programmes can be discussed. Most of these aspects will be analysed in detail in Chapters 7,

Table 2.3 Income replacement ratios in unemployment and social assistance in three Nordic countries and average for four other countries in 1994 (percentage of average production worker income)

	Denmark	Finland	Sweden	F, D, GB, NL
Unemployment compensation	58	64	70	55
Social assistance	46	40	47	27

Source: *Unemployment Benefits and Social Assistance in Seven European Countries* (1995)

8 and 9. Table 2.3 presents income replacement ratios in two programmes.

As a general rule, the income replacement ratio has been higher in the Nordic countries than in some other industrialized nations. In unemployment compensation in 1994, there was variation among Denmark, Finland and Sweden, the range being between 60 per cent and 70 per cent of an average production worker's income. As to social assistance, the compensation level was just under 50 per cent of an average worker's income in 1994, which is distinctly higher than in some other European nations.

Ageing of the welfare state's population

Different areas of social welfare have accounted for slightly different shares of expenditure in the four Nordic countries, owing either to political priorities or to differences in demographic and other structural factors. In all four countries, expenditure for taking care of the elderly has been rising along with ageing of the population.

Table 2.4 Breakdown of social spending as percentage of total social spending on major areas in 1995 (and change since 1984)

	Denmark	Finland	Norway	Sweden
Families and children	12.4(+2.2)	13.3(+0.3)	14.1(+4.2)	11.4(−0.4)
Sickness insurance and health care	17.8(−3.6)	21.2(−6.7)	26.3(−14.7)	21.7(−9.0)
Old age, disability and survivors	48.2(+3.2)	47.6(+2.4)	48.4(+7.6)	49.5(+3.0)
Unemployment	14.7(−2.6)	14.3(+8.7)	6.7(−7.0)	11.1(+4.9)
Social assistance and miscellaneous	6.9(+3.4)	5.6(+3.3)	4.5(−1.0)	6.3(+5.1)

Source: *Social Security in the Nordic Countries*, 1986, 1996.

Expenditure for compensating the unemployed and for other labour market activities has increased as a result of the recession in the 1990s, but also as an effect of structural changes in the labour market. Information on how different target groups and target areas have been developing in the last decade is presented in Table 2.4.

With respect to the distribution between major target areas of social welfare, only slight differences between countries and shifts over time are found. Ageing of the population can be seen in the fact that the rate of spending for old age has been growing in all four countries. On the other hand, the fact that these costs were changing more rapidly in Norway than in the other three nations is not related to demographic differences only, but is an indication that there was more political will in this area. The same can be said about the fact that there was a distinct decline in relative cost for sickness insurance and health care in Sweden and Norway during this period. In Sweden the decline occurred in absolute figures, whereas in Norway it was only a relative decline. In neither of the two nations, however, does the decline have anything to do with improved health; instead, it is more related to a relative shift from the sick towards the old.

Institutional profile of the Nordic welfare states

The way the welfare state caters for various groups of service recipients can be studied in different ways. Finding relevant and reliable information about the quantity and quality of public services is more complicated than finding information about transfers. This is partly because services in all four Nordic countries have been provided by local authorities rather than national authorities, but it is also partly because the quality of services cannot be measured easily in overall figures. It should also be mentioned with respect to services that the need for public services has been heavily dependent on the labour market structure and on the family structure. In all four countries, the female labour market participation rate has been extremely high, as has been the rate of single households and single parents.

There has been a rapid rise in public daycare for children but a stagnation in care for old people in all the Nordic countries (see Table 2.5). The growing numbers of children receiving public daycare was related to changing labour market participation rates and ambitious plans for expansion of children's daycare in all four countries during the 1980s. It should be mentioned that the rise in the number of children receiving daycare has outstripped the growth in personnel employed to provide children's daycare. This may indicate a decline in quality.

Table 2.5 Institutional profile of social services in the Nordic countries in 1995

	Denmark	Finland	Norway	Sweden
Children in day care (1994)[a]	77.0	58.0	57.0	64.0
Children in foster care or institution[b]	15.0	7.9	7.4	6.5
People 75 and over in institutions	13.3	11.2	16.4	23.2[c]
Recipients of home-help among people 75+	45.1	22.3	27.3	29.2[c]

Source: *Social Security in the Nordic Countries*, 1986, 1996.

Notes
a   Percentage of children 3–6 years of age in day care outside of their home.
b   Percentage of children 0–20 years of age in institutional care or foster care.
c   Age group 80 years and older

There have been distinct differences between the nations in terms of their institutional profile. Denmark has had a larger share of children in daycare and in foster care than the other three nations. It has also given home-help to a much higher proportion of its elderly citizens. Norway has had a relatively higher share of its aged population in institutions.

The growth in the number of people over the age of 75 and receiving home-help has been most rapid for the oldest people in this age group. In fact, there has been a shift over time, indicating that decreasing proportions of retired people have received home-help in the 1990s as compared to the 1980s. A growing group of people above the age of 85 need more help in the home, and the distribution of home-help and other services within the retired population has become increasingly more unequal over time. These issues are discussed in more detail in Chapter 5.

Employment and unemployment

In general, the economic development of the Nordic countries is also reflected in the figures for labour market conditions. In many respects, the relationship between employment and social welfare has been a most vital part of the structure of the Nordic model. High levels of employment and low levels of unemployment form a crucial general precondition to a number of other welfare arenas, but employment and unemployment are also strongly affected by the size and structure of the public welfare system. The work orientation has

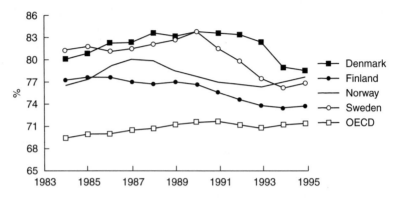

Figure 2.6 Labour market participation rates in the Nordic countries and
OECD average, 1984–95
Source: OECD 1997.

been strong with respect to how welfare benefits are distributed and
strong with respect to how the problems of the welfare state have
varied over time. Partly with the exception of Denmark, the Nordic
countries have traditionally had low unemployment rates and high
levels of labour market participation. This changed in the early 1990s
in both Sweden and Finland.

On average, the labour market participation rate has fallen by
about 5 per cent in the last decade. Compared to other OECD
countries, all four Nordic countries are still well above average
(Figure 2.6). However, as there has been a downward trend in the
Nordic countries in later years and an upward trend in most other
industrialized nations, this difference may be reduced in the future.
Norway has not had declining labour market participation rates at
all; this may be because of an increasing demand for labour and
stricter rules with regard to pre-retirement exits from the labour
market during the 1990s.

The increased levels of unemployment together with delayed labour
market entrance among the young and increasing numbers of early
exit among older workers caused a general decline in labour market
participation rates in the 1990s. Measured by labour force participation rates the decrease was rather dramatic in Denmark and Sweden
and less so in Finland. There is a general trend towards increasingly
smaller differences between the Nordic countries and the OECD
countries as well as within the Nordic countries with respect to labour
market participation.

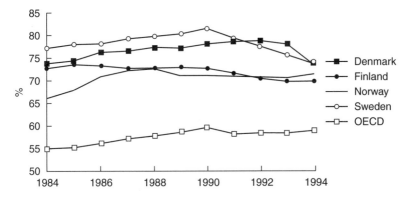

Figure 2.7 Female labour market participation in the Nordic countries and OECD average, 1984–94
Source: OECD 1997.

When the labour market participation rate is examined for women and men separately, a different picture emerges. In Norway, the rate of participation among women has been increasing, while in Denmark, Finland and Sweden, the participation rates for women have been decreasing in the early 1990s. However, the female labour market participation rate in the Nordic countries has exceeded that of other industrial nations by between 15 and 20 per cent throughout the period after 1945 (Figure 2.7). Despite the slight growth in women's participation rates that has occurred in other nations in the last few decades, and despite the slight decline in Finland and Sweden in the last few years, women in the Nordic countries continued to maintain this unique position in the mid-1990s. In Finland, the peak in women's labour market participation was reached in 1985, the corresponding peak in Denmark and Sweden being reached in early 1990s.

Closely linked with women's labour market participation is the level of public employment. Public employment has been distinctly higher in the Nordic countries than elsewhere in Europe. The growth in public employment is clearly associated with expansion of welfare state services in the 1960s and 1970s, most visible in the provision of health care services, children's daycare, education and care for the elderly.

Figure 2.8 shows that the level of public employment was almost twice as high in the Nordic countries as that in other OECD nations. Finland had a slightly lower level of public employment, partly

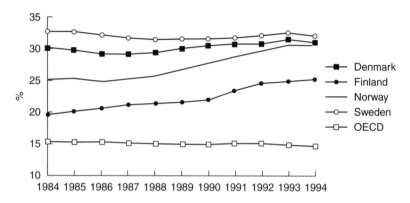

Figure 2.8 Government employment as share of total employment in the
        Nordic countries and OECD average, 1984–94
Source: OECD 1997.

because of its later expansion of welfare services. The growth in
public employment was most rapid in Norway and, contrary to the
situation in Sweden and other OECD nations, the government's
share of total employment showed no decline in Norway in the
early 1990s.

However, when we look at the annual change in government
employment, we observe that Finland and Sweden both lost a
considerable number of positions in the public sector after 1991.
In Sweden the decline in public employment was more than 10 per
cent and in Finland it was almost 8 per cent (OECD 1997). Thus,
the decline in labour market participation and the rise in unemployment during the early 1990s were not only related to the
international recession but were also partly due to decreased public
employment.

Unemployment levels have increased after 1980 in all of the Nordic
countries except Denmark, which had high levels already in the early
1980s. The most dramatic change from the 1980s occurred in Sweden
and Finland, where the unemployment rate increased by about threefold after 1991. In Finland the unemployment rate had been between
4 and 5 per cent, and it rose to over 17 per cent after 1991. In Sweden,
the rate of 2 to 3 per cent increased to almost 8 per cent in the same
period. Norway has had a more stable unemployment trend, but
there, too, an increase occurred in the 1990s (Figure 2.9).

Young people in general have higher levels of unemployment than

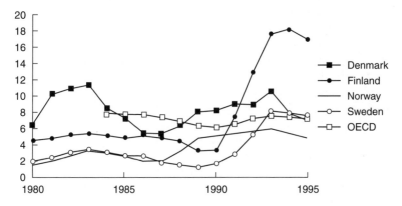

Figure 2.9 Unemployment rate in the Nordic countries 1980–95 and OECD
average 1984–95
Source: OECD 1997.

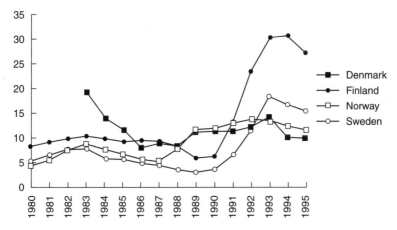

Figure 2.10 Youth unemployment rate in the Nordic countries, 1980–95
Source: OECD 1997.

other age groups. This is true for most nations and does not seem to
be determined solely by variations in the business cycle.

Inspection of unemployment rates among people under the age of
25 in the Nordic countries reveals that the figures for Denmark have
been very stable over time. The youth unemployment rate increased in
both Finland and Sweden after 1991. In Norway, the rise in
unemployment among young people had already started in the late

1980s. Thus the changes in Finland and Sweden can be seen as related to the recession, but this was not the case in Norway (Figure 2.10).

The proportion of unemployed people under the age of 25 may be used as a more sensitive indicator of the distribution of the burden of unemployment between age groups. As to this indicator, no strictly comparable figures are available for Denmark, but in the other three Nordic countries, between one in five and one in three among the unemployed are under the age of 25. However, the distribution has varied considerably between the countries. Norway has generally had a larger proportion of young people among the unemployed. It has declined only slightly, from about 40 per cent during the 1980s to one-third during the last five years. Finland, on the other hand, has the smallest proportion of young people among the unemployed. In Finland, a marked decline occurred, from about 30 per cent in the 1980s to under 20 per cent in the 1990s.

Political development

It is an understatement to say that politics matters with respect to social policy in the Nordic countries. One key feature of the Nordic countries is the state's involvement in providing its citizens with security. This means that social policy developments are closely bound to decisions made in the national parliaments and in regional and local political assemblies. The purpose of this section is to give a brief description of party politics and the parties' struggle for governmental power during the 1980s and 1990s. However, since other chapters in this book deal with specific political decisions concerning social policy, this section will focus on whether Nordic politics have undergone any significant changes during the period under scrutiny.

When analysing party politics, one obvious aspect is voter support for political parties. After all, voter support is the foundation of a democracy. Nevertheless, the executive power rests in the hands of the government. The process of forming a government has been a delicate issue in the Nordic countries during the 1980s and the 1990s, due to the fact that no party in any of the four countries has been large enough to form a majority government on its own. One alternative for resolving the ensuing situation is to form a minority government which manoeuvres from case to case. Another possible alternative is to form a coalition government. The struggle for government power has a significant impact on how parties formulate their politics. A party in a coalition government must adjust its politics in order to enable co-operation with other members of the government. A minority government must present propositions that attract enough support in the national parliament. This means that a description of politics in the Nordic countries must include both an analysis of voter support for single parties as well as an analysis of the struggle for government power.

Denmark

Voter support in Denmark after 1980 has for many parties been quite volatile (see Table 2.6). The Conservative Party gained more support in the mid-1980s, but has since then lost a considerable amount of its popularity. The trend of popular support for the Liberals, which is the other major bourgeois party, is the opposite. The number of votes cast for the Liberals has doubled since the beginning of the 1980s. Interestingly, at the centre of Danish politics there have been a rather sharp decline in votes for the Centre Democratic Party and a relatively stable trend in votes for the Radical Liberals, while the Christian People's Party has dropped out of the national parliament altogether. Support for the Progress Party, which is a populist party, has fluctuated greatly. The Social Democrats experienced a decline in voters' support in the 1980s, but have regained popularity in the two elections held in the 1990s. There was a rather sharp decline in votes for the Socialist People's Party in the late 1980s and early 1990s.

The Danish governments since the 1970s have been characterized by their weak base in the parliament; this has often led to governmental instability. In many cases this instability has called for broad

Table 2.6 Election results in Denmark, 1981–94 (percentages)

Party	1981	1984	1987	1988	1990	1994
Social Democratic Party	32.9	31.6	29.3	29.8	37.4	34.6
Conservative People's Party	14.5	23.4	20.8	19.3	16.0	15.0
Liberal Party	11.3	12.1	10.5	11.8	15.8	23.3
Socialist People's Party	11.3	11.5	14.6	13.0	8.3	7.3
Progress Party	8.9	3.6	4.8	9.0	6.4	6.4
Centre Democratic Party	8.3	4.6	4.8	4.7	5.1	2.8
Radical Liberals	5.1	5.5	6.2	5.6	3.5	4.6
Christian People's Party	2.3	2.7	2.4	2.0	2.3	1.9
Other parties	5.1	4.9	6.3	3.7	3.2	3.1
Participation	83.2	88.4	86.7	85.7	82.8	84.2

Source: Petersson 1995.

Table 2.7 Government composition in Denmark

Year	Prime Minister	Prime Minister's party	Other coalition parties		
1979	Jørgensen, A.	SDP			
1982	Schlüter, P.	Conservative	CDP	ChPP	Liberal Party
1988	Schlüter, P.	Conservative	RLP	Liberal Party	
1990	Schlüter, P.	Conservative	Liberal Party		
1993	Rasmussen, P.N.	SDP	RLP	ChPP	CDP
1994	Rasmussen, P.N.	SDP	RLP	CDP	

Source: Petersson 1995.

Notes
SDP: Social Democratic Party.
CDP: Centre Democratic Party.
RLP: Radical Liberal Party.
ChPP: Christian People's Party.

coalitions and co-operation with regard to single issues, but it has also raised questions about the definition of parliamentarism (Petersson 1995: 94). During its first six years, Prime Minister Poul Schlüter's government lost over one hundred votes in the parliament without causing the Government to fall (ibid.). The traditional definition of parliamentarism is that a government must have support in the parliament, a truth that has been challenged by Danish politics in the 1980s and the 1990s.

Table 2.7 shows the composition of Danish governments. In 1982, the Social Democrats resigned and the new government was headed by a Conservative Prime Minister for the first time in Danish post-Second World War history. Prime Minister Poul Schlüter formed a government consisting of the Conservatives, the Liberals, the Christian People's Party and the Centre Democratic Party. Schlüter's problems, stemming from the weak base in parliament, forced him to call a new election in 1983. The Conservative Party won the election and Schlüter was able to form a new government. This time the Radical Liberals joined the government, but the Christian People's Party and the Centre Democratic Party left. In 1990, Schlüter decided to call an election after a serious defeat in the parliament. He was able to form a government again, but this time with an even weaker base since the Radical Liberals decided to remain outside the government. This government was in power until 1993, when the government resigned after an investigation had shown that government ministers had been involved in shady business concerning Tamil refugees.

This time, the Conservative Prime Minister Schlüter refrained from calling an election and the Social Democrats formed a new government together with the Radical Liberals, the Christian People's Party and the Centre Democrats. In the 1994 election, the Christian People's Party lost its representation in parliament, which meant that they also left the government. In 1996, the Centre Democratic Party left the government and the current government, consisting of the Social Democratic Party and the Radical Liberal Party, was formed.

Two important observations can be made from the Danish parliamentary situation in the 1980s and the 1990s. First, Danish governments were headed by a Prime Minister from the Conservative Party during the main part of the 1980s, which was something new in modern Danish politics. Second, the Radical Liberal Party, the Christian People's Party and the Centre Democratic Party were members of governments with Prime Ministers from both the Conservative Party and the Social Democratic Party. How was it possible for the Social Democratic Party to form a government with parties having a recent history of co-operation with a conservative party? Two critical events in the early 1990s provide evidence that it was the Social Democrats who reconsidered previous standpoints and not the other three parties. The first event was the change of party leader from Svend Auken to Poul Nyrup Rasmussen. Several parties at the centre of Danish politics had indicated in 1992 that Auken was an unacceptable candidate for the post of Prime Minister (Bille 1992: 53). The election of Nyrup Rasmussen was clearly a strategic choice in order to attract parties at the centre of Danish politics. The second event was the new Social Democratic Party programme introduced in 1992. This new programme replaced the previous programme, dating back to the 1970s; it clearly indicated a shift from classic socialist thought to ideas that were more suitable for co-operation with parties at the centre of Danish politics (Bille 1993: 63). To sum up, Danish governments have experienced severe difficulties associated with their weak parliamentary base. Furthermore, Danish politics have turned to the right compared with the political situation of the 1970s.

Finland

Compared to that in Denmark, voter support for Finnish parties has been fairly stable since the beginning of the 1980s. Some changes in

Table 2.8 Election results in Finland, 1983–95 (percentages)

Party	1983	1987	1991	1995
Social Democratic Party	26.7	24.1	22.1	28.3
National Coalition	22.1	23.1	19.3	17.9
Centre Party	17.6	17.6	24.8	19.8
Left-Wing Alliance	14.0	9.4	10.1	11.2
Rural Party	9.7	6.3	4.8	1.3
Swedish People's Party	4.9	5.6	5.5	5.2
Other parties	3.8	12.0	11.0	12.3
Participation	75.7	72.1	68.4	71.7

Source: Petersson 1995; Sundberg 1996.

electoral support are, however, worth noting (see Table 2.8). Support for the Social Democratic Party declined during the late 1980s and early 1990s, but the party regained all its losses in the last election. The conservative National Coalition had stable support in the 1980s, but the 1990s has meant a decline in voter support. The Centre Party experienced a sharp increase in voter support in the election of 1991, but lost some of its gains in the 1995 election. Support for the Swedish People's Party has been fairly stable at a low level during both the 1980s and the 1990s. The result of the election of 1995 was a disaster for the Rural Party, and it ceased to exist. The Left-Wing Alliance lost a great deal of support in the election of 1987 but has experienced a slight increase in support since then.

One central character of Finnish politics after the Second World War has been governments with a weak parliamentary base. However, since the 1960s Finland must be regarded as a country with a tradition of relatively stable majority governments (Petersson 1995: 91). In many cases, this trend of majority governments has meant broad coalitions consisting of both left-wing and right-wing parties. Table 2.9 shows the composition of Finnish government since 1979.

The Social Democratic Party had a strong position after the election of 1982 and Kalevi Sorsa took over as Prime Minister after Mauno Koivisto (Jansson 1992: 162). The new government consisted of the same parties as did Koivisto's government, i.e. the Social Democratic Party, the Centre Party, the Swedish People's Party and the Communist Party. The Communist Party, however, had severe difficulties in remaining loyal to Sorsa's government, largely due to internal conflicts (Jansson 1992: 162). Sorsa decided to form a new government, without the Communist Party, later in 1982.

After the election of 1983, Sorsa decided to incorporate the Rural

Table 2.9 Government composition in Finland

Year	Prime Minister	Prime Minister's party	Other coalition parties		
1979	Koivisto, M.	SDP	Centre Party	SPP	LWA
1982	Sorsa, K.	SDP	Centre Party	SPP	LWA
1982	Sorsa, K.	SDP	Centre Party	SPP	
1983	Sorsa, K.	SDP	Centre Party	SPP	Rural Party
1987	Holkeri, H.	NC	SDP	SPP	Rural Party
1990	Holkeri, H.	NC	SDP	SPP	
1991	Aho, E.	Centre Party	NC	SPP	Christian League
1994	Aho, E.	Centre Party	NC	SPP	
1995	Lipponen, P.	SDP	NC	SPP	LWA Green League

Sources: Petersson 1995; Sundberg 1996.

Notes
SDP: Social Democratic Party.
NC: National Coalition, Conservative.
LWA: Left Wing Alliance.
SPP: Swedish People's Party.

Party as the fourth coalition party (Jansson 1992: 163). This government became long-lived and stayed in office until the election of 1987. It was also in many respects very stable despite the fact that co-operation between the Social Democratic Party and the Centre Party was not always smooth. On several occasions, signals were sent from Sorsa to the National Coalition concerning prospects for co-operation, but there was no change in government during this period (Jansson 1992: 164).

In the 1987 election, the Social Democratic Party lost support at the same time as the National Coalition gained support. Harri Holkeri from the National Coalition (Conservatives) became Prime Minister and he formed a coalition consisting of the Conservatives, the Social Democrats, the Swedish People's Party and the Rural Party. Thus, a broad left–right coalition government was created, a novel solution in Finnish politics. This government was also very stable, with the exception that the Rural Party left the government in 1990.

In the election of 1991, both the Social Democrats and the National Coalition lost voter support. The Centre Party became the largest party in the parliament. Prime Minister Esko Aho from the Centre Party formed a government together with the National

Coalition, the Swedish People's Party and the Christian League, although the Christian League left the government in 1994.

The Social Democrats regained support in the 1995 election at the same time as the Centre Party lost support. This enabled Paavo Lipponen to create a coalition government consisting of the Social Democratic Party, the conservative National Coalition, the Swedish People's Party, the Green League and the Left-Wing Alliance. This 'rainbow' coalition must of course be viewed from the perspective of Finland's severe economic crisis. However, a coalition embracing parties from left to right must be regarded as something unique in Nordic politics.

Finland has, as shown above, a strong political tradition of coalitions between left-wing and right-wing parties. This well-established tradition of co-operation has gone so far that it is possible to ask whether the left–right dimension has any substance at all in Finnish politics (Jansson 1992: 87; Lane *et al.* 1993: 219).

Norway

For several Norwegian parties, election results have been quite volatile since the beginning of the 1980s (see Table 2.10). The Conservatives realized an impressive result in the election of 1981 and obtained nearly 32 per cent of the votes. The election of 1989, however, meant a sharp decline in voter support; a decline which continued in the elections of 1993 and 1997. The Centre Party was stable at around 7 per cent during the 1980s, but gained more voter support in 1993. The election of 1997, however, meant that the Centre Party lost a

Table 2.10 Election results in Norway, 1981–97 (percentages)

Party	1981	1985	1989	1993	1997
Social Democratic Party	37.2	40.8	34.3	36.9	35.0
Conservative Party	31.7	30.4	22.2	17.0	14.3
Christian Democratic Party	8.9	8.3	8.5	7.9	13.7
Centre Party	6.7	6.6	6.5	16.7	7.9
Socialist Left Party	4.9	5.5	10.1	7.9	6.0
Progress Party	4.5	3.7	13.0	6.3	15.3
Liberal Party	3.9	3.1	3.2	3.6	4.5
Other parties	0.8	1.3	1.5	1.2	3.3
Participation	82.0	84.4	83.2	75.8	–

Source: Petersson 1995. Election results for 1997 are own calculations based on information from Stortinget.

considerable amount of its support. Between 1981 and 1993, the Christian Democratic Party had a stable support of around 8 per cent, but climbed up to around 14 per cent in the election of 1997. The Liberal Party has been fairly stable at about 4 per cent during the whole period from 1981 to 1997.

If we turn to the left of Norwegian politics, we find that the Social Democratic Party lost voter support sharply in the 1989 election. The Social Democratic Party regained some of its losses in the election of 1993, but fell back in the election of 1997. Support for the Socialist Left Party peaked in 1989, but has since experienced a decline. Finally, support for the populist Progress Party has been very volatile during the 1980s and 1990s. The Progress Party increased its voter support sharply in the 1989 election, but lost much support in the 1993 election. In the election of 1997, the Progress Party made another impressive climb in voter support, and became Norway's second largest party.

Contrary to those in Denmark, Finland and Sweden, Norwegian government coalitions have never embraced both left-wing and right-wing parties after the Second World War (Petersson 1995, 92). Furthermore, for a couple of decades, Norwegian politics has changed from parliamentary rule through majority governments to a situation characterized by unstable minority governments (ibid.). Table 2.11 shows the government compositions since the late 1970s.

Gro Harlem Brundtland followed Odvar Nordli as Prime Minister

Table 2.11 Government composition in Norway

Year	Prime Minister	Party with Prime Minister	Other coalition parties	
1976	Nordli, O.	SDP		
1981	Brundtland, G.H.	SDP		
1981	Willoch, K.	Conservative		
1983	Willoch, K.	Conservative	Centre Party	ChD
1986	Brundtland, G.H.	SDP		
1989	Syse, J.P.	Conservative	Centre Party	ChD
1990	Brundtland, G.H.	SDP		
1996	Jagland, T.	SDP		
1997	Bondevik, K.M.	ChD	Centre Party	Liberal Party

Sources: Petersson 1995.

Notes
SDP: Social Democratic Party
ChD: Christian Democratic Party

in 1981. Brundtland's government was the third Social Democratic minority government in a row since 1973. However, Brundtland took over a government struggling with multiple problems. First, the government had a weak parliamentary base (Valen and Aardal 1983: 21). Second, Norway had been experiencing economic stagnation during the 1970s (ibid.). Norway's economic problems were not as severe as they were in other countries, but clearly visible for Norwegian voters. Third, since the middle of the 1970s, the Conservative Party had been profiting from a general 'swing to the right' in Norwegian politics (ibid.; Lane *et al.* 1993: 199; Valen 1986: 177). The Social Democratic Party was unable to handle this problematic situation and was defeated in the election of 1981.

After a successful election, the Conservative Prime Minister Kåre Willoch formed a minority government with parliamentary support from the Centre Party and the Christian People's Party. In 1983, these two parties were incorporated into a majority coalition government. The election of 1985 was not particularly successful for Willoch's government. Despite a good election result for the opposition parties to the left, the Social Democratic Party was unable to form a government. Willoch's coalition government remained in office, but this time depended on the Progress Party's two seats (Petersson 1995: 92).

One year later, the Progress Party used their two seats and voted with the Social Democratic Party and the Socialist Left Party in order to defeat Willoch's government. The government crisis that followed was solved through a new minority government headed by Brundtland. Although there was a non-Socialist majority in the parliament, the Social Democratic government managed to remain in office for the rest of the election period, which ended in 1989.

The election of 1989 showed clear signs of polarization and protest (Valen 1990). The result of the 1989 election meant that Jan P. Syse formed a non-Socialist three-party government. However, disagreements on the EU issue created internal tensions and the coalition was terminated in 1990 (Narud 1995: 10). Brundtland took office as Prime Minister once again and formed a Social Democratic minority government. The election of 1993 meant continued support for a Social Democratic minority government. Again, the government's parliamentary base was weak, and it needed support from two other parties (Aardal 1994: 172). The Social Democratic government had to seek parliamentary backing partly from the left and partly from parties at the centre (Narud 1995: 11). In 1996, Harlem Brundtland resigned from her post and Thorbjørn Jagland took office as leader of the Social Democratic Party and as Prime Minister.

During the campaign prior to the election of 1997, Jagland threatened to resign if the result for Social Democratic Party was below the party's result for the 1993 election. The Social Democratic Party did not reach Jagland's target of 36.9 per cent and the government resigned as promised. A new minority government was formed by the Christian People's Party's leader Kjell Magne Bondevik, consisting of his own party, the Liberals and the Centre Party.

To sum up, the parliamentary situation during the 1980s and the 1990s has been characterized by weak minority governments (Petersson 1995: 92). Furthermore, the parliamentary situation has forced both the Conservatives and the Social Democrats to co-operate with parties at the centre (cf. Valen 1990: 288–9). Finally, during the 1980s, the Conservative Party was strong enough to claim the post of Prime Minister for the first time since the early 1960s.

Sweden

Before we scrutinize the struggle for government power, we will take a look at election results between 1982 and 1994. Table 2.12 shows that the Swedish Social Democratic Party has received a voter support well over 40 per cent in all elections with the exception of 1991. The Conservative Party has remained the second largest with around 20 per cent of the voters since 1980. Support for the Centre Party has gradually faded during the 1980s and the 1990s. The Liberal Party waged a successful election campaign in 1985, but since then it has lost voter popularity. For many years, the Left Party has been dangerously close to the 4 per cent rule, which is the minimum requirement for representation in the parliament. The Christian Democratic Party was excluded by the 4 per cent rule for many years, but managed to pass the threshold in 1991 and 1994. The Green Party entered the political stage in the beginning of the 1980s and managed to overcome the 4 per cent rule in the elections of 1988 and 1994. In the beginning of the 1990s, another new party entered the political stage. The populist New Democracy received support from almost 7 per cent of the electorate in the election of 1991. However, internal conflicts destroyed the party from inside, and it vanished from the political scene in 1994.

The election of 1976 ended a 44-year-long period of Prime Ministers from the Social Democratic Party, if the short-lived non-Socialist government of the summer of 1936 is excluded. Thorbjörn Fälldin formed a three-party non-Socialist government consisting of the Centre Party, the Liberal Party and the Conservatives. However,

Table 2.12 Election results in Sweden, 1982–94 (percentages)

Party	1982	1985	1988	1991	1994
Social Democratic Party	45.6	44.7	43.2	37.7	45.3
Conservative Party	23.6	21.3	18.3	21.9	22.4
Centre Party	15.5	9.8	11.3	8.5	7.7
Liberal Party	5.9	14.2	12.2	9.1	7.2
Left Party	5.6	5.4	5.8	4.5	6.2
Christian Democratic Party	1.9	2.6	2.9	7.1	4.1
Green Party	1.7	1.5	5.5	3.4	5.0
New Democracy	–	–	–	6.7	1.2
Participation	91.4	89.9	86.0	86.7	86.8

Source: Petersson 1995.

conflicts between the parties concerning nuclear power caused the government to collapse in 1978. Ola Ullsten, the party leader for the Liberal Party, formed a one-party minority government. After the 1979 election Ullsten's government was replaced by a new three-party bourgeois government.

The election in 1979 was a great success for the Conservative Party, but the Liberal Party and the Centre Party could not accept a Conservative Prime Minister. Thorbjörn Fälldin took office again as Prime Minister (Table 2.13). The bourgeois government was struck again by internal conflicts in 1981. The Conservatives resigned from government co-operation, owing to diverging opinions on tax policy. The election of 1982 was a disaster for the Liberal Party and to some

Table 2.13 Government composition in Sweden

Year	Prime Minister	Prime Minister's party	Other coalition parties		
1979	Fälldin, T.	Centre Party	Liberal Party	Conservative Party	
1981	Fälldin, T.	Centre Party	Liberal Party		
1982	Palme, O.	SDP			
1986	Carlsson, I.	SDP			
1991	Bildt, C.	Conservative	Centre Party	Liberal Party	ChD
1994	Carlsson, I.	SDP			

Source: Petersson 1995.

Notes
SDP: Social Democratic Party.
ChD: Christian Democratic Party.

extent also for the Centre Party. Support for the Conservative Party increased, and it was now clearly the largest party in the bourgeois camp. However, large losses for the Centre Party and the Liberal Party meant that Olof Palme was able to form a Social Democratic minority government.

The increased support for the Conservative Party meant a shift in climate in Swedish politics, and the term 'system shift' became frequently used in political debates (Hadenius 1996: 196). The Conservative Party used the term as a promise and the Social Democratic Party used the term as a threat. However, the new neo-liberal tendency in Swedish politics had little impact on the election result of 1985 and the Social Democratic Party remained in office (Hadenius 1996: 200).

Ingvar Carlsson became party leader for the Social Democratic Party as well as Prime Minister after Palme was assassinated in 1986. Carlsson was able to form a Social Democratic minority government after the 1988 election. In 1990, the government presented an austerity package which included a pay freeze, a freeze on local taxes, restrictions on trade union activities, and price and rent controls. Despite the fact that these measures were seen as concessions to the non-Socialist parties, Carlsson failed to gain the backing of a parliamentary majority for the package, and he decided to resign. The government crisis, however, was solved by reconstituting the Carlsson government and the Social Democrats remained in office.

The election of 1991 became a new 'system shift' election. During the election campaign, the Conservatives and the Liberals presented a joint election platform entitled 'New start for Sweden'. This platform argued that a fundamental change in Sweden's welfare state was necessary. Furthermore, the populist New Democracy entered the political scene, campaigning against high taxation, state bureaucracy and immigration. The election results meant great advances for the Conservatives, and the four bourgeois parties – the Conservatives, the Centre Party, the Liberal Party and the Christian Democratic Party – formed a minority government led by the chairman of the Conservative party, Carl Bildt. A Prime Minister from the Conservative Party was a new phenomenon in modern Swedish politics.

The financial market played an important role in the campaign prior to the 1994 election. Spokesmen for financial institutes argued that Sweden was close to bankruptcy and that interest rates would imminently be rising. This lack of trust in Sweden's economy had a great impact on the election campaign. It was characterized by suggested measures as to how Sweden's debt and budget deficit could be decreased. The Social Democrats also presented an austerity programme during the election campaign.

The 1994 election was a success for the Social Democratic Party. They regained all their losses in the 1991 election and were back at the same level of voter support as in the beginning of the 1980s. Ingvar Carlsson formed a one-party minority Social Democratic government. The first goal of Carlsson government was to get public finances onto a solid base. During the first period, the government sought support from the Left Party for its measures to reduce Sweden's budget deficit. In 1995, the Social Democrats decided to change partner from the Left Party to the Centre Party. This co-operation was very close, and the Centre Party was consulted prior to every major policy decision. The Social Democrats had two purposes in co-operating with the Centre Party. First, parliamentary support for policies was secured. Second, collaboration between the bourgeois parties disintegrated.

In the autumn of 1995, Prime Minister Carlsson declared that his intention was to resign from his posts as Prime Minister and chairman of the Social Democratic Party. Göran Persson was appointed to succeed Carlsson. Persson followed the same track as Carlsson, and co-operation with the Centre Party continued. Furthermore, Carlsson's austerity policy was also continued.

For a long time, politics in Sweden were characterized by relative consensus about social policy issues. There are examples of conflicts, one example being the supplementary pension system (ATP) in 1958, but once implemented, controversial policy measures were soon accepted by all political parties. The bourgeois government between 1976 and 1982 provides a good example of this relative consensus. If Swedish politics were characterized by major conflict over social policy at this time, this would have been a golden opportunity to make sweeping revisions. However, the bourgeois government showed no intentions of changing the foundations of the Swedish welfare state (Hadenius 1996: 183). Instead, the bourgeois government strove to show the Swedes that the bourgeois parties were as good as the Social Democrats in governing the country. The 1980s became a turning point. From the mid-1980s up to the present time, Swedish social policy has been fiercely attacked by right-wing parties as well as segments of the Social Democratic Party. The new spirit of the age in Swedish politics is illustrated by the bourgeois government of 1991 to 1994. This government had the explicit intention of realizing a 'system shift', which included suggestions for radical changes in Swedish social policy.

The Social Democratic Party has also been subject to ideological changes as well as strategic reconsideration. In 1981, while still in opposition, the Social Democrats supported a tax reform put forward by the Centre-Liberal government. The 'tax reform of the century' in 1989 was designed in co-operation with the Liberal Party. Finally, the strategic move to co-operate closely with the Centre Party in the mid-1990s is another indication of a re-orientation from co-operation with the Left Party to co-operation with parties at the centre of Swedish politics.

Conclusion

A number of different economic indicators show that the four Nordic countries have taken rather different paths after 1980. Finland and Sweden both experienced the effects of a deep economic crisis that followed the international recession in 1991. Denmark was affected but to a lesser degree, partly because Denmark already had higher levels of unemployment and partly because of its much earlier attempts to restructure the country's economy. Norway was the least affected, and this is largely due to its oil resources. There are signs in Finland and Sweden that the economic crisis is over now. It should also be mentioned that despite the critical problems encountered in the public economies and despite the lack of economic growth, all four countries remained prosperous on an international perspective and their export industries did rather well during the crisis.

It is evident that the Nordic countries are still different from other industrialized nations in a large number of criteria. The four differ from one another, but they differ still more from other nations. Denmark, Finland, Norway and Sweden do constitute a group that differs from other nations with respect to expenditure for social welfare, tax rates, large public service sectors, a large public transfer sector and a more active labour market policy. There are also indicators to show that the income distribution is more even and that poverty levels are lower. In most cases, the differences between the Nordic countries and other countries have not changed much. There is very weak support for the idea that there is a convergence between industrialized nations with respect to welfare state issues, despite the fact that unemployment figures are higher and welfare spending is lower in the late 1990s in the Nordic countries than they were in the early 1980s.

For several decades, political life in the Nordic countries was dominated by large Social Democratic parties. This situation changed during the 1980s. Conservative parties gradually grew while the electoral support for Liberal and Centre parties declined. For much or most of the 1980s, Denmark, Finland and Norway had coalition governments led by Conservatives. In Sweden the Social Democrats remained in office until 1991 but owing to their minority position, they had to depend on support from various partners. In the beginning of 1990, Denmark, Finland and Norway all had Conservative-led governments and in 1991 Sweden had its first Conservative administration after the Second World War. However, the situation changed in 1990 when the Social Democrats returned to office in Norway. In 1993 the Social Democrats regained power in Denmark and in 1994 the Swedish Social Democrats formed a new government. In Finland, the election of 1995 led to the formation of a broad coalition including the Social Democrats as well as the Conservative and left-wing Socialists. Consequently, Social Democratic dominance in Nordic politics has decreased and Conservative parties have made progress. Furthermore, during the 1980s and the 1990s Social Democratic parties have in many cases reconsidered their co-operation partners, changing from parties on the left of the political spectrum to parties on the right.

The emergence of new parties is another indication of a changed political structure in the Nordic countries. In Denmark the right-wing populist Progress Party had some influence during much of the 1980s. Its Swedish equivalent, New Democracy, managed to get almost 7 per cent of the votes in the election of 1991, but the party later disappeared from the political scene. In Norway, the Progress Party had a good election return in 1989, declined in 1993 and grew again in the election of 1997. The Rural Party in Finland attracted around 10 per cent in the beginning of the 1980s, but ceased to exist after a catastrophic election in 1995. Green parties have had limited influence on governmental political life in Scandinavia in general, but the Greens in Sweden and Finland have been represented in the parliament during parts of the 1980s and the 1990s. In Finland, the Green Party was also included in the Social Democratic coalition government formed in 1995.

Economic and political developments in the Nordic countries taken together, there is great potential for reform of welfare structures here. Economic pressure on the public economies, together with new structural demands, has forced governments to seek extraordinary policy measures. A clear tendency towards political reorientation together with relative government stability has offered political options for reconsidering some of the basic social welfare patterns.

However, as discussed later in this book, the extent to which social policies have undergone any fundamental changes is as yet an open question, as is the extent to which this has changed living conditions in the Nordic countries.

Notes

1 The authors wish to express their gratitude to Karolina Matti for assistance with an earlier version of this chapter.

2 The main source of information are OECD and Nordic statistics. For OECD the CD-rom version of OECD Statistics that was published in November 1997 has been used. Nordic statistics include the Yearbook of Nordic Statistics and the publication *Social Welfare in the Nordic Countries*, which has been published every three years until recently, when it became annual.

3 Changes in age structure, family stability and dependency

Mikko Kautto

Introduction[1]

In addition to problems in economic growth and labour market performance, welfare states are faced with changes in their social structure. The prominent view in the 1990s in most industrialized countries has been that age, family and employment structures especially are transforming rapidly and creating more or different social needs and risks. As social structures shift, demands on the welfare state change. Ageing alone is expected to result in more demands for income support, health care, long-term care and other services. Moreover, the traditional role of family in caring is changing as family structures change. As most visible trends imply financing pressures, most governments would go along with the conclusion reached by the OECD: 'improvements in the efficiency and effectiveness of social policies are urgent, not only because of current circumstances, but also in preparation for the future' (OECD 1994b: 12).

Yet, the interrelationship between changes in a society's social structure and its social policy is by no means explicit. There are two main reasons. First, although the starting point is that welfare state policies exist primarily to meet the needs of the population and that social structure to a great extent determines the scope of 'welfare effort', to use Wilensky's (1975) wording, there are other factors that affect the shape the policies take, such as historical legacies, cultural preferences, economic development and political choices. Second, the direction of causality obviously goes both ways; developments in the social structure affect welfare state measures, but welfare state measures surely affect developments in the social structure. A careful analysis of the implications of trends in social structure should take both of these points into account. It then becomes obvious that to draw unambiguous policy recommendations from demographic developments is not an easy task.

So the question of how changes in population and family patterns could affect welfare state priorities is trickier than most policy documents would suggest and is well worth further consideration. This chapter examines the interrelationships by first presenting the main demographic trends and then discussing some of their consequences for the Nordic welfare states. The first part of the chapter deals with two main questions. What are the changes in demographic trends in the Nordic countries? Is there convergence or divergence between the countries? The second part of the chapter discusses the consequences of factual changes in population and family patterns from a welfare state perspective. Age structure as well as family composition of a society affect the way welfare states allocate resources between different social risks. Yet, while it can be admitted that the trends affect welfare spending and welfare state development in direct and indirect ways, it is not certain how severe a 'burden' the trends entail. In analysing the implications of demographic trends other factors must be brought into the analysis.

Approach and data

The aim of the chapter is to provide the reader with a statistical overview of the demographic changes taking place in the Nordic countries and to direct the reader's attention to those areas that are of significance for welfare state development. The choice of time period in this sort of scrutiny is not without significance for interpretations. The chapter concentrates on the period from 1980 until 1995 (or to the last available year) according to the focus of this book. However, as demographic changes happen quite slowly, reference to earlier periods is sometimes needed to avoid too hasty interpretations. One should quickly add that the choice not to include projections in the analysis does not mean forecasts are meaningless. Quite to the contrary, and as will be discussed in the latter part of the chapter, it may well be that in the case of demographic developments, projections and their interpretation are more important for policy adjustments than the available evidence about actual changes in the near past.

The data for this chapter come from the four countries' Central Statistical Offices (Statistics Denmark, Statistics Finland, Statistics Sweden and Statistics Norway) and the Nordic Statistical Secretariat. Most of the statistics used in this chapter are taken from the

NOSOSCO (Nordic Social-Statistical Committee) and NOMESCO (Nordic Medico-Statistical Committee) Yearbooks, Yearbooks of Nordic Statistics and from Nordic Statistics CD-ROM, a database issued by the four Central Statistical Offices. Also Eurostat, Council of Europe and OECD statistics are used to situate the Nordic countries in a larger context.

Statistics have been compiled in the Nordic countries for many decades to show administrations the trends in social security and to make comparisons between countries possible. For instance, one of the sources used for this chapter, NOSOSCO, has existed in the Nordic countries for over 50 years, since 1946. Despite ambitions regarding comparability, the categorization of different schemes has not been an easy task because there have been enormous changes in the field of social security and because there are differences in terminology, classification rules and data collection. So one has to be aware that despite long-term work towards comparability in Nordic statistics, there still remain significant differences in practices.[2] As regards the statistics presented in this chapter, the differences in how the statistics have been compiled are probably greater for family statistics than for population data because of their different character.[3] Full comparability may never be reached, but keeping in mind the fifty-year tradition and continuing sincere work for comparability, the statistics used in this chapter should be trustworthy enough for the purpose of trend comparison.

The population grows slowly and ages surely

Before examining the trends, it has to be said that the Nordic countries have different starting points. In the future the demographic situation is expected to change most dramatically in Finland due to the postwar baby-boom experienced in the latter part of the 1940s and early 1950s, visible in the present age structure as a peak in the number of people aged around 50 years. In Denmark, Norway and Sweden the ageing of society is less pronounced than in Finland. Finland differs from the other countries also in its skewed gender balance in the elderly age groups.[4] In 1990 in the age group over 65 years there were 181 females per 100 males in Finland (Koskinen 1997). The gender balance in the other Nordic countries is more even.

As we can see from Table 3.1, the population growth in the Nordic countries has been relatively slow, between 4 per cent and 6 per cent between 1986 and 1996 (*Recent Demographic Developments in Europe* 1996). Compared to 1980, in 1995 the population in Denmark had

Table 3.1 Main population growth indicators in Denmark, Finland, Norway and Sweden, 1980–95

| | Population (thousands) | Births, deaths, migration and population changes per 1000 inhabitants | | | | | | Average life expectancy at the ages of 0 and 65* | | | |
		Live births	Deaths	Natural increase	Net migration	Population increase	Total fertility rate*	Males, 0	Males, 65	Females, 0	Females, 65
Denmark											
1980	5,123	11.2	10.9	0.3	0.1	0.3	1.65	71.2	13.7	77.3	17.5
1985	5,114	10.5	11.4	−0.9	1.9	1.0	1.42	71.5	13.8	77.5	17.7
1990	5,140	12.3	11.9	0.5	1.6	2.1	1.57	71.9	14.1	77.7	17.9
1995	5,205	13.3	12.1	1.3	5.5	6.7	1.76	72.6	14.2	77.8	17.6
Finland											
1980	4,780	13.2	9.3	3.9	−0.4	3.5	1.67	68.5	12.4	77.2	16.5
1985	4,902	12.9	9.8	3.0	0.5	3.5	1.69	70.1	13.1	78.4	17.3
1990	4,986	13.2	10.1	3.1	1.2	4.3	1.68	70.7	13.6	78.8	17.6
1995	5,088	12.3	9.6	2.7	0.6	3.3	1.82	72.8	14.5	80.2	18.6
Norway											
1980	4,086	12.5	10.1	2.4	1.0	3.3	1.77	72.2	14.1	78.7	17.4
1985	4,153	12.3	10.7	1.6	1.5	3.2	1.68	72.7	14.4	79.4	18.4
1990	4,241	14.4	10.9	3.5	0.4	3.9	1.82	73.1	14.5	79.7	18.6
1995	4,337	13.8	10.4	3.5	1.5	4.9	1.88	74.8	15.1	80.8	19.1
Sweden											
1980	8,310	11.7	11.1	0.6	1.2	1.8	1.66	72.4	14.2	78.5	17.7
1985	8,350	11.8	11.3	0.5	1.3	1.9	1.65	73.6	14.6	79.5	18.4
1990	8,551	14.5	11.1	3.4	4.1	7.4	1.95	74.4	15.1	80.2	18.9
1995	8,781	11.7	10.6	1.1	1.3	2.4	1.97	76.2	16.0	81.5	19.7

Source: Nomesco 36:1991, 38:1992, 49:1997; *Recent Demographic Developments in Europe* 1996.

Note:
* Five year averages, figures in row 1980 refer to years 1976/80, in row 1985 to years 1981/85, in row 1990 to years 1986/90 and in row 1995 to years 1991/95.

increased from 5.1 to 5.2 million, in Finland from 4.8 to 5.1 million, in Norway from 4.0 to 4.4 million and in Sweden from 8.3 to 8.8 million (NOMESCO 49: 1997: 70). These population growth figures are above the European average. The population growth can be divided into two components, natural increase and net migration, that are affected by different factors. Starting from natural population increase, one can show the growth of these populations has been largely due to increases in life expectancy rather than high birth rates. Turning to the migration component of population growth, the differences between the countries are sharp. The Nordic countries have followed different immigration policies towards migrants, with Finland and Norway taking in less immigrants than Denmark and Sweden.[5]

In most industrialized countries fertility rates have for years been too low to reproduce the population. This is the case also in the Nordic countries, although the fertility rates of the Nordic countries are among the highest in Europe. In Western Europe there has been much debate about the interlinkages between fertility rates, women's participation in the labour market and family policies. On one hand the Nordic welfare states have been criticized for being family hostile societies by debilitating traditional family values with their liberal family and reproduction policies and their emphasis on gender equality. On the other hand they have been praised for their efforts in guaranteeing equal opportunities not only in working life but in the family and society at large. Recently Esping-Andersen (1996a) has argued how the Nordic welfare regime, in contrast to other countries' regimes, allows for combining employment and family life, resulting in the Nordic countries having the highest fertility rates in Europe. While it is true that the total fertility rates in the Nordic countries are higher than in Southern Europe, the impact of social policies on fertility rates remains to be proven by research.[6] Among demographers there have been many hypotheses about high fertility rates, which have pointed out elements ranging from good economic situations, full employment and generous family policies to a reaction to the previous postponement of childbearing (Hoem 1996). There is presently no consensus on the factors affecting fertility rates and few demographers would be willing to predict how fertility will develop, even in the short run (Hoem 1996).

While the Nordic countries as a group are in the lead in European fertility statistics, there are some differences in their pattern of development, as Table 3.1 shows. The fertility rates presented are five-year averages, which evens out year-to-year changes somewhat. Starting with Denmark, one notices the drop between 1976/80 and 1981/85 and the following trend of rising fertility rates. Norway's pattern is close to that of Denmark, with a similar drop between 1976/80 and 1981/85 and a consequent rise in fertility rates since then. Finland shows a pattern of constancy between 1976 and 1990 with a sudden increase in the fertility rate in the early 1990s. Sweden experienced the increase in fertility rates earlier in the late 1980s, when the total fertility rate rose from 1.6 in 1984 to over 2 in 1990 (Hoem 1996). So while as a group the Nordic countries might look similar, in country-specific comparison their trend timing differs. This is all the more evident from a year-to-year perspective. Especially in Sweden the fertility rates have varied from year to year, showing that considerable changes can happen in a short period: In 1995 the total fertility rate in Sweden had dropped to 1.7. These fluctuations can hardly be explained by changes in family policies or in the welfare state. Unpredictable changes in fertility rates suggest it is wise to avoid unambiguous interpretations about recent trends. There might be only one acceptable conclusion: there are differences between the countries over the last two decades, but over the longer perspective (from the 1940s) we witness decreasing differences among the countries (Nord 1994: 3: 23), that clearly show a converging trend among the Nordic countries in the long term.

All Western industrialized countries show increasing life expectancies. By international comparison women and men in the Nordic countries live very long. However, in their average life expectancies the Nordic countries are somewhat different. Sweden has since early 1980s been alone at the top in average life expectancies for both women and men. The averages for the years between 1991 and 1995 show a life expectancy more than three years longer for Swedish males than for Danish and Finnish males. In the case of Denmark the difference with Sweden is also close to three years for women. In men's series, Finland has moved from the last position only during the last five-year period, leaving Denmark behind. The positions of the countries have otherwise been intact since the 1980s, with Sweden ranked first, followed by Norway and with Denmark and Finland ranking third and fourth. From a gender perspective Finland has the widest gap between the life expectancies of men and women, which in 1995 was almost seven and a half years. But again the differences are highlighted in a narrow time-perspective, as over a longer time period the Nordic countries have converged (Nord 1994: 3: 22). This convergence has taken place so that the life expectancy 'laggard',

Finland, has been able to increase life expectancies for both men and women faster than its neighbours.

Although the similarities between the countries in their internal population-growth dynamics are worth pointing out, from a welfare state perspective a decomposition of the population into shares of age groups is more important. The main indicators regarding age groups and dependency are shown in Table 3.2.

Turning first to age groups, we notice that even during this relatively short period of time between 1980 and 1995 there was a clear tendency towards ageing populations. Compared to population growth indicators, trends in this respect are more different in the Nordic countries. In absolute figures we find that during this period the size of the age group 0–14 years decreased in Denmark and Norway, while it remained stable in Sweden and Finland. In all countries the absolute size of the age groups 15–64 years and 65 years and over increased. In relative terms the picture is more complex: the size of the youngest age group decreased in all countries. The drop was sharpest, close to 3 per cent, in Denmark and Norway, and minor in Sweden and Finland (close to 1 per cent). The share of the population of working age (15–64 years) increased in Denmark and Norway, but decreased in Finland and Sweden. The ageing of society is reflected in changes in the age group 65 years and over. The size of this group has grown in all countries: the share of the population over 65 years of age increased by amounts varying from 1 per cent in Denmark to 2 per cent in Finland. The picture regarding this age group is sharpened by breaking it further into two groups, 65–79 years and 80 and over. Relative growth is mainly apparent in the 80 years and over group (Nordic Statistics on CD-Rom 1996).

For policy analysts demographic trends are of interest chiefly because they describe in a reliable and concise way the development in the numbers and proportions of population in their active or passive ages. There are basically two ways that have been used to describe this dual division of populations. The first, the crude dependency ratio, can easily be calculated from the population statistics. The dependency ratio, calculated as the share of those 0–14 years and those over 65 years of age to those between 15–64 years will give a figure of the balance between age groups. In Table 3.2 this dependency ratio is referred to as the 'age dependency ratio'. A little more elaborate dependency ratio will attempt to count as dependent all those not working, as there are people over 65 who are still working and there are people between 15–64 not working. Reaching an accurate figure for the latter indicator is a more tricky task that should

Table 3.2 Age group shares, age dependency ratios and economic dependency ratios in Denmark, Finland, Norway and Sweden, 1980–95

	Mean population (thousands)			Employed (thousands)	Age group shares, %			Age dependency ratio (0–14 + > 65)/15–64	Economic dependency ratio Employed/total population
	0–14 years	15–64 years	over 65 years	over 65 years	0–14 years	15–64 years	over 65 years		
Denmark									
1980	1,068	3,317	738	2,473[a]	20.8	64.7	14.4	0.54	0.48
1985	943	3,399	771	2,543	18.4	66.5	15.1	0.50	0.50
1990	876	3,463	802	2,604	17.0	67.4	15.6	0.48	0.51
1995	901	3,517	800	2,557	17.3	67.4	15.3	0.48	0.49
Finland									
1980	971	3,236	572	2,328	20.3	67.7	12.0	0.48	0.49
1985	952	3,339	612	2,437	19.4	68.1	12.5	0.47	0.50
1990	963	3,356	667	2,467	19.3	67.3	13.4	0.49	0.49
1995	973	3,407	720	2,068	19.1	66.8	14.1	0.50	0.41
Norway									
1980	906	2,577	603	1,913	22.2	63.1	14.8	0.59	0.47
1985	831	2,669	653	2,014	20.0	64.3	15.7	0.56	0.48
1990	803	2,746	692	2,030	18.9	64.7	16.3	0.54	0.48
1995	845	2,810	696	2,079	19.4	64.6	16.0	0.55	0.48
Sweden									
1980	1,628	5,328	1,354	4,232	19.6	64.1	16.3	0.56	0.51
1985	1,517	5,394	1,439	4,243	18.2	64.6	17.2	0.55	0.51
1990	1,535	5,494	1,522	4,485	18.0	64.2	17.8	0.56	0.52
1995	1,663	5,614	1,540	3,986	18.9	63.7	17.5	0.57	0.45

Source: Nordic statistics on CD-Rom 1996; *Recent Demographic Developments in Europe* 1996; Yearbooks of Nordic Statistics, *Aktuell nordisk statistik* nr 35, 1996; and own calculations based on their figures.

Note:
a No labour force sample survey was held in 1980 in Denmark, so the figure for employed persons is for 1979.

take into account not only age group shares but also all kinds of other factors, especially unemployment figures, labour participation rates, social security arrangements affecting job participation (such as early retirement, parental leaves, sick leaves, etc.) and their changing nature. There are many ways to calculate such dependency ratios, some being more accurate than others. Probably the easiest way to do this is to compare the share of those employed to the total population, as is done in Table 3.2. This latter ratio is referred to as the 'economic dependency ratio'.

The lower the age dependency ratio is, the 'more favourable' the age structure. The lower the economic dependency ratio is, the 'less favourable' the burden of support. When the economic dependency ratio is 0.50 it means there is one person supported for each employed person. If the ratio is less than 0.50, there are more of those being supported than those contributing to this support.

The two ways of looking at dependency ratios show interesting differences in the situations in the four countries. Looking first at the age dependency ratios we notice that in 1980 Norway had the least favourable age structure. There has been a slight increase in the share of the population of working age since then. The age structure of Denmark in turn has followed a trend of 'improving' age dependency ratios, starting from only a little better level than Norway and Sweden in 1980 but in 1995 having the most favourable age structure of the four countries. In contrast to Denmark, Finland, who had the most favourable age dependency ratio in 1980, has felt a slight increase in the share of those not of working age. Thus the age structure of Finland in 1995 is close to that of Denmark. For Sweden age dependency ratios show very minor changes during this period. Thus the countries' recent development trends move in different directions, but with the overall result of decreasing differences.

The economic dependency ratio shows a different picture, of course, as it is sensitive to the development in employment situations.[7] Here we see that the economic dependency ratio for Denmark in 1995 shows basically the same situation as in 1980, with a little improvement until 1990 and then a fall in the early 1990s. For Norway also, the situation between 1980 and 1995 remained very stable. The Swedish economic dependency ratios show in a clear way the effect of unemployment between 1990 and 1995. For Finland, with the worst unemployment rate and the sharpest drop in employment, the drop in the economic dependency ratio from 1990 to 1995 is particularly visible.[8]

Thus, the age structure in the mid-1990s seems to have been most favourable in Denmark and Finland, but when the employment situation is taken into account, Finland falls a long distance behind all its neighbours. The difference between Denmark and Finland in the mid-1990s was considerable. The leading position of Denmark despite its relatively high unemployment rates is also worth pointing out. Interestingly, Norway, with the best situation regarding official unemployment rates, does not fare better than Denmark with this measure. Further explanation for differences in economic dependency ratios can be sought from labour force participation rates. All the Nordic countries have had high labour force participation rates (see e.g. OECD 1996e), but this similarity hides the fact that the participation rates are very different for different age groups. Finland deviates from the other three countries with its high early-exit rates, especially in the age groups 55–59 years and 60–64 years. In Finland in 1995 the percentage share of pensioners in the age group 55–59 years was 32.3 per cent and in the age group 60–64 years 80.6 per cent. Percentages for the other Nordic countries for the respective age groups are 19.7 per cent and 38.7 per cent in Sweden, 24.6 per cent and 39.1 per cent in Norway and 26.4 per cent and 59.6 per cent in Denmark (NOSOSCO 6: 1997: Table 7.4. For a discussion of early retirement in the Nordic countries see Øverbye 1997). Interestingly, the arithmetical average age of early retirement in 1994 was about 58 years in Finland, Norway and Sweden (NOU 1994: 2: 303), despite differences in the prevalence of early retirement.[9]

To give a reference point, one could compare the economic dependency ratios of the Nordic countries to OECD averages. In this comparison, the Nordic countries are still above OECD average; their economic dependency ratios have all these years been more favourable due to higher than average labour force participation rates. However, one can detect in the OECD figures a gradual increase in labour force participation rates in other countries; this has affected the economic dependency ratios in such a way that the exceptional status of the Nordic countries in relation to other OECD countries has slowly eroded during the last two decades, while in intra-Nordic comparison the Nordic countries seem to have become less similar.

'Standard' family histories are over

The forces at work behind family changes are different from yet connected to population developments. The role the family plays in society affects population trends. The family, in turn, is affected by economic and social policies of the state, for instance via the standard of living, the opportunities for women to participate in the labour market, legislation concerning nuptiality, family obligations, inheritance, etc. The family is a key institution to be considered also because developments in the family sphere affect the need for social policies.

Before the examination a word of warning may be appropriate, as despite the notion of 'family' being a part of our everyday vocabulary, the concept is not as self-evidently clear. A family is supposed to share, besides life events, accommodation and income also. Yet it can be quite hard to try to draw the boundaries of family membership. Family is an institution with a changing nature. For various cultural, historical, economic and political reasons the definition of family is different in each of the Nordic countries. It is often a domain of not only blood-ties, but also of other personal ties that make it a delicate area of scrutiny. Partly for this reason statistics also gather information about households, which is a broader concept than family.

These warnings notwithstanding, it is possible to draw attention to some uniquely Nordic characteristics in the family sphere. In contrast to some other parts of Europe the concept of family in the Nordic countries is limited to two generations. It encompasses the parent(s) with children or a couple without children, but does not include grandparents, not to speak of parents-in-law. This is partly due to housing arrangements, as it is a notable exception to find three generations living in the same quarters, but also to differences in legislation as there is no maintenance liability. Of relevance to family policies is also the fact that welfare state measures in the Nordic countries are in principle based on individual claims, i.e. benefits and services are available on need for each person, not for a family as a unit. In a recent comparative study (Millar and Warman 1996) on family obligations the European countries were divided in three groups based on differences in family law, social care provision and eligibility for income transfers. Denmark, Finland, Norway and Sweden were categorized as one group that is 'emphasizing individual autonomy'.

Demographers have drawn attention to the fact that trends concerning families are very similar in all the industrialized countries. Without doing too much violence to differing realities in various countries, one could argue that since the 1960s family structures have diversified so that there are now different kinds of families, but also more people living alone. Families have become smaller, there are fewer marriages and more cohabitation, there are more divorces, there are more children born outside marriage and there are more people living on their own (Hallvarsson 1994: 45). In compiled reports about demographic development (e.g. *Recent Demographic Developments in Europe* 1997; *The Demographic Situation in the European Union* 1995) the Nordic countries are usually referred to as a single group because these trends are more pronounced in the Nordic countries than elsewhere. Yet under an intra-Nordic focus the similarities may vanish. Joachim Vogel (1991: 150) pointed out in his survey-based *Social Report for the Nordic Countries* on living conditions in the late 1980s that there are significant variations in the Nordic countries in family formation. In the late 1980s Sweden had most single persons, the lowest marriage rate and Swedish mothers gave birth older. Do these differences remain in the mid-1990s? To give an up-to-date picture of the family trends and the situation in the mid-1990s, statistics on marriages, divorces and average age of childbearing are presented in Table 3.3.

The 'crude marriage rates' obtained by number of marriages per 1,000 average population show how marriage as an institution has become weaker in the long run. Since the 1940s marriages in the Nordic countries have decreased to a third, as in Denmark, or nearly halved as in the other countries (Yearbooks of Nordic Statistics). The development trends from the latest 20 years show that the decrease in marriage rates has continued in Finland, Norway and Sweden. However, in Denmark there has been a revitalizing trend since the low in 1980. Marriages have become rarest in Sweden, where the crude marriage rate was only 3.8 per 1,000 in 1995. A more sophisticated measure is the 'total first marriage rate for females below the age of 50'. This measure highlights the development in Denmark, as the rate has increased from 0.53 in 1980 to 0.67 in 1995. Meanwhile there have been rate drops of similar magnitude in Finland (from 0.67 to 0.57), Norway (from 0.65 to 0.55 in 1990) and Sweden (from 0.53 to 0.44) (*Recent Demographic Developments in Europe* 1996).

During the same period, divorces became more common. After a significant leap in the early 1970s, divorce rates continued to increase in Finland and Norway. Meanwhile, the development in divorce patterns during the last 20 years has been relatively stable in Sweden and Denmark. Overall, the four countries show remarkably similar crude divorce rates in the mid-1990s. A look at the statistics on divorces per 1,000 married women in the Yearbook of Nordic Statistics 1996 (Tables 38, 68) and at total divorce rates in the *Recent Demographic Developments in Europe* 1996 (Table 2: 5) confirms the development trend in Finland and Norway. However, in this latter measure Sweden is similar to Finland and Norway. These figures also

Table 3.3 Marriages, divorces and mean childbearing age in the Nordic countries, 1980–95

	Crude marriage rate (marriages per 1,000 average population)	Total first marriage rate for females below the age of 50	Crude divorce rate (divorces per 1,000 average population)	Total divorce rate	Mean childbearing age
Denmark					
1980	5.2	0.53	2.7	0.40	26.9
1985	5.7	0.57	2.8	0.46	27.7
1990	6.1	0.60	2.7	0.44	28.3
1995	6.7	0.67[a]	2.5	0.44[a]	29.1[a]
Finland					
1980	6.1	0.67	2.0	0.28	27.2
1985	5.3	0.59	1.8	0.28	27.9
1990	5.0	0.57	2.6	0.41	28.4
1995	4.6	0.57	2.7	0.47	28.8
Norway					
1980	5.4	0.65	1.6	0.25	26.7
1985	4.9	0.57	1.9	0.33	27.4
1990	5.2	0.55	2.4	0.40	28.0
1995	4.8[a]	n.a.	2.5[a]	n.a	28.8
Sweden					
1980	4.5	0.53	2.4	0.42	27.8
1985	4.6	0.53	2.4	0.45	28.5
1990	4.7	0.55	2.3	0.43	28.5
1995	3.8	0.44	2.6	0.50	29.1[a]

Source: *Recent Demographic Developments in Europe* 1996: Tables T2:1, T2:2, T2:4, T2:5 and T3:5.

Note:
a Figure for 1994.

bring further, although weak, evidence that divorce was becoming less common in Denmark in the 1990s than in the 1980s. It is too early to say whether this heralds a comeback of marriage in Denmark or whether it is just a temporary phenomenon that can be detected only in the statistics, but anyway these trends in both marriage and divorce are different from those in the other Nordic countries. In comparison to Western Europe the Nordic countries have the highest divorce rates (surpassed only by the UK) (*Social Portrait of Europe* 1996: 50).

Marriage and divorce statistics are very closely tied to legislative changes.[10] Divorce has been made much easier than it was not long ago. The most widespread 'new' form of family life is cohabitation. It is difficult to assess the importance of marriage and divorce trends, as cohabitation blurs the picture obtainable from the statistics on family changes. It has been pointed out that cohabitation can often be regarded as a pre-stage of marriage (e.g. Melkas 1993; Hoem 1996) and that when a couple have a child, cohabitation is usually super-seded by marriage. Owing to its recent origins and witnessing of generational differences, cohabitation is also much more popular in younger age groups than among older age groups. Although trends in marriages seem to be very similar in the Western countries, cohabita-tion as its 'substitute' is not a universal phenomenon for different reasons. In Europe the Nordic countries seem to be the 'front-runners' in the popularity of cohabitation. In Southern European countries a phenomenon called 'living-apart-together' is more com-mon (Nikander 1997). As there is no reason to believe pair-making should be more common in Northern Europe than in Southern Europe, one is drawn to conclude that in the Nordic countries marriage is no longer the norm for making couple relations public. Since the mid-1970s it has become common and acceptable to live together without being married. Aksel Hatland and Anne Skevik (1996) point to this trend saying that over a remarkably short period of time, cohabitation has changed from being a social scandal to being a normal and widely approved family type.

Since the 1970s, the Nordic countries seem to have followed a similar pattern of women having children at a later age, and in the case of several children, at shorter intervals (Hallvarsson 1994: 46). Having children at a later age has meant that the time period for a couple to be childless has become longer (Nikander 1997). It is also worth noticing that the number of couples without children has increased, partly because of postponing childbearing and increased time spent together after children have moved out, but partly also because the number of couples who cannot have children is increasing (Ritamies 1996). Historically new also is the fact that couples decide not to have children. Furthermore, notice should be made of the fact that marriage and having a child are no longer strongly correlated. The main difference at the turn of the decade between the countries seemed to be in the number of extramarital births. According to earlier surveys on statistics, almost half of newborn babies were born outside marriage in Denmark and Sweden (Hallvarsson 1994: 50; Vogel 1991: 154). In 1990 there was a big difference between Sweden with the highest rate of extramarital births (51.8 per cent) and Finland with the lowest (22.9 per cent); Denmark and Norway had rates of 46.1 per cent and 38.6 per cent, respectively (Therborn 1995: Table 14.8). However, since then the Finnish rate has rapidly increased, showing a converging trend for the Nordic countries here, too (Nikander 1997; *Recent Demographic Developments in Europe* 1997).

The trends in marriage and divorce are very much connected to the two other family trends selected for investigation in this chapter, the types of family and the structure of dwelling households in terms of number of members. Table 3.4 shows how similar the four countries are in terms of family types. Only a cross-sectional picture presenting the situation in 1994 is available here. The table presents family compositions by counting families with children under 18 years as families with children. In interpreting the table one should notice differences in the countries' age structures, e.g. Sweden's population with its older age structure naturally has fewer families with children.

The percentage of families without children ranges from 23.4 per cent in Norway to 26.7 per cent in Denmark. For families with children the order is reversed with 18.3 per cent in Denmark and 21.9 per cent in Norway. At least one third of the family units are married: the lowest figure for married couples (34.4 per cent) is found in Sweden, and the largest in Norway (41.7 per cent). Norway also has the largest share (6.0 per cent) of single-parents.

Looking at the statistics on population by type of family, the countries show similar trends in the decrease of the share of married couples among families with children (NOSOSCO 2: 1995, 1993). In just three years from 1990 to 1993 the share dropped by 3 per cent to 4 per cent in Denmark, Finland and Norway. In Sweden the share remains the same. Increases have occurred both in the share of cohabiting couples and in singles. In a European-wide comparison there are many more single-parents in the Nordic countries (*Social Portrait of Europe* 1996: 51). However, the figures presented in

Table 3.4 Family units by living arrangements and number of children under 18 years of age in Denmark, Finland, Norway and Sweden, percentages, 1994

Family unit	Denmark	Finland	Norway	Sweden
All family units, thousands	2,858	2,680	2,019	4,736
Married cohabiting couple without children	21.0	19.5	23.4	20.0
Married cohabiting couple with children	14.4	17.2	18.3	14.4
Unmarried cohabiting couple without children	5.7	5.1	n.a.	4.6
Cohabiting couple with children	3.9	2.8	3.6[a]	3.1
Women not living in couple without children	25.3	27.1	48.6[b]	27.2
Men not living in couple without children	25.1	24.3		26.7
Women not living in couple with children	3.7	3.5	5.3	3.3
Men not living in couple with children	0.5	0.5	0.7	0.6
Other living arrangements	0.5[c]		0	
Total, %	100	100	100	100

Source: Figures from Yearbook of Nordic Statistics 1996, Table 23 and own calculations.

Notes:
a   Unmarried, cohabiting couple with at least one biological child.
b   Total figure for women and men not living in couple without children.
c   Includes registered partnerships (couples of the same sex) and children under 18 years of age not living with either of their parents.

NOSOSCO statistics and in the Eurostat publication differ considerably, probably due to differences in how cohabiting couples are treated in the statistics (Miettinen 1997). The distribution within single-parent families shows women are more often single-parents than men, as is the case also in the rest of Europe (*Social Portrait of Europe* 1996). The share of single-parent men in the four countries ranges from 12 per cent in Finland to 15 per cent in Sweden. The NOSOSCO statistical yearbook emphasizes that the number of children living with only one adult in reality is smaller, as many single-parents cohabit with someone (NOSOSCO 2: 1995: 30).

The changes in household structure are closely linked to developments in family trends. From statistics about household structures we can also detect the gradual withering of the 'traditional nuclear family', if understood in terms of a family composed of a mother, father and child(ren).

There were many more households in the mid-1990s than in 1980, and the growth in the number of households has been quicker than the population growth.[11] The growth in the number of households varies from 9 per cent in Sweden to 11 per cent in Denmark, 13 per cent in Norway and 16 per cent in Finland calculated from 1980 to the last available year. The growth has been concentrated among one-person households. In Denmark and Finland also the share of two-person households has grown a little. In all countries the growth in one-person households has been about the same, close to 6 per cent. In 1990 four out of ten Swedes lived alone. Other countries followed closely, with one-third of the households being one-person households. In Table 3.5 one can also detect the shift to smaller households in all Nordic countries; although the total number of households has grown, in relative terms the number of households with three or more members has declined.

After this statistical examination it should now be possible to answer the question whether the Nordic countries have followed similar development patterns. Most demographic indicators show similarities and increasing convergence between the countries, so the answer to the first question posed in this chapter would be yes, notwithstanding the fact that the way convergence has occurred is not uniform in all areas. For instance, although the direction of change in most areas is indeed similar, there are small variations in timing. Also, the trends may at times head in different directions, but owing to different starting points the overall result could still be diminished differences between the countries.

The main difference between the countries can be found in net migration owing to different immigration policies, but beyond this the rest of the major trends are alike. The Nordic populations are becoming older due to increased life expectancies and declining birth rates. This trend also has a gender dimension, as there are more women than men in the elderly age groups (e.g. Nord 1994: 3; NOMESCO 49: 1997). Recent family trends have been much sharper than population trends, yet they have attracted less attention than ageing. Regarding family trends the patterns are also very similar in all countries: people marry less often and later, and if they do so, the marriages tend to be less durable. Being single is more common than before, so is cohabitation. Furthermore, divorced people set up new families. The borderline between being single and being married has become less distinct and it has become clearly and widely accepted that family histories do not follow a standard path. These developments are also reflected in the statistics on household composition.

Table 3.5 Dwelling households by number of members in Denmark, Finland, Norway and Sweden, 1980–95

| | Number of households, thousands | Total population in dwelling households, thousands | Households by number of members, % | | | | | |
			1	2	3	4	> 4	Total, %
Denmark								
1980	2,069	5,027	29.5	31.4	15.8	16.0	7.3	100
1985	2,121	4,984	31.2	32.2	15.5	15.1	6.0	100
1990	2,229	5,028	33.5	33.0	15.1	13.4	5.0	100
1995	2,315	5,109	35.3	33.1	14.3	12.3	4.9	100
Finland								
1980	1,782	4,708	27.0	25.7	19.4	17.6	10.2	100
1985	1,888	4,840	28.2	27.3	18.4	17.2	8.9	100
1990	2,037	4,927	31.7	29.4	16.3	14.8	7.8	100
1993	2,120	5,004	33.8	29.5	15.4	13.7	7.6	100
Norway								
1980	1,524	4,046	27.9	25.8	16.3	17.9	12.0	100
1990	1,751	4,206	34.3	26.3	15.2	16.0	8.2	100
Sweden								
1980	3,498	8,132	32.8	31.2	15.0	14.7	6.3	100
1985	3,670	8,168	36.1	31.4	13.6	13.4	5.5	100
1990	3,830	8,181	39.6	31.1	12.3	11.8	5.2	100

Source: Yearbook of Nordic Statistics 1996, Table 104 and own calculations based on the figures.

Note:
Years presented are different because in Denmark and Finland data can be obtained from population registers; in Norway and Sweden, from population censuses.

There are more households today than 20 years ago and they are smaller in size.

What are the consequences of demographic trends?

Turning now to the second area of interest in this chapter it may be asked what kinds of consequence these trends have for the welfare state. This is a broad question which is often posed, but where no unambiguous scientifically-based answers exist because some of the parameters are simply not known. As policy-makers should always try to design policies that prepare for the consequences of known trends, it is important that at least some issues are raised for discussion, despite the fact that the data presented in this chapter about *what* the changes are does not allow for making conclusions about *how* exactly trends affect the welfare state.

The implications of changes in the age structure for resource allocation can be summed up in two ways. First, the decrease in the number and share of children during the last 15 years should, other things being equal, mean *less* social spending on families and children. The rise in the number and share of people over 65 years of age in turn should lead, again other things equal, to *increased* expenditure on pensions, health care and social care services if the present standard of benefits and services is maintained, let alone improved. The net impact of ageing increases costs because people are dependent on the welfare state longer at the end of their life cycle than at the beginning. Thus ageing still seems to be the key challenge, as is well known. Financing pressures are caused not only because bigger cohorts reach pensionable age, but also because the time spent in retirement has become much longer due to increases in life expectancy. The falling fertility rate, which is one of the most important aspects of demographic change shaping the age structure of the population, slowly results in an increase in the proportion of pensioners to working-aged people, which, in turn, puts pressure on pay-as-you-go pension systems (on the relations between ageing and pensions see, for example: Hougaard Jensen and Nielsen 1995 on Denmark; Kruse 1995 on Sweden; and Forss 1997 on Finland). Furthermore, the pension systems are maturing, i.e. the average pensions are growing larger.

Pay-as-you-go funding has part of its rationale in intergenerational solidarity, but there have been warnings about conflicts between generations, as it seems the pension burden for those employed will be significantly heavier in the future. In discussions about the ageing of society, it is not just a question of the proportion of elderly and possible pension financing problems. It is also a question of welfare state priorities and about the way society will take the elderly into account. This is something David Thomson (1996) has called the 'ageing of the welfare state'. The prominent discussion in international organizations like the OECD, the WHO and the EU about ageing is much concentrated on changes in the numbers of young people and old people. This is just one side of the picture, the other being that welfare state priorities have in the long run shifted from prioritizing children and youth to prioritizing the elderly (Thomson 1996). One good motivation for continuing debate on ageing and intergenerational relations could come from becoming aware of the changing nature of social risks,[12] not solely from cost-oriented calculations about the number of benefit receivers and contributors that is most visible in today's talk about dependency ratios.

Assessing the future burden of care seems to be even more difficult than calculating the sustainability of pension schemes. It is certainly true that the old are not a single homogeneous group (Schulte 1996; Walker and Maltby 1997). With more careful scrutiny one could see that population trends are different with regard to subgroups in the category of persons over 65 years of age. In some countries ageing means a bigger group of active 'young old persons', in others ageing means an increase in 'old persons in need of care'. From this viewpoint ageing (in the sense of reaching the age of 65) is not the point; rather the issue is functional abilities and the way old people participate in society.

Family trends also have consequences for social needs, posing some challenges for the welfare state. There are both economic and ideological concerns over this development. Single parents are more often in need of support for housing, income and care. Hatland and Skevik (1996) argue that single people are more vulnerable to social problems – the fewer you are to share the risks, the greater the possibility you need help from outside. Single-parent families cause most concern as they are more prone to experience economic disadvantage; besides, most single parents are women, which adds a gender dimension to the problem (for a focused discussion on developments in single-parenthood and public policy concerns see OECD 1990b). Smaller households imply that care may be needed from outside the household.[13] The weakening role of the traditional family in the Nordic countries would thus increase the demand for both income transfers and services.[14] Gustafsson *et al.* (1997) investigated the economic well-being of single parents and the consequences of growing up in a single-parent family in Sweden. They found that the economic level of single parents in Sweden was good in the sense there were remarkably few below the poverty level. This is the success side of the Nordic income transfer policies. While investigating possible long-term consequences they found that women and men who had grown up in single-parent families, although not earning less than those growing up with both biological parents, were over-represented among recipients of social assistance (Gustafsson *et al.* 1997). Although there are some indications that new family patterns tend to raise social spending, there are hardly any calculations or systematic research available about this relationship. This could be an area for further research.

In European discussions about family trends there is a moral dimension that is missing in discussions about ageing. Many would like to return the family to its idealized state, where the family is a solution to social ills rather than a source of social problems (Smart 1997). Smart has argued that in England the New Right criticism recognizes only one kind of family organization as legitimate. 'Broken homes produce social misfits who, in turn, produce broken homes', goes the argument (Smart 1997: 304). Depending on whether policy-makers see family trends as being irreversible or not, they have a choice in policies. Smart argues that in England policies affecting the family have been introduced in terms of how they will restabilize the family, or how they will reinforce parental responsibility (Smart 1997). It could be argued that in the Nordic countries the family trends are widely accepted and therefore present a starting point for social policies rather than an issue to be fought against. If the trends are accepted, policy-makers face very different sorts of questions. Referring to the trends presented in this chapter, it might be asked how the social policy designer could plan universal family policies that guarantee equal treatment of different family and household types with the existing wide variety of couple relations. Hatland and Skevik (1996), at least, have argued that the welfare state can not rely on registers to reach the redistribution goals because the boundary between cohabitation and single-parenthood has become blurred.

A conclusion about the net impact of population and family trends for the Nordic welfare states is that both trends have increased welfare state dependency and expenditure. The prognoses do not suggest any immediate relief in sight.

Discussion

From a policy-maker's perspective demographic changes pose difficult questions. The changes are slow enough to allow for careful planning, but then again, not all parameters are known. Policy-makers have been aware of ageing and the consequences of demographic trends for a long time, as can be detected from policy documents (for relatively recent policy documents expressing this worry see, e.g. St.meld.nr. 35. (1994–5) for Norway and STM 1994: 9 for Finland). The direction of trends and consequent problem areas were up-dated in this chapter, but they are not particularly new (see, e.g. Rogoff Ramsøy 1987 and Østby 1993 for earlier descriptions). Possible difficulties, such as financing of pensions, the related crowding out of other schemes and the increasing number of elderly needing care frequently appear in policy documents as issues to be addressed. These are areas where cost projections have been attempted. Intergenerational solidarity, reference to changing social risks or the capacity of 'old' welfare state arrangements to respond to new risks, however, are problem areas that seem to attract less emphasis in the literature.

The examination of dependency ratios showed why it is also important to take into account factors other than demographic trends. Classification of countries according to the ageing of their populations, as was done with the age dependency ratios, can be totally overturned when we take into account the employment structure, as was the case for the four countries in this examination. It was argued that the economic dependency ratio is more important for welfare state development than the age structure and the considerable differences between the countries were pointed out. First, the economic dependency ratios are more favourable in the Nordic countries than elsewhere in the OECD group. Even Finland, with one of the highest unemployment rates in the industrialized world, is still above the OECD average. Second, in the Nordic group Finland and Sweden have followed a different path from Denmark and Norway. One would think that the policy preoccupations of countries with differing realities would not be the same, but in examining the policy documents one finds the worries seem to be similar for all. Regardless of major differences in their economies and economic dependency ratios, the sustainability of pension schemes is a hot issue both in Finland and Norway. It could well be that unfavourable scenarios about tomorrow are more important for policy-making than the factual situation today.

If this is the case, one could ask how accurate the projections are in assessing the future burden of support. Population projections, especially in the peaceful Nordic countries, can be done with quite high certainty. The conclusions to be drawn from them are not simple, though. Population and family trends can move in different directions; it is hard to assess their consequences; needs are not determined by these trends alone and, besides, the way needs are answered depends on a variety of other factors. Demographic changes are not an advantage or disadvantage *per se* for the welfare states, although they naturally provide the starting point for analysis. The demographic projections have to be complemented with other projections from a number of other areas, and it is in these other areas that most uncertainty lies. Employment projections, especially, are notorious for going wrong, as the recent history of the Nordic countries shows. But there are also factors we do not know yet, such as the effects of new technology and improvements in the quality of care and changes in productivity that affect the 'welfare burden'. So, while it is undoubtedly the case that the numbers of those over 65 years have risen in relation to those of working age and will continue to do so, it is not at all easy to assess how light or heavy the task of supporting the elderly, or the 'passive' population at large, will be.

Nevertheless, and despite all the uncertainties involved in projections and their interpretations, policy-makers have to prepare for the future. What policy-makers can do to make the economic dependency ratios less pressing is to operate within domains other than demographic factors. The welfare state itself is one of the crucial factors. It is possible to alter the coverage and compensation rates of cash benefits. 'Institutional incentives' can be adjusted so that work becomes a favoured alternative to receiving benefits. The right to receive care services might be adjusted. Policy-makers could emphasize activation measures to help the young to enter labour markets sooner and to prevent older workers' early exiting. The scope and nature of these solutions are examined in the following three chapters.

Notes

1 The author wishes to thank Johan Fritzell, Björn Halleröd, Aksel Hatland, Seppo Koskinen, Juhani Lehto, Pirkko-Liisa Rauhala, Juho Saari and Hannu Uusitalo for their valuable comments during the writing of earlier versions of this chapter.
2 The recent example of how statistics have to be reformed comes as a result of European integration. EU membership has affected the way Sweden and

Finland compile their statistics since 1993. In the field of social affairs they now categorize social spending according to the ESSPROS system, developed by Eurostat and Member States' authorities. This will affect future time-series comparisons. For an overview of these changes see NOSOSCO 6:1997.

3 For instance, it is harder for the registration systems to catch phenomena such as cohabitation than those such as births.

4 The explanation for Finland's different population pyramid can be found in the losses caused by wars against the Soviet Union between 1939 and 1944 and the following birth-boom, but also in the fact that especially between the 1920s and 1960s deaths among Finnish men were at a disproportionately high level compared to deaths among Finnish women, and compared to deaths among men in the other Nordic countries.

5 Besides differences in immigration policies, other explanations for the difference, ranging from geographical location to employment situation, could be sought. Explaining this major difference is outside the scope of this chapter.

6 That family policies could or should affect population trends is not a new idea. Gunnar Myrdal's ideas not long ago about the role of social policy were heavily influenced by considering its effect on population development. However, one can argue, as Meisaari-Polsa and Söderström (1995) did in the case of Sweden, that there have not existed official policies with respect to the *number* of children, but instead, the policies are concerned with the *quality of life* of children. If the policies did affect the number, then that outcome would be quite unintentional. Notwithstanding, official policies may deem it desirable to have more than two children per family.

7 There are limits to this measure, too, as it cannot take into account e.g. differences in part-time work and in work done outside measured GNP.

8 The employment figures presented in Table 3.2 are Nordic statistical secretariat figures. Using OECD figures the economic dependency ratios are a little different. Although the choice of source affects the results, the overall picture of the position of the countries and trends does not change.

9 This point was made by Helka Hytti from the Social Insurance Institution, Finland.

10 The sudden increase in marriages in 1989 in Sweden illustrates the effect of legislation. Marriages per thousand average population increased from 5.2 in 1988 to 12.8 in 1989 because of the changes introduced in the pension system and dropped to 4.7 in 1990 (*Recent Demographic Developments in Europe* 1996: 329).

11 For instance, in Finland the proportional growth in the number of dwelling households between 1960 and 1995 was 65 per cent, while the proportional growth of the size of the population during the same period was 15 per cent (Statistics Finland).

12 Some decades ago becoming old posed a special risk of income poverty and lack of care in all countries. Today the situation with regard to poverty in old age is very different in the Nordic countries than in the rest of Europe (Eurostat 1996). According to recent research on income poverty in the Nordic countries, in the 1990s one can say that poverty in

old age has become almost nonexistent (for the situation in Sweden see Hedström and Ringen 1990; for Finland see Kangas and Ritakallio 1996). While demographic development may direct our interest to the situation of the old and to elderly policies, a social-risk perspective would pose very different questions to policy-makers, guiding their attention probably more to the situation of the young and unemployed.

13 The extent of public care services often leads one to think that the role of family-based care is smaller in the Nordic countries than elsewhere. Unfortunately there is not much comparative evidence on the amount of care provided by families in different countries. In the Nordic countries, it has been shown that despite wide-spread services that are largely available, the family still is clearly the main care provider.

14 It is important to be aware that demographic changes consist of population changes and family changes that are two distinct phenomena not necessarily having parallel consequences. So, contrary to the expected reduction in expenditure that should result from the decline in the number and proportion of young people, the family trends result in more needs for social services, such as child care. The end result has been that expenditure in the category of families and children has not decreased (see NOSOSCO yearbooks for expenditure trends).

4 Cuts in and reform of the Nordic cash benefit systems

Niels Ploug

Introduction[1]

The purpose of this chapter is to describe the development of the cash benefit systems in the Nordic countries from the beginning of the 1980s to the middle of the 1990s, paying particular attention to changes made to their institutional structures. During this period, the social security systems of the Nordic countries have been subject to transition and ongoing reforms which have challenged traditional thinking with regard to the Nordic model of the welfare state.

Some years ago, at least some scholars thought that the Nordic countries had found an unexpectedly simple solution to the basic societal problem of combining social equality and economic efficiency. Subsequent to the Second World War, these countries had developed into welfare states, based in principle on citizens' rights and featuring universal coverage, liberal criteria for eligibility, comparatively high income replacement levels, comprehensiveness of services, etc. From the late 1950s, generous welfare benefits were developed in a context of rapid economic growth, low unemployment and high levels of participation in the labour force, particularly among women. These developments both contributed to, and were caused by, the gradual transformation towards a service-intensive welfare state. The apologists for the Nordic-style welfare state argued that the Nordic countries in general, and Sweden in particular, had developed a unique capacity to introduce social reforms while simultaneously managing the economy in an effective way.

The idyllic picture had already started to crack in the mid-1970s. Following the first oil crisis, the Danish unemployment rate began to rise from a low 0.9 per cent in 1973 to 5.1 per cent in 1975 and continuing to a peak of 11.4 per cent in 1983. The OPEC oil price increase of 1973 did not affect the other Nordic countries to the same extent. Thanks to the country's huge oil reserves, Norway was in a stronger position. On the other hand, the Norwegian economy was, and still is, suffering from a number of defects which are only partly masked by revenues from the State's oil sector. During the 1970s, the Governments of Sweden made use of a time-honoured 'Swedish-style' counter-cyclical policy supported by extensive active labour market policies combined with industrial policy measures. The corollary, however, was mounting public budgetary deficits, which proved to be the Achilles' heel of the Swedish economy entering the 1990s. Finland was situated in the middle, with unemployment rates below those in Denmark but above the levels in Norway and Sweden. Finland's economic growth during the 1980s, however, was spectacular – the late 1980s being a particularly prosperous period.

During the early 1990s, both the Swedish and Finnish economies had severe problems. In Sweden the unemployment rate started rising, and peaked at an unprecedented 8.2 per cent in 1993; this figure does not include those participating in active labour market measures. Growth halted and then took a negative turn over the years 1991–3. Developments in Finland were even worse. The unemployment rate rocketed, hitting its peak of 17.7 per cent in 1993, and economic growth rates for the first years of the 1990s were strongly in the negative. Finland was extremely hard hit by the collapse of the former Soviet Union, but structural problems in the Finnish economy, caused in part by the intensive growth experienced in the late 1980s, are the basic reason for the severe economic and social problems that have faced Finland from the beginning of the 1990s. The currency policies of Finland, Norway and Sweden failed and all were eventually forced to let the currency float.

It is outside the scope of this chapter to investigate the economic policies of the respective Nordic countries in depth. The above sketch serves only to illustrate that the Nordic model, much praised in the past, seems to be less effective today. The economic problems associated with the issue of macroeconomic stability and the related fiscal pressure call for re-evaluation of many of the arrangements worked out and developed in the prosperous years of the past. The need for re-evaluation is especially keen because most Nordic politicians do not consider it likely that unemployment rates will return to the low levels of former years, at least not in the near future. This makes it rather difficult to adhere to the institutional set-up devised in the past. Most schemes date back to the 1960s, a decade characterized by low unemployment and high growth rates; they were amended during a period that most policy-makers considered to be only a temporary downturn.

The generous benefit schemes of the past are causing increasing alarm. There is anxiety regarding their effects on incentives and their impact on the structural problems of the labour market. There is also concern regarding the consequences that generous benefit schemes may have for public budgets in a situation where growing numbers of people collect benefits. As unemployment rises, an increasing number of people become dependent on public support; in consequence, the tax base shrinks. Ultimately, an issue that started as an unemployment problem has evolved into a problem for the entire cash benefit systems.

It is hard to predict the consequences that the ongoing reform of the cash benefit systems will have on the Nordic model of the welfare state in the future; thus, this chapter strives mainly to describe what has happened by looking at two development trends. First, the trends of expenditure for different kinds of cash benefits, and the recipients of these benefits, are examined for the period extending from the beginning of the 1980s to the beginning of the 1990s. Second, major changes that have been made to the institutional framework of the cash benefit systems in the 1990s are described. Among these are, e.g. revision of allocation criteria, changes in benefit levels and changes in the length of the period for which benefits are paid. The chapter concludes with an interpretation of how these cutbacks and reforms have affected the Nordic model of the welfare state.

Development of cash benefit systems from 1982 to 1993[2]

This section describes the development of cash benefits from 1982 to 1993 in relation to the main social contingencies of unemployment, sickness, maternity, disability, old age, family and need. The trend for each benefit is analysed by the number of recipients and the amount of expenditure. These graphs tell a very simple but illustrative story; namely, that compensations have been decreasing if the curve for recipients overtakes the curve for expenditure over time, while compensations have been increasing if the opposite occurs. The trends in old-age pensions, being largely due to maturation of the system, are an example of the latter story.

In some of the countries and for some of the benefits, the changes that have taken place in the numbers of recipients and in expenditure are dramatic, while in other countries and for other benefits the trends have been quite stable. All in all, knowledge of the development that occurred during the period of 1982 to 1993 – and not least the trend for the latter part of the period – is important if one wants to understand the changes in the institutional structure of the cash benefit systems that either have been carried out in recent years or are being discussed at present in the Nordic countries.

Unemployment

Throughout the 1980s, the Nordic countries were famous and praised for their low level of unemployment. In reality, only Sweden and, in part, Norway were able to live up to this picture, with unemployment rates not exceeding 5 per cent; unemployment in both Denmark and Finland remained above 5 per cent in most years of the decade. Entering the 1990s, unemployment rose sharply in all the Nordic countries, the most dramatic changes occurring in Sweden and Finland (Figure 4.1, see also Chapter 2, Figure 2.9)

In Denmark, unemployment fell from the beginning to the middle of the 1980s, owing mainly to a domestic economic boom. Major deficits in the balance of payments in 1985 and 1986 curtailed financing of private consumption through borrowing, and meant the introduction of tax reforms in 1986. The consequence was a substantial decline in domestic consumption and a sharp rise in unemployment. In the period 1982 to 1988, the individual maximum benefit level was fixed, i.e. it was not adjusted in accordance with either price or wage developments, which explains why the number of recipients exceeds the index for expenditure in that period. The scheme was revised in 1988; since then, unemployment benefits – and all other cash benefits – have been adjusted in accordance with wage development.

In Finland, unemployment became a major problem at the beginning of the 1990s. The structural problems created in the Finnish economy at the end of the 1980s led to severe economic problems in Finland. Unemployment rose from 3.4 per cent in 1990 to 17.7 per cent in 1993. This explains the sharp rise in the number of recipients of, and in expenditure for, unemployment benefits after 1990. Most attempts to ease the economic burden by revising the unemployment benefits system have failed – in fact, expenditure has risen somewhat more than the number of recipients. Since 1993 unemployment has been falling slightly.

In Norway, unemployment more than doubled from 2.1 per cent in 1987 to 4.9 per cent in 1989, and the rising trend continued into the 1990s. This development resulted mainly from the fall in oil prices that took place in 1986 – as the Norwegian economy is highly dependent on exportation of oil – and from the economic difficulties

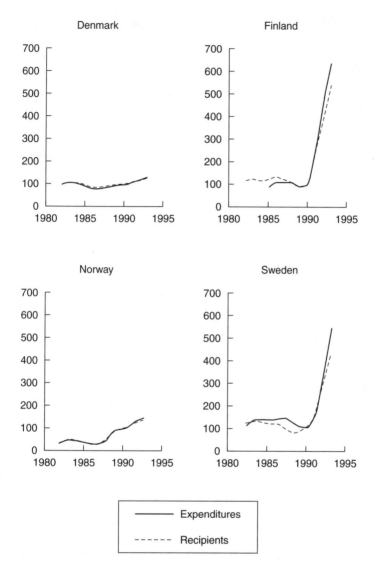

Figure 4.1 Expenditure on and recipients of unemployment benefits in Denmark, Finland, Norway and Sweden from 1982 to 1993; fixed prices, 1990 = 100

experienced in Sweden and in the UK, which account for more than 30 per cent of Norwegian exports. Tax reforms also played a role here, as they led to a decline in private consumption and private investment. In the 1990s, Norway has taken over Sweden's role as the Nordic country with the lowest rate of unemployment.

In Sweden, unemployment was at a very low level throughout the 1980s. Owing, however, to the nation's heated economy, overvalued currency and major public deficits, which led to negative economic growth from the beginning of the 1990s, Sweden's policy of full employment could not be continued into the 1990s. Unemployment rose from 1.3 per cent in 1989 to 8.2 per cent in 1993. The rate has been decreasing slightly in recent years, though it is still at a high level compared with that in the 1980s.

Sickness

Quite typically, expenditure for sickness benefits is relatively higher in the countries with the lowest rates of unemployment – i.e. Sweden and Norway – than in the countries with the highest rates of unemployment – i.e. Denmark and Finland. In Sweden and Norway, expenditure for sickness benefits amounted to between 1 and 2 per cent of GDP in the period 1982 to 1993, while the corresponding expenditure in both Denmark and Finland was below 1 per cent of GDP.

In Denmark, the sickness benefits system has undergone a number of reforms, which have meant changes in the number of sickness days financed by the State, as shown in Figure 4.2. The so-called 'employer period' was extended to 13 weeks in 1983 and cut to five weeks in 1987. In 1988, the period was further cut to one week for private employers and extended to 13 weeks for public employers. The period is now two weeks for private employers and it is unlimited for public employers. In the period 1983 to 1987, the sickness benefits system had a waiting period of one day. The trend in the number of recipients and in expenditure shown in Figure 4.2 partly reflects these changes; both decreased after the 'employer period' was extended in 1983 and increased after the 'employer period' was cut in 1987 and 1988 and after abolition of the waiting period in 1987.

In Finland, the sickness benefits system is quite generous, with benefits typically amounting to 70 per cent of former wages. The scheme is stepwise, implying a lower percentage of compensation at higher incomes; but there is no maximum in the scheme. The number of recipients has been fairly stable during the period. The increase in

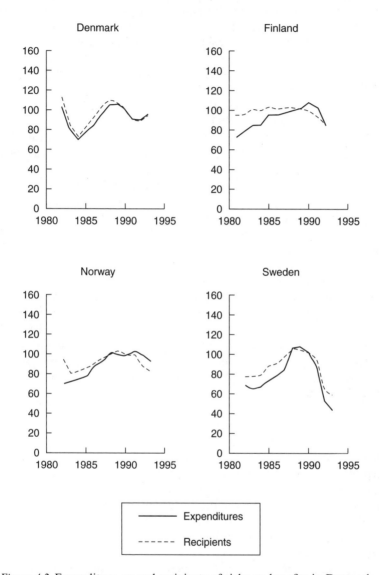

Figure 4.2 Expenditure on and recipients of sickness benefits in Denmark, Finland, Norway and Sweden from 1982 to 1993; fixed prices, 1990 = 100

expenditure reflects, on the one hand, the general wage development and, on the other hand, the fact that as of 1990 those unemployed were guaranteed a sickness benefits level of no less than 86 per cent of their unemployment benefits. The downward trend in expenditure observable since 1992 derives from changes in the benefits level for wage-earners, which was cut from 80 per cent to 70 per cent in 1992 and to 66 per cent in 1993. The waiting period was extended from seven days to nine days in 1993.

In Norway, an increase occurred in the number of recipients of and expenditure for sickness benefits. The rise in expenditure was slightly higher than the increase in the number of recipients, reflecting, among other things, the fact that the average sickness benefit period rose from approximately 44 days in 1983 to 49 days in 1988. Since 1988, the expenditure for sickness benefits has been quite stable.

In Sweden, expenditure for sickness benefits, measured in fixed prices, rose by 25 per cent from 1982 to 1991. Among other things, the rise stemmed from changes made to the system in 1987, when the waiting period was abolished and compensation for short-term sickness was increased. This led to an 18 per cent increase in the number of sickness benefit days from 1986 to 1988. As of 1991, a number of changes were implemented, including a reduction in the level of compensation. Also, in 1993 the one-day waiting period was reinstated. At the end of the period under review, there was a sharp decline – approximately 40 per cent – in the number of sickness benefit periods.

Maternity

While some major benefit schemes, e.g. unemployment and old-age pensions, have been – and still are – subject to debate in the Nordic countries, maternity benefits have been widely improved without much debate. For instance, the length of the benefits period has been extended and the possibilities for fathers to take leave have been improved. The major features of the maternity benefits are shown in Figure 4.3.

In Denmark, the maternity leave period was extended from 14 to 24 weeks after delivery in 1984–85. The last ten weeks of the period is in principle reserved for the father, but it can be shared between the parents or taken solely by the mother. At the same time, a two-week leave period immediately after delivery was introduced for fathers. The dramatic increase in the number of maternity leave weeks that occurred from 1984, however, is not due only to these changes. The

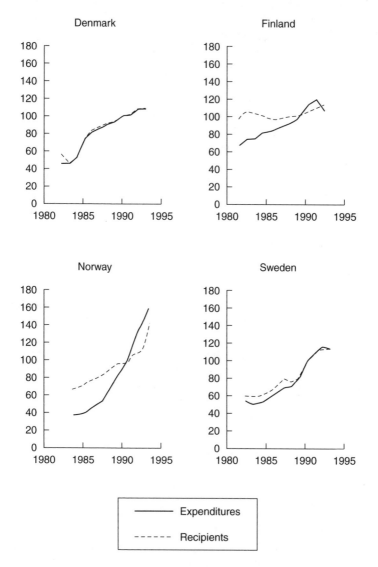

Figure 4.3 Expenditure on and recipients of maternity benefits in Denmark, Finland, Norway and Sweden from 1982 to 1993; fixed prices, 1990 = 100

number of newborn children rose steadily from 51,000 in 1983 to 68,000 in 1993. At the same time, the number of women entitled to maternity leave increased, owing to an increase in women's labour market participation, the rate rising from 74 per cent in 1983 to 78 per cent in 1993.

In Finland, both employed and non-employed parents are entitled to maternity leave. Mothers and fathers are entitled to separate rights. The combined benefit period cannot exceed 263 days. The rise in expenditure for maternity in the period 1983 to 1993 to some extent stems from an increase in the benefit period and to some extent from an extension of the eligibility rights to include partners of either mothers or fathers.

In Norway, the increase in expenditure for maternity leave has been even more dramatic than in Denmark. The factors explaining the increase are parallel to those for Denmark, but the changes have been more pronounced. From 1987 to 1993, the leave period was extended from 18 to 33 weeks – or to 42 weeks if one opts for only 80 per cent of the compensation. Women's labour market participation rose from a rate of 64 per cent in 1983 to 71 per cent in 1993; simultaneously, the number of births has increased from around 50,000 per year in the middle of the 1980s to around 60,000 per year in the beginning of the 1990s.

In Sweden, developments have been somewhat more conservative. The only noteworthy change – which explains the slight increase in both expenditure and the number of recipients from 1988 to 1989 – was an extension of the leave period from 360 days to 450 days. For, the last 90 days, however, only a low, flat-rate compensation is paid.

Disability

In order to understand the development of disability pensions, one needs to take into consideration interactions with other parts of the cash benefits system because the development of disability pensions is intertwined with developments on the labour market – and with the existence of different types of early or part-time retirement schemes. Differences between the Nordic countries in this respect explain some of the differences in the trends of expenditure for and recipients of disability pensions in the period 1982 to 1993. Figure 4.4 shows the development of expenditures and numbers of recipients in the Nordic countries from 1982 to 1993.

In Denmark, the disability pension system underwent reform in 1984. This reform introduced the possibility of granting a pension on

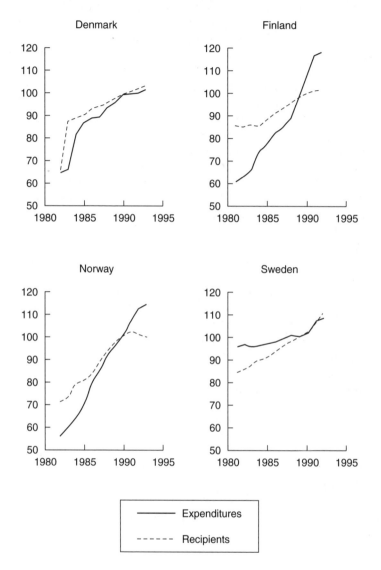

Figure 4.4 Expenditure on and recipients of disability pension in Denmark, Finland, Norway and Sweden from 1982 to 1993; fixed prices, 1990 = 100

the basis of social as well as medical reasons. In consequence, a number of long-term social assistance recipients, e.g. drug addicts, could be transferred to disability pension. In general, the number of recipients of disability pension increased from 167,000 in 1982 – i.e. two years before the reform – to 237,000 in 1986 – i.e. two years after the reform. Since then, only a slight increase in the number of recipients has taken place.

In Finland, there is both a state disability pension scheme and a labour market disability pension scheme. While the increase in recipients has been only 18 per cent in the period – from 262,000 people in 1982 to 310,000 people in 1993 – expenditure has risen by 95 per cent. This increased expenditure stems from the fact that more people have become entitled to benefits through the labour market disability pension scheme during the period. In 1982, this system paid out 55 per cent of all disability pensions; while in 1993, this figure had increased to 71 per cent. As the labour market scheme pays higher benefits than the national scheme, expenditure has increased more than the increase in the number of recipients.

In Norway, the number of recipients of disability pension increased by 41 per cent in the period 1982 to 1993; contrary to Denmark, however, no major reforms that would explain this increase were implemented in Norway. One possible explanation may be that Norway is the only Nordic country without any early retirement scheme which makes it possible to leave the labour market around the age of 60. All the other Nordic countries have had such schemes throughout the period of 1982 to 1993.

In Sweden, a slow but steady increase in the number of recipients of disability pension occurred during the period 1982 to 1993. No major reforms of the system were carried out in that period, but the high level of recipients of sickness benefit has a direct influence on the disability pension system, as prolonged periods of sickness benefit are often terminated by granting a disability pension. The scheme expanded considerably when unemployment started to rise.

Old age

Old-age pensions constitute an area of income transfers that has been and will continue growing in importance in the Nordic countries. The demographic development and projections are somewhat different among the countries (see Chapter 3), but all of them will experience an increase in the number of old-age pensioners in the future.

In Denmark, there has been a very moderate rise in the area of state old-age pensions, the increase in expenditure mainly reflecting a rise in the number of recipients. The change in expenditure level from 1988 to 1989 reflects a one-off increase in pensions, the increase being 5 per cent for single pensioners and 7 per cent for couples. The central changes in Denmark's old-age pension system during the period have not occurred in relation to the state pension scheme, shown in Figure 4.5, but in the increasing importance of collectively-based labour market pension systems. These changes, which will have a considerable impact in the future, have altered the traditional picture of the Danish old-age pension system as being a flat-rate state pension scheme financed through taxes.

In Finland, there is both a state old-age pension scheme and a labour market old-age pension scheme. The increase in expenditure for old-age pensions is explained by demographic factors and by the interplay between these two schemes. Expenditure rises as more people become entitled to old-age pension through the labour market scheme, which pays out greater pensions. A 25 per cent increase in the number of old-age pensions recipients has occurred in the period. The proportion of old-age pensioners receiving pension through the labour market pension scheme has risen from 45 per cent in 1982 to 72 per cent in 1993.

Norway also saw steady growth in the number of old-age pensioners during the period, the increase amounting to 15 per cent from 1982 to 1993. Expenditure has risen somewhat more because of an increase in the number of recipients entitled to higher pensions.

The situation in Sweden is a combination of those in Norway and Finland, i.e. Sweden has experienced a moderate increase in the number of old-age pension recipients, as did Norway, the rise in Sweden totalling 11 per cent from 1982 to 1993, and a shift from state pensions to labour market pensions, as occurred in Finland. In consequence, old-age pension expenditure in Sweden grew by 44 per cent.

Major changes in the Swedish pension system were introduced after 1993, but only some of these changes have been implemented. Some changes have also been carried out in Denmark. These are discussed in the third section of this chapter.

Family

As was the case with maternity benefits, family benefits, too, have been increasing in most of the Nordic countries, without this provoking much debate. These are small segments of the cash benefits

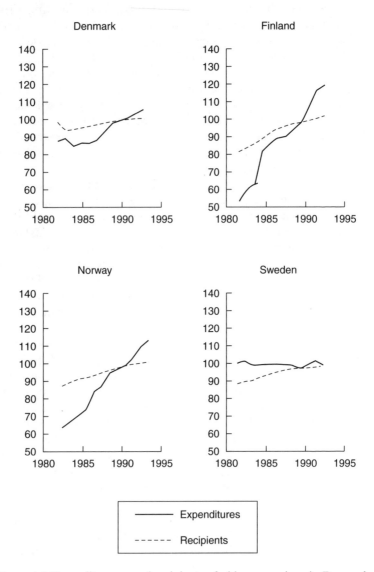

Figure 4.5 Expenditure on and recipients of old-age pensions in Denmark, Finland, Norway and Sweden from 1982 to 1993; fixed prices, 1990 = 100

system, typically accounting for less than 1 per cent of GDP; thus it has been possible to realise significant improvements with small amounts of money. Figure 4.6 shows the salient developments from 1982 to 1993. Denmark had no general family benefits in the first half of the 1980s, only minor means-tested benefits. In 1987, a general family benefit for all children below the age of 18 years was introduced, and both the number of recipients and the level of expenditure increased dramatically.

In Finland, there have been no major changes in the number of recipients of family benefits. However, a change in the tax system – which reduced deductions for families with children – was combined with an increase in direct benefits, which explains the increase in expenditure that occurred during the latter part of the period.

In Norway, expenditure for family benefits has risen, owing to an increase in the amounts granted. A special amount for very small children was also introduced.

In Sweden, no major changes were made to the family benefits system in the period 1982 to 1993. The increase recorded in expenditure during the latter part of the period stems mainly from increases in the number of recipients. A number of changes were made to the family benefits system after 1993; see the presentation later in this chapter.

Need

In all the Nordic countries the social assistance scheme is the lowest level of the cash benefits system, i.e. the social assistance scheme looks after the needs of people not entitled to benefits by virtue of other sectors of the cash benefits system analysed so far. Changes in eligibility for cash benefits, for example, as well as general changes in the labour market are reflected in the social assistance scheme. See Figure 4.7 for developments from 1982 to 1993.

In Denmark, expenditure on and recipients of social assistance have followed the trend in unemployment – which is understandable, as most social assistance recipients are granted benefits because they are unemployed without being eligible for unemployment benefits. A number of changes made in 1989, when some new types of benefits were included in the social assistance scheme, have led to an increase in expenditure that is greater than the increase in the number of recipients after 1990.

In Finland, two events have caused major increases in the number

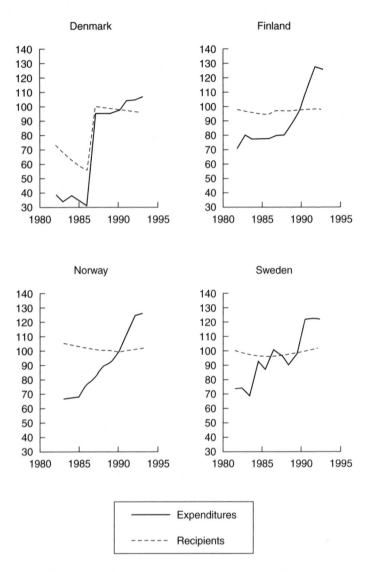

Figure 4.6 Expenditure on and recipients of family benefits in Denmark, Finland, Norway and Sweden from 1982 to 1993; fixed prices, 1990 = 100

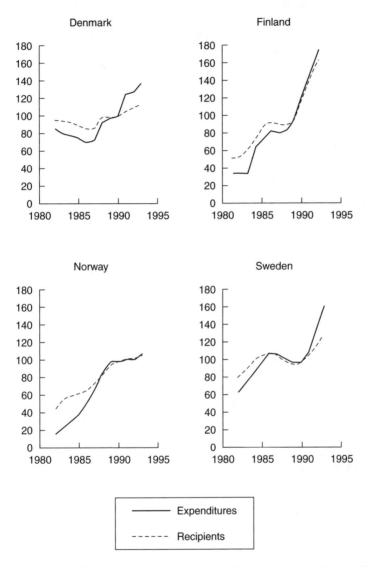

Figure 4.7 Expenditure on and recipients of social assistance in Denmark, Finland, Norway and Sweden from 1982 to 1993; fixed prices, 1990 = 100

of people receiving social assistance. First, the social assistance scheme was reformed in 1984, when it was simplified and access to benefits was made easier. The number of recipients thereafter increased, but levelled out within a few years. Since 1990, the number of recipients has increased dramatically, owing to changes in Finland's economic situation.

In Norway, the increase in recipients of social assistance has to some extent followed the increase in unemployment. The rise in expenditure, in turn, is explained by an increase in the level of benefits, which doubled from 1981 to 1986, the average benefit period being increased by 42 per cent during the same period.

As Sweden did not have any major unemployment problems until the beginning of the 1990s, both the recipients of and expenditure on social assistance were very low. The increase that occurred in the beginning of the 1990s is mainly explained by the rise in unemployment.

Major changes in the institutional framework of the cash benefit systems

The political response to developments in the cash benefit systems has been to implement a number of changes in the systems. Because the changes that have been introduced do not share a general pattern, it is difficult to present an overall description of the effects of the many changes that have been made to the welfare systems in the Nordic countries. The main purpose of this section is to describe major changes that have taken place in the institutional framework of the cash benefit systems in the Nordic countries during the 1990s, and to discuss the potential implications of these changes with regard to understanding the Nordic model of the welfare state.

Denmark

Of the Nordic countries Denmark has had the longest experience of an employment crisis. Unemployment in Denmark has been at a fairly high level ever since the mid-1970s. For this reason, different parts of the cash benefits system – especially unemployment benefits and the social assistance scheme – have undergone a long chain of increments, partial revisions and amendments extending into the 1990s. The labour market reform of 1994, the tax reform of 1994 and the social security reform of 1997 brought a halt to this line of increments and partial revisions, and all in all have led to the establishment of a new institutional framework on which the cash benefits system will be based in the coming years.

The labour market reform of 1994 had, among others, the following institutional implications:

● The duration for which unemployment benefits could be granted was limited to seven years in 1995 and to five years in 1996.

● Eligibility for unemployment benefits, including eligibility for a new five-year period presupposes six months of non-supported employment in 1995 and twelve months of non-supported employment as of 1996.

● Members of unemployment benefit funds, whether employed or unemployed, were granted the right to take educational, parental or sabbatical leave lasting a maximum of 52 weeks.

Before the reform, the unemployment benefit period had in practice been nine years. Before the reform it had been possible to become eligible for unemployment benefits through subsidized work as opposed to non-supported employment; this had unintended effects, because it enabled the municipalities to make social assistance recipients eligible for primarily state-financed employment benefits. The reform did not introduce changes to benefit levels. Greater emphasis was placed on active labour market policy, including an obligation for those unemployed to take part in employment measures and training programmes.

The tax reform of 1994 had, among others, the following implication:

● Social assistance and state old-age pension, which previously were partly exempt from taxation were made taxable benefits. Benefit levels were, on average, raised more than correspondingly.

Another relevant point should be mentioned here. The basic amount of the state old-age pension hitherto received by anyone reaching the age of 70 became income-tested in relation to earned income.

The social security reform of 1997 has no major institutional implications when it comes to eligibility, benefit level, etc. for social assistance. However, it places greater emphasis on active employment measures, e.g. job training and education for recipients under the age of 30.

To sum up, these reforms have created a more transparent system with regard to the benefit level for persons of working age. All benefits are now measured as a percentage[3] of the level of unemployment benefits, and they are all considered part of taxable income. The Government has called this revised system a system of 'obligations and rights', meaning that the system incorporates both an obligation to participate in active labour market measures – e.g. job training and education – and the right to do so in accordance with what is called the personal plan jointly drawn up by the individual unemployed person and the labour market office.

In the early 1990s Finland[4] experienced severe economic difficulties. In the beginning of the 1990s, no cuts where made to the cash benefits system. In 1991, increases based on decisions taken in the 1980s were still implemented. As unemployment climbed rapidly from 1991 to 1992 and onwards need arose to adapt the system to the economic reality.

Finland

Initially, most changes took the form of cost-cutting measures, only some of which can be mentioned here. The budget for 1992 made cuts to the unemployment benefits and the earnings-related sickness benefits; the latter indirectly led to cuts in the level of maternity, paternity and parent benefits, as these are linked to sickness benefits. Also, the level of means-tested housing allowance was cut by not taking the cost-of-living index into account in the limits of earned income. In 1993, additional cuts were made to sickness benefits and thus also to the related benefits (see above), and the waiting period was extended. The duration of the payable period for parental benefits, which had been increased to 275 working days in 1991, was reduced to the original level of 263 working days. The level of unemployment benefits was reduced, and eligibility was tightened by extending the waiting period for newcomers on the labour market.

After three years of rising unemployment and cost-cutting measures, it was realised in 1994 that the explosion of costs could not be curbed only by lowering the level of support. Therefore a new – a third – scheme for the unemployed was introduced. 'Labour market support' was to function as a basic livelihood for those entering the labour market for the first time – and for those who had collected earnings-related benefits for the maximum period of 500 days. It proved difficult to implement further cuts in the sickness benefits system, but a child supplement associated with this benefit scheme was abolished.

After the spring general election held in spring 1995, the cuts continued and a new target was found – the child allowance, which had been untouched by the cuts until that time. In 1996, cuts were targeted at minimum-security benefits; for the first time, a whole group of people was excluded from support. People whose income fell below the 'approved' level were excluded from sickness benefits altogether. This meant, in practice, that housewives and students – who had been entitled to collect sickness benefits at the minimum level – were excluded from the scheme. A group of people under the age of 20 who had been included in the newly introduced labour-market support scheme, lost their entitlement to national pension. The benefit level was also lowered and the child supplement related to labour-market support was lowered. The cuts also included a reduction in the levels of pensions payable in the future. Social assistance was not incremented for the cost-of-living index, and means-testing for persons living with their parents and refusing work or training was tightened.

In 1997, eligibility for earnings-related benefits and basic allowances in the unemployment security scheme was restricted by extending the period of work required during the previous two years from six to ten months and by changing how the benefits were calculated so that earnings during the previous 10-month qualifying period only were included. Eligibility for labour-market support was made stricter by introducing a waiting period. Sickness benefits were not incremented for the cost-of-living index. Pensions were untouched by the cuts made in 1997 and housing allowance was improved slightly following yearly cuts that had been made from 1992 to 1996.

Norway

As mentioned in the introduction to this chapter, the economic situation in Norway[5] is somewhat different from that in the other Nordic countries. State revenues from oil production mean that the public budget shows a surplus. On the one hand, economic necessity is not prompting reforms and cuts in the cash benefits system in Norway in the same way as in the other Nordic countries. On the other hand, Norway to some extent faces present and future problems in relation to its cash benefits system similar to those of the other Nordic countries; the current problems pertain to ensuring full employment, and the problems in future stem from the expected increase in the number of old-age pensioners. But all in all the Norwegian system has not been subjected to as many cuts and changes as have the corresponding systems in the neighbouring countries, even though

Norway has also introduced reductions and restrictions in certain areas, e.g. indexation of benefits and replacement rates.

One important feature of development in Norway is the great emphasis on the so-called 'work line' materialising in the strengthening of qualifying conditions for unemployment, disability and sickness benefits and in greater efforts for rehabilitation. Great expansion of maternity leave has taken place. The benefit period has been extended from 18 weeks in 1986 to a total period of 52 weeks, if the level of compensation is 80 per cent of wages, or alternatively to 42 weeks at full compensation of wages.

Sweden

Sweden[6] experienced an economic recession at approximately the same time as Finland, i.e. in the beginning of the 1990s; but expansion of the Swedish welfare state came to a halt some years earlier, in 1988. During the election campaign of that year proposals were made to extend the parental leave period from 12 to 18 months and to provide access to public daycare for all children over 18 months, but neither of these proposals was ever achieved. Changes made to the Swedish welfare system since then have primarily been in the form of cutbacks.

The first cutback was announced in 1990 and implemented in the beginning of 1991. As absence due to sickness had been a major problem in Sweden in the 1980s, cash benefits for sickness were a natural target for cutbacks, which were implemented in three steps. In 1991, the statutory replacement rate was reduced from 90 to 65 per cent for the first three days of absence, and to 80 per cent from day 4 to day 90. In 1992, a two-week period of sick pay was introduced, obliging employers to pay sickness benefits for the first two weeks. In 1993, a waiting day was introduced and employers were obligated to pay a tax-deductible contribution, amounting to 0.95 per cent of gross wages, into the sickness benefits system.

Major changes also took place in the unemployment insurance system. In 1993, the benefit level was reduced to 80 per cent of previous earnings, and the five-day waiting period which had been abolished in 1980 was re-introduced. In terms of principles, the introduction of compulsory unemployment insurance the same year was a major change. Everyone who had not joined a voluntary unemployment insurance fund was affiliated with a government equivalent; at the same time, a personal social security contribution to the unemployment insurance funds, set at 1.5 per cent of earnings, became obligatory.

After the general election of 1994, the new Social Democratic

Government abolished both the compulsory clause and the personal contribution. The duration of part-time benefits was restricted, and the grounds for re-qualification for unemployment benefits were re-defined, making it no longer possible to re-qualify for unemployment insurance merely by taking part in training programmes and relief work. The reform of 1997 also unified the unemployment benefits system by having the existing unemployment funds, which are linked with the trade unions, take over the administration of the flat-rate basic benefits scheme called KAS, which had previously been administered by regional public authorities. Special conditions for long-term unemployed persons over the age of 60 were also introduced. Until April 1998, they will be able to collect unemployment benefits without being required to seek a new job until they reach the statutory pensionable age.

As to pension, two types of change have been made. One is a major reform *vis-à-vis* long-term development of the pension system, introducing a partly funded scheme for the future. As the technical problems associated with this reform have not yet been solved, the reform cannot be described here in detail. There is no doubt, however, that this reform would be a structural one, even though the shift will be felt by the individual pension recipient as only a small step. Second, a number of smaller changes have been introduced to the present system. A small reduction of pension benefits was introduced in 1993, when the method of calculating pensions was changed. Pensions were now calculated on the basis of 98 per cent of the so-called base amount, instead of the 100 per cent rate used earlier. There have also been cuts in the housing supplement for pensioners, and married people now receive the lower rate of basic pension even when the spouse is not a pensioner. In 1997, the widow's pension for those below statutory pensionable age was made income-tested.

As early as 1991, it was decided that disability pension could no longer be granted on labour market grounds only. More recently, the special rules applied to those above 60 have been abolished. It has also been suggested, as part of the major pension reform, that disability pension be transferred to the sickness insurance system. Owing to changes in defining the kind of work a person is expected to take, there has been a clear decline in the number of new disability pensioners; from about 60,000 in 1993 to about 40,000 per year in the following years.

Minor changes have been made to the family support scheme. In 1994, the special bonus included in the family support scheme for families with five or more children was lowered. In 1996, the monthly benefit per child was lowered from SEK 750 to SEK 640 – only to be restored to SEK 750 again in 1997.

Concluding remarks

As pointed out in the introduction to this chapter, it is hard to predict how the recent cutbacks and reforms made to the cash benefit systems will affect the future development of the welfare systems in the Nordic countries. A few observations, however, can be presented regarding the changes – or maybe even the restructuring – now taking place.

In a number of areas, cutbacks have been introduced or retrenchment has taken place. This process has involved cuts in benefit levels, tightening of eligibility criteria and shortening of benefit periods. In general, these cuts have not been radical – some of them can even be seen as symbolic – and on a macro-level the Nordic countries are still among those allocating the most resources for cash benefits. For the individual citizen, however, the cuts may have had dramatic effects. The tightening of eligibility criteria is a problem for people entering the systems, and the shortening of benefit periods is a problem for those hit hardest by long-term unemployment or sickness. In general, unemployment benefits, sickness benefits and social assistance have been the targets of immediate cuts and changes, while the changes made to pension schemes are more long-term in nature. As to family benefits, including maternity, major improvements have been made, at least in some of the countries.

The Nordic welfare states today are less generous than in the 1970s and 1980s, and social security for the individual citizen is on a lower level than it used to be, but the Nordic welfare systems are still quite generous. Compared to other welfare systems, universal coverage has been a marked feature of the Nordic welfare states. All in all, this is still the case, though some of the changes implemented in the 1980s and 1990s have added some nuances to the picture of universal coverage. Strictly speaking, the Danish old-age state pension is no longer universal but is means tested; and in Finland, specific groups have been excluded from the sickness benefits system.

As a solution to the problems of the welfare state, many economists have suggested the introduction of greater economic incentives into the cash benefit systems, especially with regard to unemployment. This consideration has surfaced in the ongoing discussion. In reality, however, not many changes in that direction have been made. Instead, there has been a move towards so-called active measures. Social rights, such as the right to income support when unemployed, are increasingly being subject to question, and there has been a shift towards requiring participation in job training or educational programmes as a condition for collecting benefits.

Pension schemes, in particular, have undergone a number of long-term reforms, the effects of which remain to be seen. But also in the sphere of unemployment, the introduction of obligations in order to be entitled to benefits has in some cases been one aspect of a major reform.

In a broad context, one can ask whether these changes, as well as the overall problems facing the Nordic welfare states, indicate that the next system to topple after socialism will be Nordic exceptionalism. Recent developments contain little to point in that direction. Not many of the changes have been systemic. The Nordic cash benefit systems in total still offers citizens universal coverage. The future of the systems will depend on two things: the ability to solve the unemployment problem; and public support for the welfare state as a model for economic and social development. Since unemployment has been declining recently and public support remains widespread, it is much too early to declare the Nordic model dead.

Notes

1 The author would like to thank his colleagues at the Center for Welfare State Research – namely Jørn Henrik Petersen, Jon Kvist and Hans Hansen – for their valuable comments and suggestions concerning earlier drafts of this chapter, and research assistant Frederik Nemeth for his help with data processing.
2 This section is based on the analysis presented in Ploug and Kvist (1997). The statistical information on each cash benefit is based on national statistics. The trend is shown as an index where 1990 = 100 and where expenditure is calculated in fixed prices, i.e. prices are deflated with the GDP deflator.
3 100 per cent or less.
4 This presentation of the changes made to the Finnish cash benefit system is based on the reports of Kosunen (1997) and Alestalo (1994).
5 This presentation of the changes made in Norway is based on the following reports: Lødemel (1994); Stephens (1996); Kuhnle (1996) and Stortinget (1997).
6 This presentation of the changes made in Sweden is based on the reports of Palme (1994) and Palme and Wennemo (1997).

5 Universal public social care and health services?

Juhani Lehto, Nina Moss and Tine Rostgaard

Introduction

One of the major characteristics distinguishing the Nordic welfare state model from other types of welfare state models is the way in which the Nordic countries have arranged their health and social care services. The Nordic welfare state is called a 'public service state', because most health and social care services are funded from tax revenue and are provided by public – either local or regional – authorities. The principle of 'universalism' is extended to include, in addition to cash benefits, also access to health and social care services. In particular, the social care services are available for and used by a significantly larger proportion of the population than in the other European welfare states (Anttonen and Sipilä 1996; Rostgaard 1996). High professional standards for the universal services have also been an important policy goal in the Nordic countries. The widening of the principle of high professional standards from health care and education to social care services is a characteristic that is not as evident in other welfare states.

The way health and social care services are arranged has a significant impact on the Nordic societies. For instance, it is an important explanation for the great proportion of public sector jobs in the total employment and, particularly, in the employment of women. The extent of social care services is often linked to the high rate of female participation in wage labour. Universal health services reduce the socioeconomic risks linked with the need for health care, and universal social care services reduce the socioeconomic risks linked with having dependent children and elderly people in the family.

The aim of this chapter is to study to what extent the actual health and social service systems in the Nordic countries have corresponded over the last two decades to the particular characteristics attributed in comparative welfare state research to the Nordic welfare state model, and to examine whether and to what extent there have been tendencies towards weakening or changing these characteristics in the late 1980s and in the 1990s. We focus the empirical analysis of changes on two main service segments. The first is health care and social care for the elderly. Dealing concurrently with the health services and the social care for the elderly is necessary, because the borderline between what is health care for the elderly and what is social care for the elderly has moved during the observation period, and changes in hospital services have been compensated for by changes in social care for the elderly. The second major segment is child day care, which, in the Nordic countries, is a social care service that is aimed at universalism, and is clearly different from arrangements for caring for small children in other welfare state models. The chapter ends with a short discussion and conclusions.

Health services and social care for the elderly

Overview of changes since the early 1980s

To a large extent, the basic structure and volume of the health services and care for the elderly were developed by the early 1980s in all four Nordic countries. They had developed primary health care and specialist and hospital services where the financing was based on tax revenue and minimal or no client fees. It was the reponsibility of local authorities to provide most of these services. The service system was not free of recognized problems such as queues for certain surgical operations, lack of qualified personnel every now and then, bureaucratic unresponsiveness to differing needs, increases in expenditure and socioeconomic inequity in health. However, the basic aspects of the system were largely perceived as being mature, appropriate and legitimate. Policy development concentrated on solving the 'remaining' problems in the basically sound system and in modernization of the services, particularly in shifting the balance of care for the mentally ill, handicapped and elderly persons from institutions to outpatient and community services (NOMESCO 38: 1992, 1996).

Towards the late 1980s and particularly in the early 1990s, new themes on these services were taken up in the political discourse. Cost expansion was defined as a serious policy problem. It was mainly related to new treatment technologies and the increasing demands of the ageing populations, but it was also due to the capacity of the system to induce ever increasing demand for its services and to the ineffectiveness and unresponsiveness of the public 'bureaucratic-professional' management of the services. These themes have also penetrated the way in which the still existing queues and other quality deficiencies are perceived in the 1990s. Although the economic situation among the Nordic countries has significantly varied in the 1990s (see Chapters 1 and 2), the policy themes have been much the same in all of them (Alban and Christensen 1995).

Trends in service expenditure

In the early 1980s, the public expenditure on health per capita was significantly higher in Sweden than in other Nordic countries (Table 5.1). During the 1980s, a cost expansion was experienced in Iceland and Norway and, especially, in Finland while both Sweden and Denmark had much more modest development in their public health expenditure. Thus, by 1990 the gap between Sweden, on the one hand, and Finland and Norway, on the other hand, had decreased

Table 5.1 Trends in the expenditure on health services and social care for the elderly and handicapped in the Nordic countries, 1980–94

Year	Denmark	Finland	Norway	Sweden
Public expenditure on health per capita in relative prices, 1980 = 100				
1980	100	100	100	100
1990	112	164	133	105
1994	124	144	159	83
Public expenditure on health per capita in purchasing power parity prices, Sweden = 100				
1994	101	91	135	100
Public expenditure on services for elderly and handicapped in relative prices, 1981 = 100				
1981	100	100	100	100
1990	108	233	688	152
1994	117	265	1075	229
Public expenditure on services for elderly and handicapped in purchasing power parity prices, Sweden = 100				
1994	100	41	117	100

Sources: OECD Health Data 1997; NOSOSCO 1993, 1997; Nordic Statistical Secretariat 1984.

significantly, and Denmark clearly had the lowest expenditure. In the early 1990s the trends diverged. Sweden and Finland succeeded in cutting their public health expenditure significantly during their economic recessions while Denmark and more so Norway increased their expenditure significantly. In 1994, Norway was clearly the top Nordic country in public health expenditure, while Denmark had reached the same level as Sweden. Finland again had the lowest expenditure in 1994, although the gap with Sweden had continued to decrease.

A very rough estimate of the expenditure on social care for the elderly can be compiled from the figures given by the Nordic Social Statistical Committee for the services for the elderly and disabled together. Finland seems to have had the lowest expenditure for these services and Norway the highest in 1994. Denmark, which had the highest expenditure in 1981, experienced the smallest increase in these costs both in the 1980s and in the 1990s, as it also did with regard to health expenditure. Norway has expanded these costs rapidly during both decades, again parallel with the changes in its health expenditure. Finland and Sweden have increased this expenditure during both decades. The increase was much slower during the economic recession of the 1990s in Finland. Sweden's elderly care expenditure rocketed during the economic recession at the same time its health expenditure decreased significantly. This can be explained, to a great extent, by the organizational shifting of the management of nursing homes from the health care administration to the social care administration (NOMESCO 1996).

Trends in service resources

The trend in health care resources seems to be towards having fewer hospital beds and towards hiring more highly qualified personnel (Table 5.2). This has also been a goal of the deinstutionalization policy adopted in all the Nordic countries. The differences between the Nordic countries have decreased both in the 1980s and in the 1990s. Finland has experienced the greatest increase in personnel and the greatest decrease in the quantity of beds, particularly in the number of psychiatric beds. In the 1980s, the public health expenditure seemed to follow the increase in the number of highly qualified personnel hired. In the 1990s, both Finland and Sweden seem to have succeeded in decreasing the public health expenditure at the same time as the number of highly qualified personnel continued to increase. It may be assumed that during the recession of the 1990s Finland and Sweden could restrict wage inflation in their public

Table 5.2 Number of hospital beds and number of health professionals per 1,000 population in the Nordic countries, 1980–94

	Psychiatric beds per 1,000 population			Beds in acute somatic care hospitals per 1,000 population		
	1980	1990	1994	1980	1990	1994
Denmark	1.8	0.7	0.4	5.6	4.6	4.1
Finland	4.0	2.3	1.5	4.9	4.3	3.9
Norway	1.9	0.8	0.8	5.4	3.8	3.5
Sweden	3.2	1.7	1.1	5.1	4.1	3.2
	Actively practising physicians per 1,000 population			Registered nurses per 1,000 population		
	1980	1990	1994	1980	1990	1994
Denmark	2.2	2.8	2.9	5.1	6.5	6.7
Finland	1.7	2.4	2.7	8.3	10.2	12.0
Norway	2.0	3.1	3.2	n.a.	14.3	16.4
Sweden	2.2	2.9	3.0	7.0	9.2	10.1

Source: OECD Health Data 1997.

services, while public sector wages continued to increase quite rapidly in Norway and Denmark. If there is a relationship between the number of hospital beds and the public expenditure on health, it seems to be inverse: a reduction in the number of beds seems to be reached normally by increasing other costs by more than that saved by reducing the number of beds.

The trend in the resources for social care for the elderly also seems to be to provide less places in institutions in proportion to the increasing number of elderly people, and to hire more personnel for social care provided for the elderly living in normal housing or in so-called service housing. Sweden made an exception in the 1990s by increasing places in old-age institutions. This may again be explained by the administrative reorganizing of nursing homes from the health to social care sector (NOMESCO 1996: 38). The home-help personnel contingent increased rapidly in all Nordic countries in the 1980s. In the 1990s the trends have somewhat diverged (Daatland 1997): Finland has restricted the expansion almost totally (Lehto 1997); Sweden has allowed only a slow increase (Socialstyrelsen 1996a); while Denmark (Hansen and Platz 1995) and, particularly, Norway (NOSOSCO 6: 1997) have continued their stable increase in home-help personnel.

Trends in service use

The trend in the use of main health services has been quite the same in all Nordic countries and over time (Table 5.3). The number of treatment periods (admissions) in hospitals has increased slowly while the number of outpatient visits to physicians has increased much more rapidly. There does not seem to be any direct or inverse relationship between changes in public health expenditure and the use of health services. The fact that the number of treatment periods has increased at the same time as the number of hospital beds has continuously decreased indicates that the content of a hospital treatment period has changed significantly. One important aspect of this development is an intensification and increased efficacy of hospital treatment attributable to new health technology. A second aspect is a separation of care from medicine: the responsibility for caring for chronically ill or 'medically treated' elderly people has been moved from hospitals to the providers of social care.

The increase in beds provided by social care does not, however, compensate for the whole decrease in hospital beds (Table 5.4). Thus, an increased burden falls on home-help and home nursing. This has been met by an increase in home-help resources in Denmark and Norway. Also Finland and Sweden significantly increased home-help resources in the 1980s. However, during the economic recession of the 1990s, Finland and Sweden radically cut the number of home-help recipients while increasing the amount of help given to the remaining recipients (Lehto 1997; Socialstyrelsen 1996a). The policy has been to tighten needs testing for home-help, to retarget it to those in greatest need.

Table 5.3 Proportion of population admitted to hospital treatment and number of outpatient visits to physicians in the Nordic countries, 1980–94

	Proportion of population (%) admitted to in-patient hospital treatment within a year			*Outpatient visits to physicians (millions)*		
	1980	*1990*	*1994*	*1981*	*1990*	*1994*
Denmark	18.3	21.2	20.4	17.0	21.8	24.8
Finland	21.0	22.4	25.1	14.0	16.2	18.4
Norway	15.5	n.a.	16.5	22.0	24.2	27.1
Sweden	18.3	19.5	19.0	n.a.	n.a.	n.a.

Sources: OECD Health Data 1997f; NOMESCO 38: 1992 and 1996; Nordic Statistical Secretariat 1984.

Table 5.4 Proportions of the elderly living in institutions and service housing and recipients of home help in the Nordic countries, 1984–94

	Persons living in institutions and service housing as percentage of population 65 years and over			Recipients of home help as percentage of population 65 years and over		
	1984	*1990*	*1994*	*1984*	*1990*	*1994*
Denmark	7.2	6.5	7.0	17.0	18.0	20.0
Finland	6.7	5.6	7.0	14.0	22.0	12.0
Norway	10.5	6.5	6.0	18.0	17.0	17.0
Sweden	9.5	5.0	8.0	24.0	18.0	11.0

Sources: NOSOSCO 1993 and 1996; Nordic Statistical Secretariat 1987.

Are the changes in health care and care for the elderly relevant to the Nordic welfare state model?

Privatization of service provision?

The provision of health care and social care has never been a total monopoly of the public sector in the Nordic countries (Table 5.5). The most expensive services, particularly hospitals, are most often run by regional or local authorities. However, a considerable proportion of outpatient services of dentists, general practitioners and specialists are provided by privately working practitioners. Pharmacies may be private enterprises. A proportion of social care services for the elderly are also produced by private providers. In addition, an increasing proportion of support services for health and social care services, e.g. cleaning, catering and transport, are provided by private entrepreneurs (Alban and Christensen 1995).

A schematic dualism between private and public provision is, however, easily misleading. For instance, most of the 'private' GPs in Denmark are working on contracts with municipalities, which puts them in a similar relationship with respect to the public sector as if they were public employees. At the same time, the private GPs, and especially the private dentists, in Finland are working in a private market much more separated from the managerial or financial controls of the local authorities. The private pharmacies in Sweden are run by a state-owned monopoly, while the private pharmacies in other countries are owned by private pharmacists. Thus, a significant proportion of the private health sector activity may be described as

Table 5.5 The role of the private sector in the supply of health care and social care for the elderly in the Nordic countries in 1994

Type of Service	Denmark	Finland	Norway	Sweden
Hospital	Only a few private	Only a few private	Only a few private	Only a few private, increased in 1990s
GPs	Most of them private practitioners contracted to local authorities	Only a small proportion private practitioners	About a half private practitioners	Only a small proportion private practitioners
Dentists	Most of them private practitioners	About a half private practitioners	Most private practitioners	Almost a half private practitioners
Pharmacies	Majority	Majority	Majority	Majority a state-owned enterprise
Old age homes	A small proportion private non-profit	About 10% run by non-profit organizations	A small proportion run by non-profit organizations	A small proportion run by non-profit organizations
Service homes for the elderly	A small proportion private non-profit	About 25% run by non-profit organizations	A significant proportion private non-profit, some for-profit	A significant proportion private non-profit
Home help services	Insignificant proportion private	About 5% provided by non-profit organizations or private entrepreneurs	A small proportion by non-profit and for-profit	A proportion by non-profit and for-profit

Sources: Alban and Christensen 1995; Lehto 1997; Socialstyrelsen 1996a.

being guided by almost the same rules as those of the public sector. The real for-profit health services sector is quite narrow, especially in Sweden. It seems to be somewhat larger, although still marginal, in Finland and Norway. A significant proportion of registered private providers of social care for the elderly are in contractual relationship with the local authorities. Most of them are run by non-profit organizations. The for-profit sector in social care is even more restricted than in health care. The largest 'private' segment in social care for the elderly is informal care: care given by spouses, children and other relatives, friends or neighbours. The number of elderly dependent on significant informal care is notably greater than the number of elderly receiving public social care (Socialstyrelsen 1996a: 158; Lehto *et al.* 1997).

There has been discussion about privatization of service production in all the countries, most of all in Sweden in the 1990s. Practical shifts in this direction have been rather cautious, at least until 1996. Sweden has implemented some significant projects to privatize hospitals, resulting in an increase in the proportion of private providers in the supply of acute hospital treatments to almost 20 per cent (OECD Health Data 1997). Sweden has also increased the proportion of private providers of residential care for the elderly, but the proportion was still only 8 per cent in 1996 (Socialstyrelsen 1996a). At the same time, Finland has somewhat deprivatized service provision by cutting public funds more from contracts with private providers than from public providers (Lehto 1997).

Although the discussion on privatization has not led to widespread privatization, it has indicated and supported a shift in the approach to the management of public health and elderly care in all the Nordic countries. It may be described as an attempt to move from traditional 'bureau-professional' administration of services to a more managerialist 'new public management' of services (see, e.g. Ferlie *et al.* 1996). Management by objectives, management by outcomes, total quality management and other management 'schools' have become familiar to service providers. Plans to create a split between purchasers and providers of the services, to encourage competition between providers and to build contract-based relationships between provider units and purchasing public authorities have been presented in all Nordic countries (Saltman and von Otter 1992; Alban and Christensen 1995).

Attempts to contain rising hospital expenditures have received particular attention in all the Nordic countries. It has been claimed that the old administrative habit of fixed hospital budgets created both professional and bureaucratic incentives for continuous cost expansion (Saltman and von Otter 1992). Most reforms and reform proposals have been based on making a hospital's income dependent on its output and demand. All countries are developing negotiation and contracting models between purchasing local authorities and hospitals. Denmark has implemented such contract strategies in three counties since 1993 and is considering applying these to other counties as well. Reimbursement incentives for hospitals to increase the number of surgical operations have been developed, particularly in some Swedish counties. Norway is planning a financing model for hospitals that is based on fixed-price-for-treatment packages defined for different diagnosis-related groups, which means that there is an incentive to make the treatment packages more efficient (Nyfigen 1997). New contract models are also being developed between municipalities and hospitals in Finland.

National legislation or regulations on 'free hospital choice' have been introduced during the 1990s. The fact that patients are allowed to choose to be treated at any hospital outside the county may be seen as an attempt to introduce regulated competition in the health care sector, in the sense that it is the choice of the patient that determines which health care provider will receive the payment. Danish results from 1994 regarding patients' use of free hospital choice show that 2 per cent of all discharged patients have used their right to choose a hospital outside their own county (Danish Ministry of Health 1995). Swedish results, however, indicate that in some areas free hospital choice has led to a considerable flow of patients across county borders (Alban and Christensen 1995). The flow of patients across county borders has further increased as a result of new legislation on guaranteed maximum waiting time, which was introduced in Norway in 1990, in Sweden in 1992 and in Denmark in 1993 (Christensen *et al.* 1996). In Finland, the guarantees introduced in the 1990s have not been legally binding but, rather, have been policy goal statements (STM 1996).

Privatization of funding?

Most Nordic health and social care services have been primarily funded by public tax revenue. However, only few services are totally free of charge for the service users. The proportion paid by the service user tends to be higher in dental care, with regard to medical drugs and in social care services (NOMESCO 1996; NOSOSCO 6: 1997).

The proportion of private consumption of the total health expenditure was about 20 per cent in Finland, from 12 to 15 per cent in
Denmark and less than 10 per cent in Norway and Sweden, until the
1990s. In the 1990s the situation changed considerably. Norway and
Denmark have kept low proportions of private consumption or even
reduced it. At the same time, the proportion has increased to 25 per
cent in Finland and to 16 per cent in Sweden (OECD Health Data
1997). Denmark and Norway decreased the proportion of user
charges in the funding of home-help in the 1990s. At the same
time, Sweden and, particularly, Finland have increased the proportion paid by the users of this service. One of the adaptation measures
to the economic difficulties in Finland and Sweden has clearly been a
slow privatization of service funding.

Universalism in access and use of services?

Nordic studies on use of health services have proved that a person's
need for medical care is the strongest determinant of the use of health
services. Other factors like socioeconomic status, numbers of GPs in
the population and social networks seem to be less important in
explaining why there are differences in the use of health services
(Fylkesnes 1993; Andersen and Laake 1983). The primary reason
why the lower socioeconomic groups use health services more
frequently than the higher socioeconomic groups seems to be
explained by the former's relatively poorer health status. There is
much evidence in the Nordic countries that persons with low socioeconomic status experience more disease than persons with high
socioeconomic status (Kjoeller *et al.* 1995; Lahelma *et al.* 1993;
Lundberg 1990; Maaseide 1990).

For some health services, however, there seems to be greater use
among the higher socioeconomic groups, when differences in need are
taken into account. These include specialist and dental care services.
Differences in use of dental care services may be explained by the low
proportion of public funding of these services, at least in Finland
(Klavus and Häkkinen 1995).

The principle of universal access implies a fair geographical distribution of services throughout the country. There do not seem to be
considerable differences in the access to primary health care services
between regions in any of the Nordic countries (Alban and Christensen
1995). There are, however, significant exceptions to this general picture. Many private services are concentrated in the more prosperous
and densely populated centres (Klavus and Häkkinen 1995). Within

the public system, different professional priorities and traditions have also been proven to cause significant regional variation in the balance between different medical activities. For instance, in regions with the highest rates the numbers of certain surgical operations may be up to five times higher than in regions with the lowest rates (Madsen *et al.* 1994). Large public service units, such as specialized hospitals, are situated in regional centres and, thus, practical access to these services is somewhat easier for people living near these units.

The universalism of social care services for the elderly is more difficult to assess than the universalism in health care. Both the testing of social needs for these services and the use of income-related client fees for most of these services in all Nordic countries create at least a tendency towards selectivism in them. The tightened needs testing in Sweden and Finland and the quite high proportion of the total expenditure of client fees in Finland in the 1990s may be described as threats against universalism in the care for the elderly. The regional variation in the supply of social care services is also rather significant (Lehto 1997; Socialstyrelsen 1996a; Hansen and Platz 1995).

The radical changes in the provision of care, such as deinstitutionalization and the separation of medicine from care in hospital treatment, as well as the need for increased prioritization due to the growing gap between what is technically possible and what is financially feasible in health care have emphasized professional discretion in the provision of health care and related social care. If universalism is understood as universal access to those services for which the professional gatekeepers assess the individual's needs, the increase in professional discretion does not threaten universalism. From the client's or citizen's perspective, however, the increased discretion may also mean selectivism. It has been claimed, for instance, that the age or the life style of a patient tends to become the discriminating criterion for exclusion from some services.

Child care

Changes in the Nordic child day care systems

The common Nordic approach to child day care has been to facilitate parents' and especially women's employment and at the same time to contribute to providing for children a stimulating and educational upbringing based on pedagogical principles. While providing public day care services, the policy has also been to strengthen the parents' right to take maternity, paternity and parental leaves, in most cases with a leave benefit. The Nordic child care system is not separated into welfare and education as is the case in many other countries, but functions as an integrated system. Overall, day care provision mainly consists of public, full-time, all-year round day care. Services are mainly tax-financed, with client fees covering approximately 15 to 25 per cent of costs.

The Nordic countries do, however, to some extent also differ in objectives regarding day care and in the means of providing day care. The strategies followed in the provision of day care also reflect differences in family values and the role of the state. The Danish and Swedish systems of day care have for a long time been characterized by high public provision. In Norway the family has stood strong and public provision of child care has increased only during the last decade. In Finland, the public provision of day care has been and still is lower than in the other countries. Here, the objective has been to provide parents with the opportunity to care for a child at home if they choose, by means of a cash benefit, and the newest development is to provide a voucher to purchase private day care. Overall, however, most children today are cared for in the public day care system (Table 5.6). In Denmark, the number of children in public day care has risen to levels unmatched by that in any other country.

Trends in expenditure

The changes in the public expenditure for child care services (see Table 5.7) mainly reflect the increasing number of children in care. However, partly it also reflects the changes in the personnel/child ratio in care institutions as well as the development of the wages of personnel. Changes in the proportion of client fees in the total expenditure also have a small impact on the changes in public expenditure. Thus, the rising child care expenditure in Denmark and Norway runs parallel to the increase in the number of children in care. The financial problems experienced in Finland and Sweden in the early 1990s have also had their impact. In Sweden, considerable budgetary cuts were made during the recession of the early 1990s, the largest of which were made in child care. Especially the big cities were hit by the recession, and expenditure for children's day care was reduced by almost 15 per cent in 1993 and again in 1994 (European Observatory on National Family Policies 1995). However, the decrease in child care expenditure in Sweden in the early 1990s was attained without decreasing the number of children in care. Thus, this was achieved by

Table 5.6 Number of children 0–10 years of age enrolled in institutional day care and family day care in the Nordic countries, 1981–95

	Denmark		Norway[a]		Finland		Sweden[a]	
	Institut. day care	Family day care	Institut. day care	Family day care	Institut. day care	Family day care	Institut. day care	Family day care
1981	176,000	64,000	83,000	2,000	79,000	54,000	148,000	131,500
1987	211,000	67,000	111,000	2,700	101,000	87,000	216,000	172,000
1990	242,000	66,000	139,000	3,500	110,000	90,000	267,000	156,000
1993	300,000	77,000	173,000	9,000	112,500	62,000	322,000	128,000
1994	332,000	76,000	183,000	11,500	118,000	63,000	338,000	129,500
1995	349,000	68,500	188,000	13,500	125,031	65,580	361,000	123,000

Sources: Sweden: Socialstyrelsen 1996b. Norway: SSB 1995, 1996 and NOSOSCO 2: 1995. Note: not including educational programmes for the 6 year olds. Finland: NOSOSCO 2: 1995 and STAKES, 1996 and 1997b. Denmark: Kampmann and von Nordheim 1995 and NOSOSCO 2: 1995.

Note
a only children 1–6 years.

Table 5.7 Social expenditure for maternity and parental leave cash benefits and formal day care as percentage of GDP in the Nordic countries, 1980–93

	1980	1984	1990	1993
Denmark				
Maternity and parental leave	0.26	0.33	0.53	0.55
Formal day care	1.46	1.47	1.64	2.05[a]
Finland				
Maternity and parental leave	0.24	0.55	0.62	0.72
Formal day care	0.59	0.77	1.44	1.15
Norway				
Maternity and parental leave	0.17	0.16	0.34	0.46
Formal day care	0.46	0.45	0.7	0.82
Sweden				
Maternity and parental leave	0.67	0.66	1.16	1.32
Formal day care	1.68	1.88	2.15	2.13

Source: OECD 1996c.

Note
a   Figure from 1992.

decreasing the personnel/child ratio, by keeping a much more modest wage development than in Norway and Denmark and by increasing the level of client fees. In Finland, the decrease in the early 1990s was attained by using the same methods as in Sweden in addition to a temporary decrease in the number of children in care in the 1992–4 period.

Trends in service resources

The provision of public day care places has expanded dramatically in all the Nordic countries during the 1980s and 1990s: this has not been so much a response to demographic changes in the number of children, which has remained relatively stable (see Chapter 3) except for in Sweden and, to a lesser extent, in Norway in which there were increases in the number of children born in the early 1990s. Rather, the expansion in provision is a reflection of a policy to provide day care for children whose parents are working and, as in Sweden and Finland, for parents who are studying.

Small differences accrue in what is considered to be the best form of day care, although this is not always reflected in the way resources are used. In Denmark, the objective in children's day care at the beginning of the 1980s was to provide family day care instead of day care in institutions. The actual expansion from the beginning of the 1990s does not quite reflect this. The biggest expansion after the announcement of the universal day care guarantee in 1993 has taken place in institutional day care. Day care places in Sweden have also increased rapidly. The number of places in family day care, however, started decreasing from the mid-1980s on.

The increase in day care places in Norway reflects an extensive expansion of kindergarten places. The latter years' increase in kindergarten places has mainly taken place in private facilities for which the municipalities do not always provide financial support.

In Finland, the number of municipal day care places started increasing from the mid-1980s onward. The rapid growth in unemployment and the cuts in public expenditure in the early 1990s did, however, lead many municipalities to stop increasing the availability of day care places, and the number of places in family day care fell by about 20,000 places from 1990 to 1994. The number of places in institutional day care remained the same during this period. From 1995 on, however, the number of places has started to increase again to meet the demands of the extension of the right to day care (STM 1997; European Commission Network on Children 1996).

Trends in the use of public day care

It is mainly children aged 3 to 6 years who make use of public day care, and especially institutional day care. Sweden and Denmark have the highest proportion of all children and, particularly, of older children in public day care. However, even they have not met the demand for services in all regions of the country and in both countries there are waiting lists for entry into day care. Family day care is mainly used by the youngest children, except for Finland where older children also are in family day care. The number of children in family day care has decreased in Sweden, Finland and Denmark even though this is a more flexible solution compared with institutional day care. The government attitude in Norway has traditionally favoured the family day care system as this is considered to be most suitable for younger children, but very few children are cared for in this system compared with the other countries. A greater proportion of part-time day care for older children is also a Norwegian characteristic. About 25 per cent of day care for the 3- to 6-year-olds is part-time care.

The Finnish characteristic is a lower proportion of children in public day care and an extensive home care allowance system, which has increased the incentive of mothers to stay outside the labour market while their children are small, particularly during the high unemployment of the 1990s. Since 1995, the number of children, particularly of 3- to 6-year-olds, in public day care has increased in Finland as a result of the extension of day care rights in legislation and of the decrease in unemployment. Table 5.8 shows these developments from 1981 to 1993.

Table 5.8 Percentage of children enrolled in day care institutions and family day care by age group in the Nordic countries, 1981–93

	Percentage of children aged 0–10 years in public day care[a]	Of which: Day care in institutions, percentage of total number of children		Family day care, percentage of total number of children	
		Aged 0–2 years	Aged 3–6 years	Aged 0–2 years	Aged 3-6 years
Denmark					
1981	33	15	39	22	8
1987	45	18	56	27	9
1990	50	19	59	28	7
1993	54	18	68	29	6
Finland					
1981	21	6	25	11	12
1987	28	12	29	14	20
1990	31	15	36	16	23
1993	26	8	35	8	16
Norway					
1981	13	5	35	n.a.	n.a.
1987	20	7	49	1	1
1990	n.a.	11	57	1	1
1993	44	17	61	3	2
Sweden					
1981	36	13	50	11	15
1987	48	18	58	13	21
1990	51	19	61	10	18
1993	52	23	63	9	14

Sources: Nord (1996: 1). Norwegian 1993 figure for percentage of total number of children 0–10 years from SSB 1995.

Note
a   The figures in Norway only include the children in institutional day care.

Trends in objectives and policy goals in child care

Whether children should be cared for in institutions or in family day care has been one issue for debate, but economic hardship has also made many municipalities introduce new forms of child care which are more flexible and therefore cost-saving. The Danish expansion has thus taken place especially in more flexible forms of day care, such as age-integrated facilities, but new types of day care such as 'forest kindergartens' add to the flexibility as they are independent of institutional facilities. The parental support for these day care arrangements has been substantial, especially in the bigger cities. In Norway, the extension of the maternity leave to 42 weeks, and the increase in services provided for 6-year-olds in the pre-school system have taken some of the pressure off the provision of municipal day care. The kindergartens, as in Denmark, have moved towards age-integrated care provision as this offers a more flexible care arrangement (Halvorsen 1996). In Sweden, family day care is more and more often organized as extended family day care where several child-minders care for a number of children in facilities provided by the municipality (Svenska Kommunförbundet 1995). Apart from family day care and kindergartens, other forms of day care include the popular open pre-school which functions as a drop-in form of pedagogical arrangement. This day care arrangement is intended for children whose parents are at home, either because they are unemployed, studying or on leave. The importance of the open pre-schools has grown with the increase in unemployment, but the number of facilities has decreased since the beginning of the 1990s. Every fourth one has been closed down since 1991, leaving 1,200 in all in 1995, and opening hours have decreased, too (Socialstyrelsen 1996b). In Finland, many children, and especially children of unemployed people, make use of playground pedagogical activities. As in Sweden, these were being cut through financial difficulties in the early 1990s. More flexible forms of day care have also been introduced, such as developing extended family day care where two or three family day carers work together (European Commission Network on Childcare 1996).

Child day care in the Nordic sense has traditionally been a mixture of social care and pedagogical activity. It seems that in the 1990s the pedagogical aspects of day care policy goals have been given more emphasis. Sweden has implemented an administrative move of child care from the social service sector to the primary education sector and Norway moved the responsibility for day care for the 6-year-olds to the primary education sector in 1997 (Rauhala *et al.* 1997).

Finland was preparing a partial reallocation of the responsibility for the 6-year-olds in 1997. The Finnish move was postponed for financial reasons, but the increased emphasis on a pre-school orientation can clearly be identified.

Are the changes in child care relevant to the Nordic welfare state model?

Rights to day care – a move towards further universalism?

The Nordic model is characterized by local responsibility for provision of social services, but the individual right to receive services has not previously been emphasized. In later years, however, the right to some services has been made explicit, especially within services for children.

Sweden established a right to day care by Parliamentary decision in 1985. All children aged between one and a half years and school age were to be entitled to a place in municipal day care by 1991. For children of working parents or parents who are studying this right encompasses a place in a day care centre, in parental co-operative day care or in family day care. For children already in family day care or children who have parents working at home, the right encompasses a place in open pre-school or a place in part-time day care.

Finland established a subjective right to day care for children under 3 years of age by a Parliamentary decision also passed in 1985. It was a political compromise in which the Social Democrats supported an expansion of public day care and the right and centre parties favoured at-home care. The solution was then to offer the right to day care as a choice between a (public) home care allowance, given to parents caring for their children at home, or a place in municipal public day care. The right to public day care has, from 1996 on, been extended to include the 3- to 6-year-olds also. This was not complemented by an extension of the right to the home care allowance.

In 1992 and 1993 the Danish government announced that a public day care guarantee for all children aged 1 to 5 years was to be introduced from the beginning of 1995, ensuring each child's place either in a kindergarten or in another form of care.

The Norwegian municipalities are charged with developing and running day care for children, but no explicit right to day care has been articulated, except for handicapped children who are secured a place by law. The government has, however, stated that child care should be made available for all children during the 1990s but that is not to be considered a legal right (Halvorsen 1996).

The municipalities have, however, had problems in fulfilling day care rights or guarantees, and local differences prevail. Although the day care guarantee in Denmark was only a recommendation to local authorities, this has been taken very seriously, and the national government has provided extra funding for additional staffing costs. There are still children on day care waiting lists, although the lists are the shortest they have ever been. Children of unemployed people in some municipalities are placed at lowest priority, although there are no provisions in the legislation for such discrimination (European Commission Network on Childcare 1996).

In Sweden also there are great municipal differences in the coverage rates; there is an estimated shortage of 60,000 places, and similarly to in Denmark, the children of unemployed people have limited access to day care. Eighty per cent of the municipalities have introduced a restricted right to day care for children of unemployed parents, typically by lowering hours to three hours a day or restricting access entirely (Socialstyrelsen 1996a).

The Norwegian municipalities likewise have varied priorities in the admission to day care. Some give priority to children of municipal employees, others to children of parents with special needs or to children with special needs (Halvorsen 1996). There are still high regional differences in the provision of child day care although this tends to equal out due to the increase in part-time places in the smaller municipalities (NOU 1996).

The growth in unemployment rates in Finland has resulted in a similar attempt to restrict access of children of unemployed parents to public child care. Until the summer of 1997, this debate had not led to any changes in legislation, but recent changes in the home care allowance have made home care a less tempting alternative and this has created more demand for day care.

The introduction of the right to day care has thus moved the provision of day care services closer to the cash benefit system. However, the implementation of the day care guarantee has proved difficult due to economic difficulties, so that the right in many cases is only a right to be assessed. Local autonomy creates great variation in the provision of day care, especially in the bigger cities as compared to the rural areas, and the entitlement to social care is thus less institutionalized than is entitlement to cash benefits (Leira 1993). The exclusion of children of unemployed parents is an obvious strategy for economically hard-ridden municipalities to cut costs, but also a strategy which may increase social problems for these children. The guarantees also seem to increase pressures to decrease the quality standards of day care, to increase the client fees and to create cash benefits as an alternative to exercising the right to public care.

Privatization of service provision

Child care has not been subject to any extensive for-profit privatization policies in the Nordic countries. Yet, the day care arrangements have undergone changes in the direction of opening up private provision with public support and also for privately initiated day care. This has been spurred both by the shortage in day care provision and the cuts in budgets, but also by the philosophy that parents should be able to choose between different arrangements and be able to influence the provision of day care.

Forms of privatization other than that merely for-profit have also appeared in the shape of financial support for co-operatives or for informal care of children. This displays the other side of the coin of privatization – namely the individualization of responsibility for the provision of day care with public financing but within the private sphere.

With regard to for-profit provision of services, Sweden is perhaps the country among the Nordic countries where the spirit of for-profit privatization has meant the greatest changes in the 1990s. There the significance of private providers has had its ups and downs, and the rate of private provision fell in the early 1980s from 3.2 per cent in 1970 to 0.8 per cent in 1980. In 1988, for-profit provision of day care was even banned, but soon after coming to power in 1992, the Bourgeois government ensured that it would be possible to set up for-profit provision of day care with state funding. At the same time, the municipalities have been encouraged to take on extra responsibilities, to charge higher fees and to accept alternative ways of organizing child care. More choice and competition has been the mantra, with the addendum that high standards should continue (George and Taylor-Gooby 1996).

For-profit child care services are, however, still very few. Instead, parental co-operatives have gained ground in Sweden, where this form of day care arrangement along with provision from non-profit organizations, companies and others has grown since the beginning of the 1990s. Parents' co-operatives rose to a position equalling that of municipal day care in 1991 and were from then on entitled to state support; it is the most popular private day care arrangement today. In all, the private provision of day care made up 10 per cent of the total provision in 1995. The country-wide distribution of parents' co-operatives is, however, very unequal, and they are found mainly in the southern parts of Sweden and in the bigger cities where the waiting lists have also been the longest (Socialstyrelsen 1996a).

The economic crisis in Finland has meant that ideologies of provision of welfare have started to change, and although the municipal policy response has so far rather been to de-privatize and monopolize in order to maintain the jobs of public employees (Lehto 1995), there is now more room for a market orientation in general. In 1995, private services constituted 5 per cent of all services in full-time care and 8 per cent in part-time care (STAKES 1997a).

In Denmark, privatization policies have met greater resistance in the care for the elderly whereas they have been more accepted in day care for children thanks to the traditionally high number of so-called independent child care institutions. In 1990, under the Bourgeois government, private provision of day care with public support was made possible, e.g. for parents setting up a day care arrangement or an enterprise providing day care for the children of employees. The pool arrangement can take place either in a family setting as parent-initiated day care or as workplace-situated day care. The pool schemes are considered to be part of public provision but can be negotiated to set aside a number of places, e.g. for employees. There are approximately 150 pool scheme arrangements, mainly in rural areas (European Commission Network on Childcare 1996). For-profit provision of services has so far not been an issue. However, the cleaning company ISS has recently made an agreement with a municipality to establish a for-profit kindergarten.

In contrast to the other Nordic countries, there had been a predominance of private non-profit providers of child care in Norway up until 1974. During the 1980s and 1990s this changed slightly, and by 1995, 60 per cent of the kindergartens were municipal, and the rest were owned by voluntary organizations, enterprises, parent co-operatives and church communities (Halvorsen 1996). Only 50 per cent of private kindergartens receive public funding. The recent increase in the provision of day care has mainly taken place in private day care. An important aspect in the increase in private day care is the rise in private family day care, where the children are cared for in their own home. The number of children in private family day care increased from 4,600 to 11,600 between 1991 and 1994 (NOU 1996).

Other ways of supporting the private provision of day care can be to finance the use of private care. In Denmark, a transitional measure introduced in 1994 lasting until 1997 made it possible for some municipalities to subsidize private services by giving a grant to parents of children under 3 years old attending a non-subsidized service if the child is on a waiting list for public service. It can be given for 1 year only and ceases when the child is offered a place in the public system (European Commission Network on Childcare 1996). In Finland, a similar scheme was introduced as part of the new day care system from 1 August 1997, giving parents a choice between a place in public day care, the home care allowance or a voucher for purchasing private day care services.

The improvement in the child care leave schemes in terms of the right to take time off and in some cases also the right to receive a benefit has meant improved possibilities of caring for children in the home, and along with the introduction of various care allowances this has meant cost-cutting in the provision of public day care. The introduction of the child home care allowance in 1985 in Finland was one of the first moves in the direction of improving individual choice and increasing individual responsibility for the provision of day care (European Observatory on National Family Policies 1995). A similar individualization provision was attempted in Sweden during the period 1991–94 under a Bourgeois government. This was, however, soon abolished after the Social Democrats came to power again.

The individualization of responsibility for organizing day care services which has gained momentum with the increasing number of parent-initiated day care places, and the increase in individual responsibility for providing the services facilitated by care leaves and care allowances mean that parents have also become involved in monitoring the quality and standards of the day care for their children to a higher degree than before. This is in line with new polices to involve parents in parental boards in the kindergartens and family day care.

The increase in leave benefits and home care allowances reflects the traditional boundary between service and cash benefits, where Bourgeois parties tend to favour care allowances which facilitate home care of children and the social democratic parties favour services which allow labour market participation. The compromise has been to introduce rights to care leaves and to extend the maternity benefit period at the same time as providing day care for the children of employed parents.

Privatization of funding?

The share of costs paid by the user of services has increased in all the Nordic countries during recent years, but to a lesser degree in Denmark. Along with the changes in state subsidy systems and the reduced state funding of services, the formulation of explicit rights to services within child care has placed even greater financial strain on the municipalities in order to fulfil this right. An often used strategy has consequently been to increase client fees, both as a way to increase resources and also as a means of lowering demand. Client fees for child care are income-related in all Nordic countries. Thus, they are higher for parents with higher incomes.

In Finland, the municipalities have thus tried to improve their financial situation by increasing the client fees. In 1990, client fees covered about 11 per cent of the total expenditure for child care. In 1995, the share of client fees had increased to about 15 per cent of total cost.

The Swedish ban on increases in municipal taxes has made many municipalities raise client fees. The client fees for child care have increased from 10 per cent in 1990 to about 14 per cent of total expenditure in 1995 (Socialstyrelsen 1996b). The municipal variation in fees is great, with differences of almost 70 per cent between the lowest fees and the highest fees paid (European Observatory on National Family Policies 1995).

In Denmark, a maximum level of client fees is set centrally. The maximum was reduced during the 1990s, from 35 per cent of total running costs to 30 per cent in 1993. However, municipal subsidies reduce the share paid by parents so that it is in reality lower, on average around 20 per cent in 1994 (European Commission Network on Childcare 1996). In contrast to other Nordic countries, the share of costs paid by Danish parents has not increased much (Finansministeriet 1995).

Norwegian child day care was set to be financed 40 per cent by the state in the late 1980s, and the remaining 60 per cent was to be equally shared by the parents and the municipalities. However, the changes in the composition of day care with its greater number of private providers have meant that client fees are somewhat higher today. In 1994, the client fees constituted 45 per cent of the total running costs in private day care in comparison to 29 per cent in the municipal kindergartens. The payment arrangements differ among the municipalities, where approximately half of the municipalities use income-related charges, and the other half use set fees (NOU 1996).

Changes in standards

Most of the municipalities in the Nordic countries, particularly in Sweden and Finland, have reduced the level of standards in order to save costs. A common strategy has been to admit more children into day care groups, e.g. this has happened in Sweden where the number of children is recommended to be no more than 15 per group. In 1980, 14 per cent of the kindergartens had more children in their groups, whereas in 1990 and in 1992, 38 per cent and 56 per cent, respectively, had more than 15 children (Hedengren 1994). Staff levels have also been reduced and opening hours have been cut. In 1993, the average number of staff per 100 full-time enrolled children was between 19 and 22 in all four countries, with the highest ratio in Norway and the lowest ratio in Sweden and Finland (NOSOSCO 2: 1995).

At the same time, the average length of professional education for the employees has increased. In Sweden, the training for kindergarten teachers was increased from two and a half years to three years in 1993 (European Commission Network on Childcare 1996), and in Finland this training will now be a university degree. The training has also been extended in Denmark to three and half years. When comparing Finland, Denmark and Sweden, the number of trained to untrained employees is highest in Sweden and lowest in Denmark.

Conclusion

The basic characteristics, relevant to health and social care services, of the Nordic welfare state model are universal access to services, high quality of services, public tax funding of services and public provision of services by the local authorities. The aim of this article was to study whether these characteristics can be found in the actual service systems of the Nordic countries and whether the recent and ongoing changes in economies, politics and social needs (described in Chapter 2 and Chapter 3) are moving the Nordic countries away from these characteristics.

It may be said that the Nordic countries have had and still have universalist health care systems. There are, however, some issues that may put universalism in question. First of all, some health care, such as dental care for adults in Finland, have such a high proportion of client fees in relation to the total cost that it creates an economic barrier to service use for people with low income. A second issue is an increase in the proportion of private consumption in the total health expenditure, which has become evident in Sweden and Finland during the economic hardships facing public finances in the 1990s. This might lead to an increase in private sickness insurance or other arrangements, by which better off people could gain a better access to health services than worse off people. The third issue is an increase in the professional discretion of the gatekeepers of health care. If not democratically controlled, this could lead to problems for universalism. Until now, there has been no empirical evidence that these three trends have actually created significant ruptures in universalism.

The universalism in health care, and to an increasing extent also in social care for the elderly, is in practice universal access to services that a gatekeeping professional has assessed are needed. The universalism of child care is different. There is no professional needs assessment, but rather admittance criteria are defined in legislation. All Nordic countries have been developing a universal right of parents to put their children in public day care. None of the countries has reached this kind of universalism, yet. Sweden and Denmark have expanded their day care systems to be the most universalistic and have given guarantees, although not legally binding, to universal access to child care. Finland has created a legally binding universal right of parents to either public child care or to a home care allowance, and tries to balance the supply and demand of public day care by offering a cash benefit alternative. Norway started its expansion of child care latest but is reducing the gap between itself and Sweden and Denmark quite rapidly.

Universalism in a service that is only needed if parents cannot take care of their children themselves does not seem to be clearly accepted in the Nordic countries. This is illustrated by the attempts to exclude the children of unemployed people from the universal right and by the Finnish arrangement and the Swedish attempt to establish a similar arrangement of home care allowance as an alternative to public day care. However, it may be assumed that the Nordic countries have been moving in a direction that could establish child day care as a right similar to public primary education for older children. A significant difference seems, however, to remain: while primary education is free of charge for parents, there are substantial and income-related client fees for day care in all Nordic countries.

It seems that social care for the elderly and social care for children are developing along lines based on different forms of universalism. Child care is adopting the model of primary education while care for the elderly seems to be adopting the model of health care. This may also lead to these two branches of social care having closer linkages to these service models – and to a dissolution of the general idea of social care.

There has never been a total public monopoly in the Nordic health and social care services. It seems that the role of private providers is increasing somewhat in all four countries. This role has been largest in Norway and the increase seems to be fastest in Sweden in the 1990s. Denmark seems to be the country with the least interest in moving away from the public service model in the 1990s. In Sweden part of the increase in the role of private providers has been attained by privatization. Most of the increase in all four countries, however, is a result of a greater role for private providers in the new services that are needed for expansion of the service supply or for reforming the service structure in the process of deinstitutionalization.

Public funding – and through funding arrangements, public control – of social and health care services is more extensive than public provision. Denmark seems to be the most Scandinavian with regard to low private funding of health and social services. Finland had the highest proportion of private health care funding in the 1980s, and it even increased in the 1990s. It has also had comparatively high private funding of social care. Sweden previously had a low proportion of private funding, but increased it in both social and health services in the early 1990s. Norway has had quite high private funding of social care but seems to be decreasing it in the 1990s, and has kept the traditionally low private funding of health care unchanged. Finally, there was a tendency in Sweden and Finland to increase private funding during the economic recession of the early 1990s. It remains to be seen whether this increase is a temporary adjustment to financial difficulties or something more persistent.

The principle of high quality in universal public services seems to have resisted the economic pressures of the 1990s rather well. It seems, however, that some quality standards of child day care have been given up when the need for rapidly expanding the service supply has been more important.

A general conclusion is that the Nordic model of social and health services has not significantly weakened in the 1990s. As a matter of fact, the model is providing even better child care. The differences between the Nordic countries decreased, in the 1980s. There are some areas where the economic hardships of Sweden and Finland in the 1990s seem to have led to an increase in differences between them and the better off Norway and Denmark. In particular, they have restricted the cost expansion of services. It remains to be seen whether this has been only a temporary gain due to the weak negotiating power of the public sector trade unions during the recession. Sweden and Finland have also increased the role of clients in the funding of health and social services. In this sense, they have somewhat weakened the implementation of the Nordic model. But even this weakening seems to be rather marginal in comparison to other trends which indicate that the Nordic model is still strong and even gaining in child care.

Discussion

International comparative welfare state research has been developed mainly by analysing similarities and differences in labour markets, income transfers, cash benefits, income differentials and poverty (see, e.g. Esping-Andersen 1996b). There also are many studies that compare health service delivery, financing and management systems internationally (see, e.g. WHO 1996), although there is not very much discussion between these two strands of comparative social policy studies. The social care services have been rising in the focus of some international comparative social policy studies only during the last few years (see, e.g. Anttonen and Sipilä 1996, Kautto 1997).

There are some significant difficulties in applying the concepts and approaches of general comparative welfare state research to health and social care services. For instance, the role of professional discretion and needs testing is much larger with regard to these services than with most cash benefits. The accessibility of cash benefits does not normally vary too much within a country, while the variation in access to and the quality of services may be extensive between different parts of a country. User charges for services funded mainly by public money may restrict the actual exercise of rights to services in a way that makes rights to services quite different from rights to cash benefits. Thus, a basic concept of international comparative welfare state research such as universalism or universal social right is much more difficult to operationalize with regard to services than with most cash benefits. It may be said that universal rights to cash benefits are unrestricted by professional discretion or the limit that the budget for a given year creates. Rights to services are often restricted by professional discretion. They may also be restricted by budget – the number of surgical operations or the quality of home-help is limited by the budget of the public provider. Education, at least primary education, is an example of a public service where users have an almost unlimited right to receive the service. The development of the right to child day care in the Nordic countries is an interesting attempt to extend unlimited rights to social services as well. The fact that extending of this right is being at least partially financed in a couple of the Nordic countries by increasing the number of children per staff member indicates that the service right is not even in this case as unlimited as universal cash benefits.

In addition to universalism, also the principle of equality may be more complicated with regard to services than with regard to the compensation rates of cash benefits. Should we focus on the distribution of supply, availability, access or use of services? How can we estimate the impact of variation in the quality of the services, or in the variation in priorities between different measures – should there be equality in access to surgical operations in general or in access to all different types of operations? Or should we focus on the distribution of conditions that are supposed to be outcomes of service use, such as distribution of health and sickness or of dependency/ independency? We have not been able to answer these questions although we have indicated there are clear cases of inequality behind the general picture of rather developed equality, in terms of those with equal service needs having unequal access to services.

6 Activation policies in the Nordic countries

Jon Anders Drøpping, Bjørn Hvinden and Kirsten Vik

Introduction

Faced with the challenge of controlling the increasing costs of their cash benefit systems, the Nordic governments have had several major options at their disposal. The most obvious policy would have been simply to make straightforward cuts in the income maintenance scheme, e.g. by introducing stricter eligibility criteria, lower levels of compensation and shorter duration of benefits. This is the hard option, primarily associated with the retrenchment policies adopted by conservative governments in other parts of the Western world (Pierson 1994). Another, softer, option has involved more socially acceptable alternatives to public income support, first of all by encouraging and assisting recipients to become self-sufficient through work. To the extent that more vigorous efforts in this direction are successful, there will be less demand for income support and reduced pressure on public budgets, while the material and social well-being of the individuals remains at the same level or is possibly even enhanced.

The strong tradition of institutional comprehensive welfare (Titmuss 1974) or of policies with a distinctly social-democratic character (Esping-Andersen 1990) would seem to make it probable that Nordic governments would prefer the activist option, as it is obviously the solution that is most compatible with their image and perception of themselves as socially responsible, inclusive and caring. But knowing what one wants to achieve is a different matter from being capable of achieving it. Increasing the emphasis on activation, help-to-self-help or work approaches as foundations of practical policies will in the short run entail larger – not reduced – public expenditure. Nor is it obvious that such approaches will be equally successful under all circumstances. Furthermore, their anticipated effectiveness is based on a set of underlying assumptions that may or may not be substantiated in practice.

In this chapter, we will examine the Nordic experience with activation policies in the period 1980 to 1995. First, we will clarify the meaning of activation and the way in which it is related to the concepts of active labour market policies, the work approach, workfare and work incentive. Next, we will discuss the official rationale for activation policies. We will then ask to what degree a stronger emphasis on activation became a practical reality in the Nordic countries in the course of the period under review. Was it adopted only as a rhetorical or ideological device to distract attention from cuts in the income maintenance system or to make official unemployment statistics look more favourable? We will go into some greater detail in the case of two areas of activation policies:

1   measures to assist young people experiencing difficulties in entering the labour market; and
2   attempts to prevent premature exit from the labour market in the case of people with disabilities.

Finally, we will comment on some of the many ambiguities and unresolved issues in the field of activation policies.

What is activation?

In this chapter, the term activation refers mainly to a broad range of policies and measures targeted at people receiving public income support or in danger of becoming permanently excluded from the labour market. Often the aim is to assist the target group to enter or re-enter the labour market through various forms of education, vocational training or retraining, group processes, coaching and practice programmes, and even through the channelling of financial resources. However, the specific objectives of individual measures may vary, as they depend on the starting point of the person concerned. Some have insertion or re-insertion in work as their immediate goal, while others are focused on more limited subgoals such as developing qualifications, theoretical knowledge, technical skills, self-confidence or social competence, or socialising the participant in the routines and expectations of working life. Measures may have entry or re-entry into the mainstream labour market as their ultimate goal, while in other cases the aim is to involve the person in some sort of constructed or quasi-labour market or cultural or voluntary social activity. Thus some measures are aimed at helping the participant compete for existing and vacant positions in the regular labour market, while in other cases there may be a significant element of job creation, e.g. through the setting up of new special positions, sections or whole firms, or by providing wage subsidies for a shorter or longer period in order to give ordinary employers financial incentives to employ the person in question.

Defined in this broad sense, activation is associated with a number of other key terms describing current attempts to meet welfare state challenges:

- *Active labour market policies (ALMP)*: In the Nordic countries, active labour market policies have been closely related to the commitment to maintain a high level of employment and preferably full employment. The relative prominence of this particular objective has been perceived as a key indicator in terms of identifying models of welfare states (see, e.g. Erikson *et al.* 1987; Esping-Andersen 1990). Sweden, in particular, has been perceived as having a strong ALMP tradition, but in Finland and Norway, too, such policies have been used as a principal means of combating rising unemployment – or the threat of rising unemployment. ALMP has mainly been used to refer to public programmes, which seek to qualify and (re)train participants in order to make them more attractive on the labour market and – ultimately – to enable them to find gainful employment. Through ALMP, 'workers are re-equipped to deal with market forces' (Janoski 1994: 56). The opposite, passive labour market policies primarily consist of dispensing unemployment compensation, e.g. a daily allowance provided by social insurance schemes, or means-tested social assistance. As already indicated, ALMP is directed not only towards the supply side of the labour market, e.g. through the provision of better or more relevant qualifications among the unemployed and others at risk; it may also to some extent modify the demand side, e.g. by providing subsidies. Of the two concepts, activation is the broader and more comprehensive, as it also includes measures that are not directly geared towards participation in the labour market – at least not in the short run.
- *The work approach*: Ideas associated with the term 'arbets-/arbeidslinjen' have played an important role – at least in Sweden and Norway – in discussions about the desired guiding principles behind income maintenance schemes. According to this

approach, there should be a direct link between the social secur-
·ity system and labour market services, in the sense that it is an
official task of the income maintenance scheme to maximize
labour market participation. No person should be granted
long-term public income support until all possibility of making
the person self-sufficient through employment had been
exhausted (Hvinden 1994). Although many of the practical implications of the work approach and ALMP are the same, the
former makes the linking of social security and labour market
services more explicit than does the latter – both as a policy
principle and as an administrative arrangement.

- *Workfare*: The term workfare originated in the United States of
America, although the reasoning behind it dates back many
centuries to public concerns in most Western countries about
how to deal with the able-bodied poor (De Swaan 1990; Midre
1995). In its modern version, workfare has recently come to play
a prominent role in European policy debates. Broadly speaking,
workfare refers to attempts to introduce work requirements for
recipients of public income support. Cash benefits are reduced or
withdrawn if recipients are not willing to participate in some sort
of work or training programme (e.g. Pierson 1994). As not all
recipients will automatically wish to participate in such programmes, there is an element of pressure and diminished freedom
of choice in a workfare arrangement. We can also find examples
of a linkage between short-term income maintenance and participation in some activation programmes. In this sense, activation
and workfare overlap, but again activation is a broader (and
vaguer) concept.

- *Work incentive*: Over the last 15 years, this term has become a
catchword in the public debate on income maintenance and wage
levels – in particular, in the debate on minimum-wage arrangements. Again, the underlying thinking is not new but can be
found at many points in the history of social policy. One of the
basic ideas has been that the level of public cash benefits –
relative to the level of income that the person in question would
be able to earn on the labour market – makes it less rational and
advantageous from the person's point of view to engage in gainful employment. It is further assumed that this relationship will
also effectively diminish the person's motivation to work. On the
basis of this reasoning, it may for instance, be recommended that
benefits should be made less generous or that the length of the
eligibility period should be reduced. At first glance, this concern

for disincentives appears to be a clear alternative to the emphasis on activation, as it seems to suggest straightforward cuts in the income maintenance system (see Introduction). But activation schemes may also be faced with the problem of disincentives: potential participants may be reluctant to take part as long as they are in receipt of a benefit, the amount of which is the same or greater than the amount they will be paid as participants in the scheme and/or for the kind of job which they expect to obtain afterwards. Because of this, activation policies may in practice be combined with policies designed to improve financial incentives to work. A concern for incentives may also lead to an arrangement whereby the cash benefits received by participants while out of work are not reduced to the same extent as their incomes from work increase – at least for a transitional period.

The activation discourse in the Nordic countries

For governments, opting for comprehensive activation policies is not without its economic and political risks. Even if such policies work as intended, they will be quite expensive, at least in the short run. Financial resources may for instance be required for salaries paid to administrators, gatekeepers and instructors and for physical facilities for courses; private providers of training, wage subsidies for employers, travel expenses for participants, etc. As already indicated, some varieties of activation measures may be viewed as representing constraints affecting the freedom and autonomy of potential participants and even the prerogatives of the partners in the mainstream labour market (employers and trade unions). Finally, doubts have been expressed about the economic soundness and effectiveness of activation measures. In view of this, governments are faced with the challenge to provide a rationale – reasons and justifications – for any widespread application of activation measures. This rationale will in practice amount to what Scott and Lyman (1968: 1) have called 'an account . . . a linguistic device employed whenever an action is subjected to valuative inquiry'.

Accounts of activation policies have been presented in a wide range of documents and statements from the Nordic governments. We will summarize some of the key elements in these accounts. We will limit the explicit references to few examples from the Norwegian Government's long-term programmes and key White Papers on the need to redirect welfare policies. Many similar references to policy documents and statements from the governments of the other Nordic countries, large interest organizations and the mass media could also have been presented, but to do so would have been to go beyond the scope of this chapter.

Broadly speaking, accounts of activation policies have been formulated in terms of considerations concerning the individual or in terms of the interests of the society as a whole (the community, the economy). Not surprisingly, these two sets of considerations have tended to be presented as non-conflicting; activation measures are claimed to be in the interests of both the individual participant and society (see, for instance, St.meld.nr.4 (1992–93): 128). For the individual, it has been assumed that activation measures help to:

- maintain or even increase the person's skills and qualifications, improving his or her opportunities and long-term chances in the labour market;
- prevent the assumed negative effects of non-participation in regular gainful employment (i.e. diminishing self-confidence, passivity, destructuring of the day, temptation to become asocial, etc.) which may impede a return to the labour market when demand increases again;
- encourage active job-seeking; and
- realize the person's right to work, thus providing a sense of meaning and of contributing to society instead of being or remaining a passive social benefit recipient.

For society, it has been claimed that activation measures:

- prevent a depreciation of skills and qualifications, instead raising the level of competence and flexibility of the labour force and increasing the long-term supply of qualified labour to industry and the public sector;
- contribute to the economic integration or re-integration of the jobless, thus alleviating problems of social exclusion; and
- reduce the pressure on public budgets for income maintenance, at least in a medium to long-term perspective, and improve the basis for economic growth.

These claims may, however, be challenged in various ways. First, some activation measures appear to have been based on the assumption that people are out of work because of a temporary slump in demand and not as a result of longer-term structural problems in the labour market. When the upswing comes, it may turn out that many of the unemployed lack the more fundamental type of qualification required by employers. Short, intensive vocational training courses are unlikely to provide such qualifications.

At the same time, concern has been expressed that longer, elementary courses will make participants temporarily unavailable to the labour market; and that there should be a clearer division between the courses provided by the labour market services, on one hand, and the regular educational system, on the other hand (e.g. St.meld.nr.4 (1996–97): 54). Official discussion of these issues has, however, tended to overlook the fact that many of the long-term unemployed have had unfavourable and discouraging experiences with the education system. Another, generally neglected, consideration is that there are likely to be numerous barriers – motivational and practical – to a return to the classroom.

Second, the official activation discussion has tended to play down the less beneficial effects for the individual targeted. These may include:

- less autonomy and freedom of choice (as participation in measures is obligatory and the relevant types of measures are determined by agency regulations or decided upon by agency officials);
- less income security and predictability (as the level of benefits may be reduced or entitlements made more conditional); and
- new failures and disappointments (as participation in activation measures may ultimately create unfulfilled expectations concerning enhanced opportunities on the labour market).

Indirectly, the activation discussion may entail a message to the target groups that others know better than they themselves what is in their best interest. This paternalistic message may be given a moralistic overtone: participating in activation measures and eventually in paid work is a moral or even semi-legal duty for all citizens. The Norwegian Government's Long-Term Programme 1994–1997, for instance, states that: 'There is also broad agreement that employment is a right and duty for everybody of working age and fit for work' (St.meld.nr.4 (1992–93): 25). According to Plovsing (1994: 31) the philosophy behind the active line in Denmark is a new social policy ideology, exemplified by slogans such as 'there is a need for everyone'; 'from passive to active'; and 'give and take'. The main thrust of this view is that when the State aims only to support the unemployed and otherwise to let them arrange their own affairs, this is detrimental to the individual as well as to society. The active line means that the unemployed are obliged to accept offers of work, education and other measures. In Finland, means-tested social assistance has been changed in such a way that the payment is reduced by 20 per cent if recipients do not accept the offer of a training course or job (Kosunen 1997: 63). Arguably the introduction of such requirements and conditions may serve the more or less latent function of disciplining the affected sections of the population (Burtless 1989; Midre 1995). Thus, a consequence of the activation discussion is that the causes of unemployment are individualized: the focus on the duties and motivations of the unemployed person may become so strong that structural causes are pushed into the background.

There has also been a tendency for the official rhetoric of activation to play down the potential weaknesses of activation measures in terms of efficiency. One of the major objections to measures aimed at promoting employment among disadvantaged groups is that these measures have displacement effects: in helping some people, they put others in a less advantageous position. Two of the main forms of displacement are dead weight and substitution effects: some participants would probably have found employment without the measures; and employers may be given incentives to replace other employees with persons participating in schemes (Layard *et al.* 1991: 476–7). When such risks are mentioned, governments have tended to argue that they can counteract them through the design of measures (e.g. St.meld.nr.4 (1992–93): 129).

Third, the reasons presented by governments to justify an emphasis on activation measures have contained several ambiguous points, for instance:

- It is seldom clear whether integration or cost saving is the most important issue, or which of them should be given priority if the pursuit of the one objective does not automatically lead to the achievement of the other.
- Many accounts of activation policies more or less implicitly claim that being in receipt of some type of long-term cash benefit can be considered equal to being passive and socially isolated in general. Thus they do not allow for the possibility that many people in receipt of income maintenance support may be active and socially integrated in arenas other than the workplace, e.g. in family and neighbourhood networks or in cultural or voluntary social activities. In this context, it is striking that whereas the Danish 'active line' has adopted a rather broad definition in terms of activity, the Norwegian work approach emphasizes

regular and gainful employment as both the means to and the end of the shift towards active measures.

In some versions of the activation discourse, it is more or less taken for granted that social integration through activation is achieved most effectively through participation in paid work within the mainstream labour market. While it may be the case that participation in regular employment is one of the major links between the individual and the society at large, it is far from obvious that insertion in the mainstream labour market is a realistic objective for all the target groups of activation measures. On the other hand, if activation measures take the form of job creation, the result may be a separate labour market.

But even if the official activation discourse has been based on at least partially unsubstantiated assumptions and has played down potential weaknesses and ambiguities, it may still have provided the Nordic governments with significant political symbols and justifications for other, simultaneous shifts in their policies. One factor here has been the increasing concern over financial disincentive effects resulting from the existing level and duration of cash benefits. It has even been claimed that generous cash benefit schemes have contributed to the exclusion of people from the labour market (e.g. St.meld.nr. 4 (1992–93): 125). Nordic governments have therefore sought to reduce the level and duration of some benefits in order to make participation in paid work – and consequently in activation measures – relatively more attractive (see Chapter 4). Other measures have made the granting of cash benefits more or less explicitly conditional on the recipient's willingness to participate in activation measures. Some Nordic governments have in fact emphasized the combination of cuts in benefits, more stringent assessment procedures along with expansion of activation measures as a particular strength of a renewed work approach. For instance, in one of its long-term programmes, the Norwegian Government stated: 'It is therefore a central element of the Government's strategy to combine a restrictive application of the income support system with a stronger and more efficient labour market policy' (St.meld.nr.4 (1992–93): 128). The same point was made in the next long-term programme four years later (St.meld.nr. 4 (1996–97): 54), but at this point it was put less bluntly.

The Organisation for Economic Co-operation and Development (OECD) appears to have been an important source of inspiration and even pressure in the Nordic countries' shift towards a greater emphasis on activation policies. For instance, according to the OECD, 'unemployment benefits may be too easily available without concomitant obligations on the recipient to take active steps to re-enter employment' (OECD 1995a: 25). In line with this, the OECD Secretariat has argued strongly in favour of a switch from passive to active measures on the basis of the following rationale: 'Helping the unemployed to become competitive in the labour market is preferable to providing them only with income support' (ibid.: 27). On the basis of a review of labour market policies in member countries at the end of the 1980s (OECD 1990a), the organization launched a programme, under the heading The OECD Jobs Study, to reform the members' policies. Two of the policy recommendations from this study are directly relevant for the relationship between activation measures and cash transfer systems:

> 7. Strengthen the emphasis on active labour market policies and reinforce their effectiveness.

> 9. Reform unemployment and related benefit systems – and their interaction with the tax system – such that societies' fundamental equity goals are achieved in ways that impinge far less on the efficient functioning of labour markets.

> (OECD 1995a: 15)

One implication of the combined approach recommended by the OECD and largely adopted by the Nordic governments is that to the extent that some types of expenditure on cash benefits have been reduced, it is difficult to judge whether this is to be attributed to the activation measures as such or to other, parallel changes in public policy. For this and other reasons, we need to be careful in not taking actual reductions in some or all forms of expenditure on cash benefits as evidence for the success of activation policies. As a first step, we need to ascertain that the greater emphasis on activation in the Nordic countries has not been merely a rhetorical device but has also been matched by practical reality.

Activation as a practical reality in the Nordic countries

In order to provide better instruments for assessing and monitoring the situation in each member country, the OECD has collected and standardized statistics on active labour market measures. Even though these statistics have some limitations, we will use them to obtain a first indication of whether there has been a shift towards activation in practice in the Nordic countries.

All in all, the Nordic countries have performed comparatively well in terms of unemployment levels throughout most of the postwar period. However, as shown in Figure 2.9 (Chapter 2), the Nordic countries have not been able to avoid increasing unemployment rates since 1980, and the trend of the early 1990s posed a special challenge to national governments. The exception was Denmark, where the unemployment rate reached high levels earlier and remained high for a longer period than in the other countries. As a consequence, expenditure for unemployment compensation was consistently higher in Denmark than in the other countries, fluctuating between 4 and 5.5 per cent of GDP in the period 1980 to 1996 (see also Chapter 4). In the other three countries, expenditure remained considerably lower until the early 1990s. After that period, Finland approached Denmark's level of expenditure, while Sweden and Norway reached maxima of 2.8 and 1.5 per cent of GDP, respectively.

As a response to this development, the Nordic governments spent more resources on active labour market measures during this period (Figure 6.1). There was a remarkable growth in the volume of activation measures in terms of participant inflows in the early 1990s, with inflows reaching maxima of 20, 12 and 16 per cent of the labour force in Denmark, Finland and Sweden, respectively (data for Norway are not available). However, especially in Finland and Sweden, the costs related to unemployment compensation grew more rapidly than the investment in active measures. The degree of policy activism (measured as the ratio of active programme expenditure to total labour market expenditure) declined over the period as a whole in Finland and Sweden, fluctuated in Norway, but showed a clear upward trend in Denmark (Figure 6.2).

Although there was an upward trend in expenditure for activation measures in all four countries in absolute terms, the most striking aspect is the difference in starting points and diminishing differences in the degree of activism during the period. At one extreme, Denmark started from a remarkably low level compared with the other countries. At the other extreme, Sweden distinguished itself as the country with the most activist profile from the outset, with the other two countries in between. Towards the end of the period, differences in the degree of activism had become significantly reduced, but Denmark and Finland displayed the least favourable balance between expenditure related to active measures and that involved with passive measures.

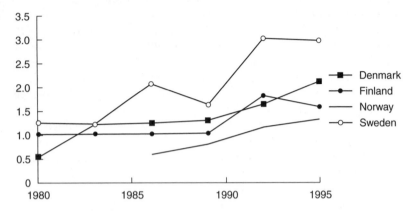

Figure 6.1 Active labour measures as percentage of GDP in the Nordic
countries, 1980–95
Sources: OECD (1994a: Table 1.B.2); OECD (1996c: Tables 2.9, 2.10); OECD (1997a:
Table K).

Notes
For Sweden, the subperiods are 1980–1, 1983–4, etc. Data are not available for 1980
and 1983 for Norway.
Active measures: expenditure on public employment services and administration,
labour market training, youth measures, subsidized employment and measures for
the disabled, as percentage of GDP. *Passive measures*: expenditure on unemployment
compensation and early retirement for labour market reasons, as percentage of GDP.

One can thus draw a provisional conclusion that a greater emphasis
on activation became a practical reality in the Nordic countries
during this period, but that Finland and Sweden, in particular,
have fought an up-hill battle against the rising costs of passive measures. But this conclusion must be tentative, as there are some limitations regarding the indicator of policy activism adopted here. The
main problem with an activism rate of this sort is what to put in the
denominator. Should the expenditure figures for so-called passive
benefits merely include those directly related to unemployment and
early retirement benefits from labour markets reasons, or should one
include all figures relating to public income maintenance for people
of employable age (e.g. 15–64)? The possibility of internal substitution in the income maintenance system may be regarded as an argument for the latter option. Often there will not only be one particular
cash benefit payable to a given person in a situation of economic
hardship, as the person may, for instance, be unemployed, partly
disabled and a single provider at the same time:

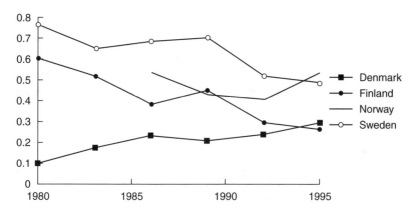

Figure 6.2 Activism rate 1, Nordic countries, 1980–95
Sources: OECD (1994a: Table 1.B.2); OECD (1996c: Tables 2.9, 2.10); OECD (1997a: Table K).

Note
See notes to Figure 6.1.
Activism rate 1: expenditure on active measures divided by total expenditure on labour market programmes (as classified by OECD).

> Sometimes invalidity schemes and early retirement programmes are used to support those who would otherwise be receiving unemployment benefits, so poor labour market performance can also increase such spending.
>
> (OECD 1996a: 27, n. 9)

There are thus reasons to expect that the trends and the cross-national differences in policy activism between the Nordic countries might have come out differently had the denominator included all cash transfers for people of employable age. If we add up all income maintenance related expenditure for people of employable age registered by OECD (1996c) and use this as the denominator, we get the results shown in Figure 6.3. The degree of activism still showed an upward trend in Denmark; it declined only slightly in Finland and was stable in Norway, while it fluctuated in Sweden, though at a comparatively high level.

Thus, if we take the total income maintenance related expenditure for people of employable age in 1980–93 into account, it is less obvious that there was a clear downward trend in the degree of activism in any of the Nordic countries in the period under consideration.

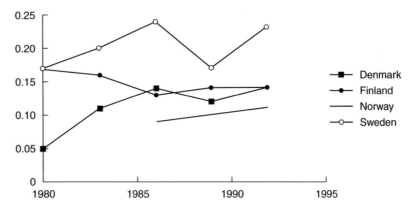

Figure 6.3 Activism rate 2, Nordic countries, 1980–95
Sources: OECD (1994a: Table 1.B.2); OECD (1996c: Tables 2.9, 2.10); OECD (1997a: Table K).

Notes
For Sweden, the subperiods are 1980–1, 1983–4, etc. Data are not available for 1995 (all four countries) and for Norway for 1983 and 1986.

Income maintenance includes all forms of public income maintenance for people of employable age; that is, early retirement, disability pensions, occupational injury pension, sickness benefits, survivors' pensions, single-parent benefits, unemployment compensation and social assistance in cases of low income.

Activism rate 2: expenditure on active measures divided by expenditure on all income maintenance for people of employable age plus expenditure on active measures.

Activation policies targeted at different groups

The general arguments in favour of activation policies tend to be given different forms when the discussion involves policies aimed at groups with particular characteristics, for instance:

- people who experience difficulties of entry or access to the labour market (e.g. school-leavers, young people with disabilities);
- people who have had stable employment for some time, but who are seen as temporarily out of work (e.g. middle-aged wage earners);
- people who have been away from the labour market for a considerable period because of family roles (e.g. single parents);
- people who have been marginal in the labour market for a greater part of their lives (e.g. people with long-term illnesses or problems of social adjustment); or
- people who have had stable employment for some time, but who

are perceived to be in the risk zone of permanent exit from the labour market (e.g. people who develop disabilities as adults).

Even if such differences in specific reasoning exist, there will be substantial similarities in the design of practical measures aimed at these diverse categories. Again there is likely to be room for internal substitution: for instance, young people or people with disabilities may be involved in and may benefit from general measures for the mainstream unemployed. It may even be claimed that this practice has an advantage over special and targeted measures, in terms of arguments about normalization and integration. But it is still worthwhile investigating whether there have been parallel or divergent trends in the specific measures aimed at these two important subcategories of the target population.

Policies aimed at alleviating entry problems: youth activation in the Nordic countries

For several reasons, activation and training measures targeted towards young job seekers constitute one field of particular concern for policy-makers. First and most fundamentally, in labour markets where participants are frequently recruited and evaluated on the basis of previous work experience as well as their objectively defined skills, the move from education to the first job is seen as a particularly critical transition period. The fact that it is hard to obtain a job without experience and impossible to acquire experience without some kind of job poses an obvious potential Catch 22 situation for the majority of young people leaving school, completing apprenticeship or finishing some other sort of training. Recognizing and acknowledging these problems, governments thus aim to make the long transition shorter.

Second, programmes are designed so as to adapt and prepare the (future) labour force for a labour market in permanent transition in terms of the skills and competence in demand. Here, labour market programmes are perceived as adjusting to the ever-changing cyclical demands posed by the market. From the mid-1970s onwards, however, unemployment has had more of a structural than a cyclical nature (cf. Grytten 1995; Schwanse 1997). In particular, increasing labour costs, negative demand shocks and a general relative decline in competitiveness have confronted Western European countries with a situation of peaking unemployment rates; this has led to new and higher unemployment equilibria (Grytten 1995: 215–20). These trends are also observed and commented upon by Layard *et al.* (1994), who maintain that rather than being related to general (cyclical) shifts in demand or supply, the differences in unemployment rates between age-groups (and occupational groups) are 'essentially equilibrium phenomena' (ibid.: 67). Considering that we are facing a situation of presumably structural problems, it is thus not surprising that traditional counter-cyclical policies have performed less than adequately across a range of countries. Among unemployed young people, one finds a disproportionate number with low formal educational qualifications.

Third, if a substantial proportion of today's young people does not manage to become established on the labour market, this can be regarded as representing a double problem. In the foreseeable future, they will represent a burden for public income maintenance schemes, especially for means-tested social assistance schemes. Moreover, it is assumed that the longer they are out of work, the more likely is it that they will be permanently disqualified from participation in the labour market, and that that they will not even be absorbed by it when future demographic changes create a shortage of labour.

For these reasons, youth unemployment has been perceived as especially sensitive to the poorer conditions on the labour market. Youth unemployment rates have therefore been a matter of considerable concern for the Nordic governments. The Nordic countries have had strikingly different experiences in the area of youth unemployment and labour market participation over the last 15 years:

● In Denmark, youth unemployment fell markedly from the early 1980s to the end of the decade and increased again up to 1993, though not to the level of the early 1980s. The level of labour market participation among young people appears to have stayed surprisingly high throughout the period.

● In Finland and Sweden, youth unemployment increased temporarily in the early 1980s, but after this peak it fell until the end of the decade. This was followed by a dramatic increase in the early 1990s, especially in Finland. There has been a clear downward trend in the labour force participation of young people in both countries.

● Norway also experienced a temporary rise in youth unemployment in the early 1980s. There was a new increase from the end of the 1980s onwards, and in this latter part of the period Norway had about the same youth unemployment rate as Denmark. The labour force participation among young people in Norway has remained fairly high and stable even in the 1990s.

It is interesting that we find a certain convergence of trends for Denmark and Norway in the 1990s. This observation illustrates that youth unemployment does not vary proportionally with the total level of unemployment in a given country. If for a moment we disregard the total unemployment level, the ratio of youth unemployment to total unemployment was particularly high in Norway and Sweden. Norway scored 2.33 on this particular indicator in 1994 (OECD 1995b). By contrast, Sweden, Finland and Denmark had youth unemployment ratios of 2.08, 1.68 and 1.05, respectively. Altogether, Denmark's achievement in the area of youth unemployment emerges as the most surprising, as unemployment rates generally tend to be higher among young people than in the general population (Julkunen 1996: 1).

The OECD figures for special labour market programmes for young people indicate that the resource input remained fairly stable in Finland and Norway, but that it fluctuated in Denmark and Sweden during the early 1990s (Figure 6.4). In Denmark the participation inflow also showed fluctuations, but in both Finland and Sweden there was a remarkable increase in the participation inflows (the OECD statistics do not present figures for Norway). Again we need to emphasize that the possibility of internal substitution means that these figures do not tell the whole story about the Nordic governments' efforts *vis-à-vis* the unemployed young. We will therefore briefly review the national strategies of the period.

Denmark

One reason for the high youth labour force participation is the long tradition of the apprenticeship system, although a problem has been that the number of apprentices has exceeded the demand for labour (Bjørn 1996). The apprenticeship scheme offers vocational training suited to the needs of the industry, with wage costs amounting to around 40 per cent of the ordinary adult wage. Persons dropping out of vocational training or higher education, or stopping at the level of basic education (about 30 per cent of each cohort), represent a relative concentration of labour market problems within the youth population. Outside the apprenticeship scheme, the starting wage is high, which makes it difficult to gain access to ordinary jobs. Participation in government-sponsored schemes has therefore become a fairly normal path into the labour market for young people with only basic education (OECD 1996d). New measures – mainly an education programme – aimed at assisting young people

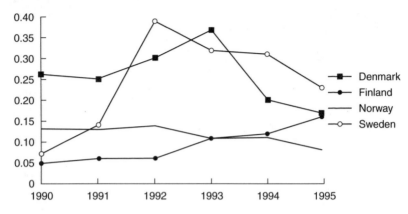

Figure 6.4 Labour market measures for youth as percentage of GDP in the
Nordic countries, 1990–5
Sources: OECD (1994a: Table 1.B.2); OECD (1997a: Table K).

Notes
For Sweden, the subperiods are 1990–1, 1991–2, etc. Data are not available for Norway
for 1983 and 1986.

According to OECD definitions, these measures include only special programmes for
youth in transition from school to work. Thus the category does not cover young
people's participation in programmes that are open to adults as well. It mainly consists
of remedial education, training or work experience for disadvantaged youth, to
facilitate transition from school to work. The principal target group usually comprises
those who are not in upper secondary or vocational education and who have been
unsuccessful in finding work.

were adopted in the 1996 Finance Act Agreement, and they build on
the principle of rights and obligations. Actually, the number of young
people involved in the new youth schemes is lower than expected,
partly because of increased incentives for the unemployed young to
accept work or start ordinary education (Ministry of Labour and
Ministry of Finance 1996). Young persons who have been in employment for at least two years may choose to participate in job training
instead of education/training (Ministry of Labour 1996).

Finland

Youth unemployment and the exclusion of young people from the
labour market have emerged as a special problem in Finnish society.
Annually, almost 20 per cent (or about 10,000 young people) of those
who have completed comprehensive school do not apply for further
education or are not accepted. The duration of unemployment

among young people with a vocational or university qualification is substantially shorter than among young people without such qualifications and skills. Priority is given to projects that are targeted at young people without vocational skills who are threatened by long-term unemployment, young people with multiple problems and young people who have dropped out of school. Several measures are to be implemented in Finland by means of YOUTHSTART (a community initiative programme), especially designed to promote access to the labour market for young people under the age of 20 (Ministry of Labour 1995). The decline in the youth unemployment rate in Finland since 1994 can be explained by an increased enrolment in vocational education coinciding with a rise in private sector recruitment of young workers (OECD 1997b).

Norway

The main labour market programme for young people in Norway is the Vocational Training Programme, which was introduced in 1985. From 1994 onwards, young people aged 16–19 no longer received payment while taking part in the programme. This was part of a strategy to encourage teenagers to choose upper secondary education instead of labour market programmes. Since 1994, the 16- to 19-year-old age group has had a statutory right to upper secondary education or an apprenticeship lasting three or four years. With this reform, young people under the age of 20 were guaranteed education or training, a job, or participation in a labour market programme (Bjørn *et al.* 1996). The guarantee of a place in a labour market programme for persons aged less than 20 years who did not have a place in school or a job was to be continued. Unemployed persons aged 20–24 have been given priority with regard to labour market programmes since the second half of 1995. In order to monitor the unemployed in this age group systematically, individual plans of action were to be set up (Report to Parliament 1996).

Sweden

There is evidence that the high levels of youth unemployment in the 1990s can be explained by the relatively high levels of youth wages in Sweden. These wages rose between 1985 and 1990 (the opposite was the case in many other countries) and it is likely that this had an effect on the provision of youth jobs, in that young people were being priced out of jobs (SOU 1995: 39). To counteract the unemployment problem, there was a substantial increase in active labour market programmes in 1992–94, especially for young people. The most important measure introduced in 1992 was the youth practice programme, which covered the 18- to 24-year-old age group. This was replaced in 1995 by a more general programme of introduction to the workplace for young people aged 20–25 years, while from 1995 onwards the municipalities were given the responsibility of finding jobs or training for young people aged 16–20.5 years (earlier 16- to 17-year-olds). Another youth programme was introduced in 1995 in order to increase young people's computer skills. In a recent official report on youth and work (SOU 1997: 40), several measures aimed at promoting employment among youth were discussed, one of them being generation exchange, a scheme whereby a younger unemployed person may replace an older employee.

Policies aimed at preventing premature exit: activation of people with disabilities

If an increasing proportion of people already established in the labour market leave employment before statutory retirement age, this represents a double challenge for governments (see Chapter 3). Early retirement – to the extent it is seen as premature – means that the productive capacity of the economy is diminished, and that the basis for funding welfare services is narrowed accordingly. Moreover, people who have worked for the larger part of their adult life will have accumulated entitlements to earnings-related supplements to pensions, and this will increase the financial burden of providing income maintenance to this group of recipients. An important group within this category of recipients consists of people who develop some sort of disability that reduces their work capacity after a number of years in employment. If they leave the labour force and move on to a disability pension or similar schemes, the chances are high that their exit will become permanent. This fact contributes to governments' concern over the decreasing average age of new disability pensioners that has been observed in a number of countries.

It is from this perspective that one must see the greater emphasis on activation measures for people who are regarded as being at risk of becoming disability pensioners, especially people on long-term sick leave from work. But in addition to measures that seek to provide early intervention and monitoring in the case of people on sickleave, activation policies for people with disabilities include a broad range of measures providing vocational assessment, guidance and retraining for those who cannot return to their previous position or workplace, as well as measures that contain an element of job creation (e.g. wage subsidies). Furthermore, greater stress on activation in this area may also be associated with policies that seek to strengthen and clarify employers' responsibility for people with disabilities, mainly with respect to taking care of those who are already employees but also with respect to encouraging more 'socially responsible' recruitment practices. Current policies and priorities, however, have their roots in policies that go back at least 30 or 40 years.

Broadly speaking, we may distinguish between four types of measures aimed at assisting people with disabilities in finding or staying in work (Hernes 1995: 157–8):

● legislative approaches – including legislation focusing on individual rights and equality of opportunity and access (e.g. antidiscrimination legislation) and direct interventions (e.g. quota schemes);
● vocational rehabilitation, including vocational assessment and training provided and/or funded by governments;
● sheltered work and, in particular, sheltered work provided in special firms supported by the government;
● wage subsidies payable to employers in the mainstream labour market in order to promote placement and, eventually, a return to ordinary work, including recruitment of people with disabilities.

Legislative approaches have so far played a limited role in the Nordic countries, and quota arrangements have not been adopted, in contrast to the situation in many other European countries. Recently, the discussion concerning anti-discrimination legislation has reached the Nordic countries, and a public commission is reviewing the case for such legislation in Sweden. But it is the three other approaches which so far have played the key role in the Nordic countries, though in different combinations and with varying emphases. We will comment on some of these differences below.

The OECD figures on resource input and participant inflows for special measures aimed at people with disabilities suggest that during the 1990s there were significant differences of emphasis between the Nordic countries:

● In terms of resource input (Figure 6.5), Norway appeared to be the only country with a clear increase. However, the dramatic increase in the expenditure for measures from 1993 to 1994

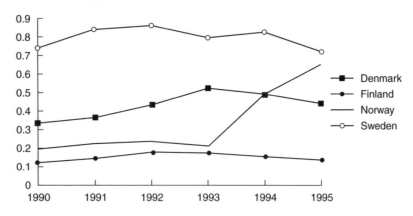

Figure 6.5 Labour market measures for people with disabilities as percentage
of GDP in the Nordic countries, 1990–5
Sources: OECD (1994a: Table 1.B.2); OECD (1996a: Table T); OECD (1997a: Table K).
Notes
For Sweden, the subperiods are 1990–1, 1991–2, etc.
  Following OECD definitions, only special programmes for the disabled are included.
Thus the category does not cover the total policy effort in support of people with
disabilities.

may to some extent be an artefact produced by a shift in the
administrative boundaries between government agencies enacted
by the Norwegian parliament as one of several means of promoting the work line. The level of input for the other three countries
was fairly stable, albeit at different levels: Sweden retained its
status as the pre-eminently activist country, with the highest level
of resource input, while Finland had the lowest level, with Denmark in between.

• The participant inflows fluctuated in all four countries, but Denmark distinguishes itself as the country with largest overall inflow
of participants. The differences here can probably be explained in
part by the divergent profiles of the activation measures. As
already indicated, Sweden has for a long time had a considerable
sector of sheltered, permanent or semi-permanent work, while in
the other countries relatively more of the resource input has been
spent on temporary measures, such as vocational retraining.

We will now briefly review the national situations in greater detail.

Denmark

The policy of integration into the workforce has been based on the principle of equality between the disabled and other citizens. No special legislation is enacted for disabled people, except where needs could not be met through mainstream provision (Thornton and Lunt 1997). The principal mainstream active employment measures adopted in Denmark have focused on the supply side, i.e. training and work habituation. Vocational training has been the favoured Danish approach, taking place predominantly in sheltered workshops (as an integrated part of mainstream vocational training), but attempts have increasingly been made to move rehabilitation from the institutions into real work situations (Lunt and Thornton 1993). Slogans such as 'everyone is needed' were adopted at the beginning of the 1990s (Ministry of Social Affairs 1990), and an emphasis on activation in the open labour market became more prominent. The *Our common concern* campaign initiated in 1994 by the Minister of Social Affairs has been used as an element of the Government's long-term policy of strengthening the responsibility of enterprises for people with disabilities (Ministry of Social Affairs 1995).

Finland

The main strategy of Finnish employment and social policy has been to integrate disabled persons and other members of disadvantaged groups into the labour market and into the mainstream employment services (Ministry of Labour 1995). Two particular problems have been identified in relation to people with disabilities: first, the situation of young persons with disabilities who have problems with entering the labour market; and second, that of the elderly disabled, who for a number of reasons are in danger of being excluded from the labour market. Current policy thus seems to be developing in the direction of earlier activation and an emphasis on facilitating work retention (Thornton and Lunt 1997). With respect to programmes directed at people with disabilities, subsidized employment has been the most important means available to the Finnish employment authorities (Mannila 1995), although since 1995 regulations governing the granting of subsidies have been tightened (Thornton and Lunt 1997).

Norway

The most striking aspect of recent social policy developments in Norway has been the focus on integration in the regular and open labour market. The objective of integration has been promoted primarily through wage subsidies and financial support to and/or counselling of employers, while special sheltered employment workshops have been seen as a supplementary provision, largely for those who would not be able to find work in the mainstream labour market even after vocational rehabilitation. According to a recent official report on labour market policy (Report to Parliament 1996), the policy towards the vocationally disabled is still to be an active one, aiming at early intervention (while persons are still employed) in order to avoid a process where people are made passive through lack of contact with their workplace.

Sweden

The three main labour market programmes for people with disabilities in Sweden have been work with wage subsidies, sheltered jobs in the public sector and employment in Samhall (a large government-owned group of companies established in 1980). According to Lindqvist and Marklund (1995), the Swedish government has recently shifted to a much stronger emphasis on the work approach, vocational programmes in general and a reinforcement of work rehabilitation for people with long-term illnesses and with disabilities in particular (SOU 1997: 40). As the provision of wage subsidies is more likely to result in integration into the mainstream labour market, and this measure is thus in line with the general principle of favouring employment rather than cash support, it has been given higher priority and has expanded in relation to work in sheltered workshops (Labour Market Studies, Sweden 1997). Accordingly, it has been proposed to place more emphasis on rehabilitation in Samhall in order to improve the chances of transition to the open labour market (SOU 1997: 64). The numbers participating in programmes for the disabled have shown an upward trend, and compared to other countries the volume has been considerable (Johannesson 1995). In addition to the special programmes for disabled workers, early intervention aimed at job retention and a return to work is likely to remain a policy priority (Thornton *et al.* 1997).

Concluding comments

Recent changes in welfare policies in the Nordic countries have been strongly influenced by external constraints such as dramatic changes in the labour market, high levels of unemployment, current fiscal pressures on the welfare state and anticipated pressures resulting from demographic changes. One of the possible responses to these constraints has been to strive towards a policy shift away from what has to a great extent amounted to a *de facto* emphasis on equity, freedom of choice and security of income for persons receiving public income support and towards a greater emphasis on efficiency and a combination of improved work incentives and practical efforts to encourage and assist people without income from paid work to take up and remain in full-time or part-time gainful employment.

Observers of social policy will recognize the significance of this new direction in the Nordic policy discourse. As noted previously, one distinguishing feature of the Nordic model in a comparative and historical perspective has been the commitment to keep unemployment at a minimum. Another related and at least equally prominent aspect has been the de-commodifying effect of Nordic welfare state policies. According to Esping-Andersen (1990), de-commodifying welfare systems render services as a matter of right, thus permitting the maintenance of a livelihood without reliance on the market. Consequently, 'a minimal definition must entail that citizens can freely, and without potential loss of job, income, or general welfare opt out of work when they themselves consider it necessary' (ibid.: 21–3). Whereas historically the Nordic welfare states have been identified as being 'consistently de-commodifying' (ibid.: 51), recent policy shifts are leading to a weakening of this tendency and appear to entail a relative *re*-commodification.

We have presented some indicators of a shift towards greater emphasis on activation at the interface between labour market and income-maintenance policies in general, and more specifically, in policies direc-ted towards the unemployed young and people with disabilities in the Nordic countries. But it would be a case of jumping to conclusions to infer that these changes have promoted the anticipated results; i.e. that they have been effective in (1) promoting a higher participation rate for people who would otherwise have a marginal position in, or would be excluded from, the labour market; or (2) diminishing the pressure on government budgets as far as passive cash benefits are concerned.

Econometric studies seeking to demonstrate the employment-promoting effect of mainstream active labour-market programmes have arrived at contradictory conclusions (e.g. Layard *et al.* 1991; OECD 1993; Scarpetta 1996). Official statistics on the employment status of participants in vocational rehabilitation have indicated that somewhere between 30 and 45 per cent of the participants are in work (full-time or part-time) immediately after their participation has terminated (e.g. Rikstrygdeverket 1991–94; Arbeidsdirektoratet 1995–97). Follow-up studies of vocational rehabilitation have reported that about equal numbers of ex-participants enter and drop out of employment in the period after the termination (e.g. Ford 1993). A study of the effects of participating in vocational rehabilitation in the period 1989 to 1993 indicated that it increased the chances of obtaining work by 5 per cent, when the figure was controlled for the impact of selection (St.meld.nr.4 (1996–97)). One explanatory factor is obviously that relatively high levels of employment combined with restructuring processes in the labour market have made it difficult to find suitable and permanent jobs for persons who have undergone a process of vocational rehabilitation.

If the pressure of so-called passive benefits on government budgets has diminished or will do so, a careful examination will be required to assess the extent to which this reduction can be attributed to a greater emphasis on active measures, training and rehabilitation. As noted, it is a formidable task to distinguish the effects of such measures from the more direct effects of the parallel tightening of eligibility rules and related changes in the income maintenance system.

Such considerations apart, it is, however, important to analyse in greater detail the normative rationale for the policy shifts that we have discussed: to what extent and in what way can one justify making income maintenance benefits conditional on participation in designated activity programmes, and demanding that members of vulnerable groups take part in measures aimed at increased labour market participation, if only a minority of these individuals will actually enter employment afterwards?

7 Changes in the social patterning of living conditions

Johan Fritzell

Introduction[1]

Theoretical discussions of and empirical investigations into human welfare have a long history in social science. In the recent past, there has been a growing interest in welfare issues from the 1960s onwards. This revived interest probably has many roots, one of the most salient being deepening concern over the consequences of economic expansion in the West. Such questions as: *Is it really true that economic growth will ultimately improve well-being among citizens?*, were formulated more and more often. There was also deepening concern over how welfare should be measured. Preoccupation with measurement of economic growth was questioned to an increasing degree, as many central aspects of welfare did not seem to be included in the GNP. Furthermore, changes in the GNP do not reveal anything about the distribution of wealth. Thus, even if one were to accept that changes in the GNP serve as a proxy for changes in welfare within a society, one could still wonder whether *all* citizens benefited from this additional affluence. Similarly, criticism was levelled against the corresponding indicator used for individuals, i.e. income. Even though most would agree that income, or economic resources more broadly, can be regarded as an important resource, many argued for a broader and more inclusive strategy for measuring welfare.

Partly in response to these issues, the first level of living survey was conducted in Sweden in 1968. It had as its aim the provision of a comprehensive picture of the welfare and living conditions of the Swedish population, in a way that would also address non-economic indicators. In the 1970s, similar studies were conducted in the other Nordic countries. Despite this common origin and the many similarities shared by the Nordic studies on the level of living, and despite the international reputation of 'Scandinavian welfare research', the various Nordic surveys have prompted surprisingly few comparative ventures, covering a broad spectrum of living conditions (see, however, Allardt 1975; Vogel 1990).[2]

Not the least due to the turbulence of the 'Nordic model', and to the diverging paths in macroeconomic conditions following the global recession in the early 1990s (see previous chapters), it seems highly relevant to conduct cross-national comparisons on changes in living conditions, targeting specifically changes in inequality of living conditions. This chapter attempts such an analysis, and is based on surveys of living conditions carried out in Finland and Sweden for the period of 1986 to 1994/95 and in Norway for the period 1987 to 1995.[3]

The fact that the welfare of individuals to a certain extent depends on changes at the macro level (overall economic performance, welfare state reforms, and so forth) is, of course, a prime reason to be interested in the macro level *per se*. On the other hand, I believe it is essential to underline that the relation between changes at the macro level and individual welfare is not necessarily a straightforward one-to-one. Furthermore, changes in the economy, in the labour market, or in welfare state programmes may indicate, but do not necessarily imply, how inequality of welfare has changed. To take just one example, if unemployment increases dramatically, as it has in at least two of the three countries under comparison here, the effects on the social patterning of living conditions depend both on how unemployment is distributed among various social categories and also on the impact unemployment has on other central aspects of life. There are no self-evident answers to these issues as, for example, recent Finnish health research has indicated (see Martikainen and Valkonen 1996). In other words, there is an obvious need to go beyond the macroeconomic and political scene, and to study the effects at the individual level.

Three central questions are addressed in this chapter. First, to what extent has the average level of welfare amongst the populations in Finland, Norway and Sweden changed when the *level* of living in various spheres of life in the mid-1990s is compared with that prevailing in the mid-1980s? Second, to what extent do these living conditions vary by age, class and gender, and are these *differentials* similar when these three countries are compared? Third, does comparison across countries reveal similar *changes* in this social patterning of welfare?

The latter two issues are strongly interrelated and are therefore analysed together, the main focus of attention being on changes. This focus on trends can be advocated, both for reasons of substance and on methodological grounds (see below). Thus, previous research has shown, for instance, that health differs by class in one country, or that both exposure to violence and economic resources vary by age in another; but less knowledge is available concerning the extent to which changes in these inequalities have occurred, nor is it known whether such changes have occurred in a similar fashion in all countries.

Research strategy, data and variables

All comparisons, whether comparisons over time, between nations or between any other aggregates, need to take a number of important methodological considerations into account. If credible conclusions are to be made, e.g. concerning changes in living conditions in a particular country, a natural starting point would be to have identical measures for different time periods as well as reasonable control over various measurement errors. If this is not the case, inferences can in some cases be made concerning changes in inequality, but these inferences most likely lead to inaccurate conclusions with regard to changes in averages for the population at large. If the main topic of interest in this chapter, for instance, were to find out whether citizens in Norway, on average, have better living conditions than citizens in Finland or Sweden, in the ideal case the indicators, the specific questions asked in the surveys and the effects of various issues related to measurement errors, all of which determine the data being compared, should be identical, not only within each country but also from one country to another.

However, if we reject comparison of this kind (as is done below), focusing instead on the extent of inequality and, in particular, on changes in this respect, these comparability requirements can be relaxed somewhat. Cross-national analyses of trends in inequality, for example, are not influenced by time-invariant errors or by issues that vary over time, but are equal in this respect cross-nationally. Similarly, even though the specific operationalization of different indicators to be studied may be slightly different from one country to another, credible conclusions can be drawn, for example, about how age differentials have changed within each country, and a cross-national comparison of these trends can be made. This, then, is the main approach followed below. It goes without saying that, as far as possible, the indicators have been made comparable between countries.

Data

The data used are derived from the nationwide Surveys on Living Conditions (Finland and Sweden) and the Level of Living Surveys (Norway), which in all three cases have been conducted as face-to-face interviews by the respective national statistical agencies, i.e. Statistics Finland, Statistics Norway, and Statistics Sweden.[4] The Norwegian data are derived from 1987 and 1995, the Finnish data from 1986 and 1994, and the Swedish data from 1986/87 and 1994/95 (in the following, the Swedish datasets are referred to as from 1987 and 1995). This study includes respondents aged 20 (for datatechnical reasons, the lowest age bracket in the Finnish data is 21 years) to 75 years, unless otherwise stated. The total non-response rates for the respective surveys were 13 and 27 per cent in Finland, 21.8 and 24.6 per cent in Norway, and 22.6 (1986), 19.4 (1987), 19.9 (1994) and 19.5 (1995) per cent in Sweden, respectively. Both the Finnish and the Swedish data are weighted, partly in order to minimise the effects of non-response differences among various sociodemographic categories.

The two datasets for each country are pooled together so as to facilitate comparisons both between the survey years and for the analysis of how differences in living condition have changed by social categories. The total number of observations in these three pooled datasets are 18,183 in the Finnish case, 6,735 in the Norwegian case, and 20,707 in the Swedish case (for further information about the data, see Ahola et al. 1995 for Finland; Statistics Norway 1996 and Teigum 1992 for Norway; and Statistics Sweden, 1991 and 1996 for Sweden).

Spheres of life and indicators

An important issue in these comparisons is, obviously, what to compare. The level of living approach has traditionally applied a multidimensional approach to welfare. Different so-called level of living components have been established in order to give a broad picture of living conditions and of variations in living conditions between different groups of the population. This is usually done by investigating a number of different areas that are seen as central to human welfare. In the Swedish case, this list includes: health; employment and working conditions; economic resources; education; family and social relations; housing conditions; recreation; security of life and property; and political resources.

This chapter cannot provide a comprehensive report on all aspects normally included in level of living analyses. Instead, attention has been focused on a few particular aspects. The areas, or spheres of life, to be analysed are the following: *economic resources; employment status; health; social relations*; and *security of life and property*. Within these areas, the interest is concentrated on negative outcomes. The choice is a normative one, but it is more likely that a consensus can be reached for certain negative consequences than for positive outcomes. The number of indicators used in these comparisons will vary in some cases, depending partly on the availability of comparable data.

Within the areas studied, the following indicators are created and then studied:[5]

- *Economic resources:* Whether or not the respondent's household faces 'economic difficulties'. This indicator is created from two questions. The first pertains to whether or not the household has a (fairly small) economic buffer set aside to deal with any unexpected costs (whether the household lacks a cash margin). The second question inquires whether or not difficulties have been encountered in paying ordinary expenses for food, rent, etc. during the last year ('trouble making ends meet'). Respondents who lacked a cash margin and had trouble making ends meet were coded as having economic difficulties. This measure can be regarded as an alternative direct measure of poverty (cf. Ringen 1987). The two Finnish surveys do not share any comparable measure of economic difficulties. Two measures of income are also analysed. One is the 'earnings of full-time employees' and the other is the household's 'equivalent disposable income'.[6] All measures of earnings and income have been adjusted for inflation, in accordance with changes in the consumer price index for each country.

- *Employment status:* Given the profound changes in unemployment rates that have occurred in these countries recently, there is clear reason to study the distribution of unemployment. Two indicators of unemployment are used for this. The first is whether or not the respondent was 'unemployed at the time of responding'. The second is whether or not the respondent had been unemployed for a total period of at least six months during the last five years ('unemployment > 5 months last five years').

- *Health:* Two measures are studied. The first indicates whether or not the respondent suffers from a 'long-standing illness'. The second health measure is 'poor self-assessed health' (not available in the Norwegian dataset), which can be said to be a measure of overall health status. These measures have been commonly used in both national and cross-national comparisons of health inequalities (for an analysis and discussion concerning the apparent high validity and reliability of the latter measure, see Lundberg and Manderbacka 1996).

- *Security of life and property:* Whether or not the respondent has been 'exposed to violence' during the last year.
- *Social relations:* Whether or not the respondent has a close friend to talk with in case of need thereof ('lacks social support').

Social differentiation

A rather restricted and standardized strategy has also been adopted with regard to which dimensions of inequality are analysed. Three basic independent variables are studied (besides survey year); namely, age, sex, and social class. *Age* is divided into four broad categories: 20–30, 31–45, 46–60 and 61–75 years.[7] A deviation from this grouping is made when the indicator studied refers to the working population. In this case, only three categories are separated, with those 46 years of age and older forming one category. *Sex*, of course, distinguishes men from women. The *social class* variable is based on present occupation, and the following categories are distinguished: First a distinction is made between the self-employed and employees. Among the former grouping, farmers are distinguished from other self-employed persons. Among employees, the usual distinction is made between manual (or blue-collar) and non-manual (or white-collar) workers. Within these groupings, a distinction is made between, on the one hand, skilled and unskilled blue-collar workers and, on the other, three categories of white-collar workers (upper, middle, and lower), distinguished in each case by the normal qualification level for the respective occupation. The analysis of class is not restricted solely to those allocated a class code (basically, those gainfully employed). For reasons explained below, people of working age but not gainfully employed, and thus without a class code, are included in some analyses and categorized into a separate group.

No doubt other dimensions of stratification could also be of great importance. Such factors include, for example, ethnicity (particularly in Sweden), regional differences and differences between single and married persons. Wider inspection, however, is beyond the scope of this chapter.

Methods

With two exceptions, all the dependent variables listed above have been dichotomised and are analysed by means of logistic regressions (see, e.g. Aldrich and Nelson 1984). The exceptions are the variables for earnings and income, which for ease of interpretation are analysed by means of the so-called semi-logarithmic OLS regressions, i.e. with ln(annual earnings) and ln(equivalent disposable income) as dependent variables. This enables easy transformation of the parameter estimates yielded by the regressions into percentage differences.

As pointed out earlier, the datasets for each country are pooled. In addition to the three basic independent variables, all analyses also include the survey year as an independent variable. The first question stated above concerned the changes in the levels of welfare that had occurred during the period of review. This is explored by analysing whether the independent variable survey year is significant and, if so, in which direction. The second question is studied through the estimates yielded by the other three variables. The third question concerned whether or not the age, class, and gender differentials had changed. Technically, this is analysed by including three interaction terms – year*sex, year*age, and year*class – in the regressions.

Changes in levels

The first question raised above concerned the extent to which average living conditions within each country have improved, deteriorated or remained constant during the period under study. Or, given the focus on negative outcomes: to what extent have different kinds of welfare problems increased, decreased or remained constant? In view of the macroeconomic changes reported in earlier chapters, as an initial hypothesis it might be argued that it would be a surprise to find that several aspects of living conditions had not deteriorated in Finland and Sweden, at least relative to Norway. It should be noted that according to standard indicators – such as growth in GDP and unemployment rates – the economies of both Finland and Sweden outperformed the economy of Norway in the late 1980s. The dramatic reversal of this cross-national variation which occurred in the 1990s, however, supports this basic hypothesis.

Table 7.1 shows the results from a large number of regressions in which only three independent variables were included: age, sex and a year variable.[8] In so far as the estimates for the year variable differ

Table 7.1 Changes in the levels of living conditions that occurred between survey years in Finland (1986–94), Norway (1987–95), and Sweden (1986/87–94/95). Results of logistic regressions (standardized for age and gender)

Spheres and indicators	Finland	Norway	Sweden
Economic resources			
Economic difficulties	Not available	Higher odds in 1995	Higher odds in 1995
Earnings, full-time workers[a]	Increase	Increase	Increase
Equivalent disposable income[a]	Increase	Increase	Increase
Employment status			
Unemployed at the time of response	Higher odds in 1994	Higher odds in 1995	Higher odds in 1995
Unemployed, > 5 months last five years	Higher odds in 1994	Higher odds in 1995	Higher odds in 1995
Health			
Long-standing illness	No signif. change	Higher odds in 1995	Higher odds in 1995
Poor self-assessed health	Lower odds in 1994	Not available	No signif. change
Social relations			
Lacks social support	Lower odds in 1994	Lower odds in 1995	Lower odds in 1995
Security to life and property			
Exposed to violence	No signif. change	No signif. change	Higher odds in 1995

Note
a This indicator is analysed by means of OLS-regressions, with the logarithm of the variable serving as the dependent variable. The independent variables are the same as in the logistic regressions, i.e. age, gender and survey year. An increase in these cases means that the earnings/income are higher in the latter survey year.

significantly from each other, the direction of the change is given in the table.

Starting with Finland, and for a moment leaving earnings and income aside, it comes as a surprise that, in most cases the situation did not deteriorate. Apart from the dramatic increases in the unemployment indicators, a betterment was detected for one of the measures of health (and actually a slight though non-significant improvement also in the other health indicator), as well as a rather substantial decrease in the prevalence of lacking social support. In Norway, the occurrence of most welfare problems was either unchanged or it was more common in 1995 than in 1987. For the population at large, the indicators for which increases were detected are the prevalence of economic difficulties, both unemployment indices, and long-standing illness. The last-mentioned trend may be more surprising than the others, but is supported by other research (see, e.g. Ramm 1997). Here, too, a significant betterment was found for one indicator, namely social support.

Finally, in Sweden, too, the prevalence of economic difficulties among the population increased between the survey years (and the magnitude of this increase was much higher in Sweden than in Norway, the relative odds in 1995 as compared to 1987 being 1.73 for Sweden versus 1.23 for Norway). As was expected, dramatic increases were found for both measures of unemployment. As in Norway, there was an indication in Sweden of a slight increase in long-standing illness (note, though, that the other health indicator did not indicate a worsening of the health status between survey years). Moreover, unlike the findings for the other countries, an increase in the exposure to violence was detected in Sweden. As regards social support, the trend was similar to the ones in Finland and Norway. Thus, no indication whatsoever was found to support the popular myth that people in modern societies are becoming more and more socially isolated; quite the contrary, this is the only indicator for which a significantly and substantially lower odds was detected for all three countries in the mid-1990s as compared to the 1980s. At least for both Norway and Sweden, this result is in line with findings covering an earlier, though partly overlapping, period; evidently, this trend has continued (see, e.g. Fritzell and Lundberg 1994; NOU 1993). The fact that fewer people in all countries lack a close friend is probably even more important given the trend that single households have become more common (cf. Barstad 1996, see also Chapter 3). Still, overall the findings for Sweden must be seen as indicating an impairment in terms of the levels of living.

However, the tendency for a lower level of welfare – i.e. the occurrence of welfare problems remaining either constant or increasing (with the exception of lacking social support) – was not reflected in the findings on earnings and income. It is important to realise that these measures do not focus upon negative welfare outcomes in the same way as all the other indicators do. What is reported is the change in real *average* earnings and equivalent income, as given by the regressions. Even so, given the macroeconomic conditions prevailing in these three countries for the past few years, it is noteworthy that real average income has increased substantially in both Finland and Sweden, and not only in Norway.[9]

In sum, the outcomes reported as to how different indicators of living conditions have changed or remained constant in these three countries are similar in several respects. Looking across the countries, most indices reveal changes in the same direction. Having said this, it should be noted that the magnitude of these changes varies cross-nationally. In particular, unemployment has become a far more common experience especially in Finland but also in Sweden as compared to Norway. The indices for which some evidence of cross-national variation in directions were detected are the measures of health status. Surprisingly, the cross-national variation indicates that the trend is most positive in Finland and most negative in Norway, i.e. quite the opposite to what would be expected on the basis of the general changes in prosperity that occurred within these countries.

The social patterning of living conditions and their changes

The fact that our societies are stratified – implying that our chances in many spheres of life, and thus our living conditions, are systematically different and depend in part on whether we are young or old, female or male, or work as a blue-collar or white-collar worker – is a statement that hardly surprises anyone. In this section we shall look into some of these differences, focusing mainly on changes that have taken place from the mid-1980s to the mid-1990s. The questions raised are:

1   Are there cross-national similarities in these age, gender, and class differentials, or are there nation-specific regularities in this respect?
2   Have recent changes in the Nordic countries altered the gender, age and class differentials?

3   Are the changes of these differentials similar cross-nationally, or are there nation-specific developments in each country?

The results will be presented with the same strategy as above but now focusing on age, gender, and class differentials – and, in particular, on changes therein – one by one, starting with the distribution of living conditions by age.

Age differentials

Welfare and well-being change over the course of life, and people born in different birth cohorts experience different contextual surroundings in different periods of their life-cycle. Owing to these circumstances, it is natural to expect that most welfare indicators are age-related. This is also the case in fact.

Table 7.2 presents the results obtained from a series of logistic regressions, carried out in the same manner as for Table 7.1 but now scrutinizing whether or not the prevalence of the dependent variable varied by age groups.[10] If age is significant (as it is in all cases), the most disadvantaged age group (the category with the highest odds or lowest earnings/income) is reported in the left-hand column below each country, which basically indicates whether the outcome was found to be most common among young people, among any of the 'middle-aged' groups, or among the oldest group. The second column for each country reports any significant changes that were detected in these differentials. As was said earlier, this is done by including an interaction term in the regressions, namely year*age. If this interaction term is significant, the direction of the change is reported in the table. In most cases, the wording 'increasing' or 'decreasing' is used for this purpose in Tables 7.2 to 7.4. In some cases, the changes cannot easily be interpreted along this dichotomy; in such a case, explanations are given in notes to the table. If we take the indicator 'long-standing illness' in Table 7.2 as an example, the left-hand column, not surprisingly, shows that long-standing illness is a more common state among the oldest age category in all countries. However, as indicated by the right-hand column, this age differential has decreased in Finland, increased in Norway but no significant change in this respect was detected in Sweden.

As seen in Table 7.2, all indicators in all the countries were most common among either the youngest or the oldest segments of the respective population. A more unexpected result, perhaps, is that in many cases these age differentials have also changed

Table 7.2 Age differences in the living conditions and changes thereof in Finland, Norway and Sweden. Results from logistic regressions (standardized for gender)

Spheres and indicators	Finland Most disadv. age group	Signif. changes	Norway Most disadv. age group	Signif. changes	Sweden Most disadv. age group	Signif. changes
Economic resources						
Economic difficulties	–	–	20–30	Decreasing	20–30	Decreasing
Earnings, full-time workers[a]	21–30	Increasing	20–30	No change	20–30	No change
Equivalent income[b]	21–30	Increasing	20–30	Increasing	20–30	Increasing
Employment status						
Unemployed at the time of response	21–30	Yes[c]	20–30	No change	20–30	Yes[c]
Unemployment > 5 months last five years	21–30	Increasing	20–30	No change	20–30	No change
Health						
Long-standing illness	61–75	Decreasing	61–75	Increasing	61–75	No change
Poor self-assessed health	61–75	Decreasing	–	–	61–75	Decreasing
Social relations						
Lacks social support	61–75	No change	61–75	Increasing	61–75	No change
Security to life and property						
Exposed to violence	21–30	Decreasing	20–30	No change	20–30	No change

Notes
a In this variable the age group given in the left-hand column for each country is the category with the lowest earnings as revealed by OLS-regressions, controlling for gender differentials.
b In this variable, the age group given in the left-hand column for each country is the category with the lowest equivalent disposable income as revealed by OLS-regressions, controlling for gender differentials.
c There is a significant change between the survey years, a finding which basically implies that those aged 31–45 in 1994(5) have higher odds of being unemployed at the time of the interview relative to both younger and older age groups as compared to the age distribution of those unemployed in 1986(7). However, the odds are still highest among the young.

rather dramatically during this relatively short period. Furthermore, a different pattern in these changes is revealed in the cross-national comparisons. With a few exceptions, the changes are, relatively speaking, to the disadvantage of young people in both Finland and Sweden, whereas in Norway, the age differentials increased in most cases, but this increase was sometimes to the advantage of elderly but according to other indicators to the advantage of younger age groups. For example, long-standing illness in Norway, which of course is more common among the elderly, had become even more sharply differentiated by age in the mid-1990s, and the same outcome was detected for a lack of social support. In contrast, a decrease in health differentials by age was found in both Finland and Sweden.[11]

Overall, the findings reported in the table suggest that, as regards levels of welfare, the highest number of problems were detected among young people, and this finding was common to all of the countries but was most pronounced in Sweden.[12] As regards changes in living conditions, in Finland and Sweden, young people in their twenties experienced different welfare problems to a much higher degree, even when compared to the situation prevailing in the mid-1980s. Here it seems safe to argue that people in the age group 61–75 years had the most positive trend.[13] It is harder to pinpoint winners and losers in the Norwegian case.

The most profound changes in age differentials revealed in this study occurred with regard to equivalent disposable income. Figure 7.1 shows how the relationships by age have developed in this respect.

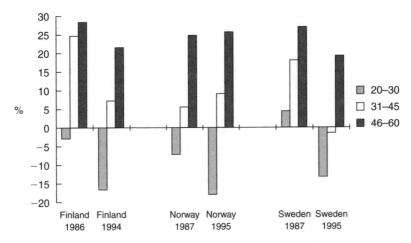

Figure 7.1 Changes in relative equivalent income by age groups (those aged 61–75 = 0) in Finland, Norway and Sweden

The figure illustrates the relative income for the young and middle-aged groups, as given by the regressions, as compared with the elderly in the respective year studied.

A dramatic relative deterioration occurred among the youngest age group in all three countries. The changes were the most radical in Sweden, and were almost as great in Finland. In Sweden, young people aged 20 to 30 had an average equivalent income that was about 4 per cent higher than that of people aged 61 to 75 in 1987 but 14 per cent lower eight years later. Perhaps even more surprising, in the mid-1990s those aged 31 to 45 had a slightly lower(!) equivalent income than those above 60 years of age, whereas the difference had been around 17 per cent in favour of the former age group in the mid-1980s (and would have been even greater if we had extended the time-span still further into the past).[14] The relative deterioration for those aged 31 to 45 was also evident in the Finnish case. Thus, one outcome of the economic turbulence and of the sharp increases in unemployment which occurred in both these countries was a striking change in the age distribution of economic well-being, the direction being in favour of elderly people and to the disadvantage of younger age groups.[15] Evidently, this change is not restricted solely to the youngest segment of the population, but also affects age groups in which 'needs' are likely to be highest, since the presence of dependent children is most common among those 31 to 45 years old.

In the case of Norway, no such significant change among the 'prime-aged' versus the elderly was detected, though those aged 20 to 30 have lost relative income in Norway, too. They already had a somewhat lower equivalent income compared to the elderly in 1987, but the magnitude of this difference was substantially greater in 1995.

It can be claimed that the findings concerning the youngest age group merely reflect educational expansions and/or changes in the economic situation of students. In order to test this suggestion, the same analysis was performed again, excluding everyone coded as students in the data. It is clear that changes affecting students cannot explain the relative deterioration noted for those aged 31–45, but to what extent does it explain the *changes* between the youngest age group and the oldest age group shown in Figure 7.1? (It goes without saying that the exclusion affects the income level of the youngest age group.) In Sweden, the relative change was about 13 per cent smaller, whereas in Finland, the change actually increased somewhat. In Norway, however, where the relative deterioration noted for the youngest as compared to the oldest age group was the least dramatic, the direction of the deterioration persisted but became insignificant as a result of the exclusion (the relative decline of the young vs. the middle-aged group was still significant). Accordingly, given the imperfect measurement of educational status during the income year, this factor seems to be of some importance, but the bulk of the changes persisted even when students were excluded from the analysis.

It should also be pointed out that this trend is not seen in the indicator of earnings (except for Finland) because of the focus on full-time employees for this analysis.[16] Among those who managed to remain fully active on the labour market, no significant changes were detected between the age groups, but the likelihood of remaining gainfully employed full-time varied strongly by age (among our three younger age groups).[17]

Gender differences

The findings indicate that despite their reputation for being 'women-friendly societies' (e.g. Hernes 1987a), the Nordic countries are considerably structured also in terms of gender, the structuring in nearly all cases being in the same direction. In the same manner as the age differentials were presented in Table 7.2, Table 7.3 gives an over-view of differentials between men and women and shows the extent to which these have changed. If no significant changes were found between men and women, 'N.S.' (not significant) is written in the table.

In all three countries women, in relation to men, are much more likely to have economic difficulties and lower annual earnings. Women also have a lower disposable income, which is solely an effect of differentials among non-cohabiting/married households since the disposable income of married and cohabiting men and women by definition is the same. Men have an expected disadvantage when it comes to social support and being exposed to violence. In contrast to what was reported concerning age, the gender differences are rather stable over time. Hence, in most cases we find either meagre or no change in the various spheres of life studied.

In the case of economic difficulties and earnings differentials among those with full-time employment, the relative gender differ-ence increased somewhat in Sweden, whereas a slight equalization of earnings differentials was detected in Norway and no significant change was found in Finland (though the estimate suggested a slight equalization). It is important to stress that this outcome is not

Table 7.3 Differences in living conditions between men and women and changes thereof in Finland, Norway and Sweden. Results from logistic regressions (standardized for age)

Spheres and indicators	Finland Disadv. category	Signif. changes	Norway Disadv. category	Signif. changes	Sweden Disadv. category	Signif. changes
Economic resources						
Economic difficulties	—	—	Women	No change	Women	Increasing
Earnings, full-time workers[a]	Women	No change	Women	Decreasing	Women	Increasing
Equivalent income[b]	Women	Decreasing	Women	No change	Women	Decreasing
Employment status						
Unemployed at the time of response	Women	Reversed	Women	No change	N.S.	No change
Unemployment > 5 months last five years	Men	No change	N.S.	No change	N.S	No change
Health						
Long-standing illness	N.S.	No change	N.S.	No change	Women	No change
Poor self-assessed health	N.S.	No change	—	—	Women	No change
Social relations						
Lacks social support	Men	No change	Men	No change	Men	No change
Security to life and property						
Exposed to violence	Men	Decreasing	Men	No change	Men	No change

Notes
a In this variable, the given category in the left-hand column for each country is the category with the lowest earnings as revealed by OLS-regressions, controlling for age differentials.
b In this variable, the given category in the left-hand column for each country is the category with the lowest equivalent disposable income as revealed by OLS-regressions, controlling for age differentials.

necessarily produced by relative changes in wage rates for men and women, but may be caused, e.g. by gender differentials in labour supply, even though the focus on full-time employees aims at minimizing this latter effect. In fact, if the analysis includes all persons with positive earnings, a slight gender equalization is revealed in all countries. Hence, the lower overall employment rate, particularly in Finland and Sweden, in the latter year has not led to a widening of labour supply differentials between men and women.[18]

The experience of unemployment has of course increased for both men and women, but with one exception the data revealed no significant change in this respect. The exception is the prevalence of unemployment in Finland at the time of the interview. In Finland, women were over-represented in the mid-1980s but a reversal of this difference was observed a decade later, when the probability of unemployment had become greater among men than women. It is important to note that this trend does not necessarily coincide with changes in unemployment rates, since all individuals of working age are included in these analysis.

Surprisingly enough, only in Sweden do we find the otherwise common result that women report more health problems than men. This finding, added to the increasing differentials in economic difficulties and earnings, may indicate that Swedish women face a more problematic situation than their sisters in Finland and Norway. It should be stressed, according to most indicators, however, that differentials between men and women revealed only slight changes (if any), especially in comparison to the corresponding changes in age differentials.

Class differences

The first analysis of class inequalities included all persons below 65 years of age with a class code, according to the criteria outlined earlier. This means that the number of observations in the following are somewhat lower, both because old-age pensioners were excluded and because those not working for a variety of reasons other than age were also excluded. The class differences stem from logistic regression, when both age and sex differentials are controlled for. The fact that most indicators studied here have a class gradient is not surprising to those familiar with earlier research on the level of living in the Nordic countries. On the basis of Table 7.4, a higher incidence of welfare problems was particularly common among farmers and unskilled blue-collar workers, albeit in some cases also among skilled

Table 7.4 Social class differences in living conditions and changes thereof in Finland, Norway and Sweden. Results from logistic regressions (standardized for age and gender) including class-coded individuals below 66 years of age

Spheres and indicators	Finland Most disadv. class	Signif. changes	Norway Most disadv. class	Signif. changes	Sweden Most disadv. class	Signif. changes
Economic resources						
Economic difficulties	–	–	Unskilled, Lower w-c	No change	Unskilled	Decreasing
Earnings, full-time workers[a]	Unskilled	Decreasing	Unskilled, Lower w-c	No change	Unskilled	No change
Equivalent income[b]	Farmers	Decreasing	Unskilled, Lower w-c	No change	Farmers	Increasing
Health						
Long-standing illness	Farmers, Unskilled	No change	Unskilled, Self-empl.	No change	Unskilled, Farmers	No change
Poor self-assessed health	Farmers	Decreasing	–	–	Farmers, Unskilled	No change
Social relations						
Lacks social support	Farmers	Increasing	Skilled	Decreasing	Farmers, Unskilled	No change
Security to life and property						
Exposed to violence	N.S.	No change	N.S.	N.S.	Skilled, Unskilled	No change

Notes
a In this variable, the given category in the left-hand column for each country is the category with the lowest earnings as revealed by OLS-regressions, controlling for age and gender differentials. Only employees included.
b In this variable, the given category in the left-hand column for each country is the category with the lowest equivalent disposable income as revealed by OLS-regressions, controlling for age and gender differentials.
N.S. = No significant class difference

blue-collar workers. Thus, with some cross-national variations, these classes have the lowest earnings and incomes, they are in poorer health, they more often lack social support and they are, in Sweden only, more exposed to violence.

Have class inequalities then increased, remained unchanged or decreased? Or to rephrase the question: is the recent recession something that was felt by white-collar and blue-collar workers to the same extent? As a general hypothesis we should, of course, expect that those with lower levels of skill to be in a more vulnerable position on the labour market and therefore to experience the hardest problems in bad times.

As to economic resources, a somewhat contradictory finding was revealed in Sweden. In terms of the risk of economic difficulties, a decrease in class differences was noted. However, this finding is not replicated in our measure of individual earnings or equivalent disposable income. The latter measure instead revealed a rather profound relative increase for the higher echelons of the white-collar classes. Once again (see note 9), this apparent anomaly can partly be understood on the basis of the innate property of the odds ratio. In instances where a phenomenon is fairly uncommon but has become more common, the relative odds differential between categories often has a tendency to decrease even though our perception of the changes is the opposite. Thus, the fact that the differences in odds for economic difficulties between unskilled workers and white-collar workers has decreased does not necessarily imply that, for example, the percentage difference between those categories has become smaller.

For most other indices, and in Norway for almost all of the indices, the stratification of living conditions by class was found to be stable over time. Surprisingly, the earnings and income differentials between social classes have decreased in Finland. A substantial decrease had occurred between unskilled workers and the upper white-collar class. It is, however, important to realize that this finding may to some extent be influenced by a selection process, since the measurement of class inequalities adopted here implies that those not participating in the labour market are excluded from the analysis. If this were the case, however, the results should indicate the same equalization in Sweden, but instead, an opposite result is obtained for equivalent income. Nevertheless, this discussion highlights the importance of adopting a more inclusive strategy in order to study class differentials and it is to this issue that we now turn.

A new division line?

Since the analysis of class differences shown in Table 7.4 is mostly based on those currently employed, one could argue that most of the substantial differences in living conditions are concealed. In many recent discussions concerning class, and divisions more generally, it is often hypothesized that the major division line in modern post-industrial societies in fact lies, and increasingly so, between those having a steady job and those excluded from the labour market (see, e.g. Dahrendorf 1987; Van Parijs 1987). In some cases, this hypothesis also includes diminishing and negligible differences between, for example, blue-collar and white-collar workers. In general, this latter statement can surely already be rejected on the grounds of the results presented in Table 7.4. Still, also within the Nordic countries, one can find empirical results supporting the hypothesis that a major shift has occurred in the social patterning of living conditions. Hence, Dahl and Birkelund (1996) report that health inequalities in Norway are increasingly found between those participating in and those outside the labour market, whereas class inequalities among those with jobs are decreasing. They relate their finding to the post-industrial class structure and the increase in selection effects, particularly among blue-collar jobs (a so-called healthy worker effect).

At any rate, the hypothesis has not been tested properly in the analyses conducted so far. For that reason, all the above analyses were tested from another angle. Also included in this new analysis are those of working age who did not receive a class code according to the criteria defined earlier, i.e. in practice those who, for various reasons, were not participating in the labour market and were put into a separate category, labelled 'others'.[19] The above hypothesis would then stipulate that the living conditions of this category should have fallen behind substantially. To what extent is this hypothesis supported by the data?

In most cases, the data suggest that, in all three countries, this latter category has a higher prevalence of welfare problems than other categories. This is, of course, expected and may even be a prime reason explaining their labour market status. More interesting is the extent to which their situation has declined relative to other social classes. Table 7.5 presents the position of this category relative to the two extremes of the ordinary class schema, i.e. unskilled blue-collar workers and upper white-collar workers. In so far as the relations have changed significantly, estimates for both years are given;

Table 7.5 Relative differences (odds) in living conditions and changes thereof between unskilled blue-collar workers (reference category = 1.0), the upper white-collar class, and 'others' (not working), below 66 years of age. Calculated from regression models including age and gender

	Indicators	Unskilled blue-collar	Upper white-collar	'Others'
Finland	Equivalent income, 86[a]	100.0	146.7	80.0
	Equivalent income, 94[a]	100.0	140.8	86.6*
	Long-standing illness	1,0	0.63	2.27
	Poor self-assessed health	1,0	0.42	1.9
	Lacks social support, 86	1,0	0.7	1.06
	Lacks social support, 94	1,0	1.19*	1.65*
	Exposed to violence	1,0	0.77	1.37
Norway	Economic difficulties	1,0	0.45	2.37
	Equivalent income[a]	100.0	124.9	82.6
	Long-standing illness, 87	1,0	0.53	1.31
	Long-standing ilness, 95	1,0	0.96*	2.70*
	Lacks social support	1,0	0.55	1.14
	Exposed to violence	1,0	0.88	1.53
Sweden	Economic difficulties, 87	1,0	0.11	1.53
	Economic difficulties, 95	1,0	0.27*	1.74
	Equivalent income, 87[a]	100.0	126.7	80.1
	Equivalent income, 95[a]	100.0	138.7*	87.6*
	Long-standing illness	1,0	0.52	2.58
	Poor self-assessed health	1,0	0.31	2.33
	Lacks social support	1,0	0.71	1.25
	Exposed to violence	1,0	0.42	0.78

Note
a   The reported figure is the relative percentage difference from the equivalent income of unskilled blue-collar workers, set at 100 for respective year. Calculated from OLS-regressions, controlling for age and gender.
* = The estimate is significantly (5% level) different from the corresponding estimate in 1987.

otherwise the estimates presented are derived from regression models, excluding interaction effects.

As seen in Table 7.5, the regressions indicate that the relations between the categories are unchanged in most cases, but that changes were detected in five (out of 17) cases. Only one of these changes, however, is exactly as suggested by the above hypothesis. That particular change refers to long-standing illness in Norway, where a significant relative impairment was detected for 'others' in relation to unskilled blue-collar workers. A remarkable decrease was also found in the differential between the upper white-collar workers and the

unskilled blue-collar workers. Hence, this rather crude analysis repli-
cates the findings presented by Dahl and Birkelund (1996) discussed
above. More important for the discussion here, though, is the fact
that similar relative changes were not detected for health inequalities
in Finland or Sweden. Nor were corresponding relative changes
found for any other indicator analysed, either in Norway or in the
other two countries.[20]

In the Swedish case, the data revealed significant changes in economic resources but not in any other area. The trend in economic
difficulties was discussed above. As regards equivalent income, Table
7.5 shows that, in Sweden, the upper white-collar workers had substantially higher relative incomes in 1995 compared to 1987, all in
relation to blue-collar workers; whereas no significant change in this
respect occurred in Finland. But in both Finland and Sweden, a
significant change in equivalent income occurred for 'others' relative
to unskilled blue-collar workers. The direction of this change is,
however, opposite to that anticipated on the basis of the above
hypothesis.

Apparently, then, the analysis provides little support for the
hypothesis. There is one specific, but interesting, exception to this
general finding; namely, the distribution of long-standing illness in
Norway. In my opinion, however, this general rejection of the hypothesis is not very peculiar. In line with earlier discussions, this 'resting'
category is clearly a very selective one and in so far as more and more
people are placed into such a category – as would be suggested by the
increase in unemployment – they ought to become a less selective
group. Here selection difference over time is also, for example, in line
with the cross-national variation in trends in equivalent income seen
among this category. It should also be noted that the above analysis
has a rather short time-span, and the possibility that the hypothesis
may receive support in the future cannot be ruled out.

Concluding discussion

The first question asked in this brief exposé of changes in living
conditions in the Nordic countries concerned how welfare, in general,
has changed from the mid-1980s to the mid-1990s. This was a period
of great economic turbulence and the trajectories of these three
nations differed sharply. According to standard economic indicators,
both Finland and Sweden outperformed Norway in the late 1980s;
the trends were dramatically reversed in the 1990s (see Chapter 2).

Given this macroeconomic background, the findings are somewhat unexpected. When the changes that occurred within each country are compared, the most positive picture seems to be painted for Finland. In contrast, many indicators of welfare problems that were studied here were found to be increasing in Norway. In all of the countries, however, average real earnings and real equivalent disposable income increased. Improvement was also detected in more immaterial resources important to the welfare of individuals, such as social support.

The second question raised concerned cross-national commonality and variation in the social patterning of these living conditions in terms of age, gender and class. In general, the findings suggest that a profound cross-national similarity does indeed exist. In all the countries, the young – and in some instances the old, too – have more problems than the middle-aged categories. In all the countries, gender differentials follow the same pattern and in most spheres of life class differentials are structured along the same lines. This is not to say that there are no cross-national variations. Class differentials, for example, seem to be somewhat smaller in Norway than in Finland or Sweden. Still, the living conditions in these three Nordic countries are, in similar fashion, influenced by processes leading to differentials by age, gender and class – some of which are widely known.

These differentials, especially their magnitude, are not so predetermined as to be uninteresting to study. In many respects, important and substantial changes have occurred – and not all of them have been in expected directions. In particular, variations in living conditions by age are changing rapidly in all three countries. In Finland and Sweden, these changes are mostly to the benefit of the older segments of the populations, whereas a substantial relative deterioration has occurred for younger age groups. This relative change is most evident in economic resources, but in Finland we also find an equalization of health status by age that conforms to this pattern. This general trend is not so evident in Norway.

The changes in living conditions between men and women and between social classes are more modest in all three countries. But here, too, interesting results pointing in different directions were noted. For example, the upper white-collar workers' relative advantage in income has increased in Sweden, whereas no such evidence was detected in either Finland or Norway. In contrast, the change seems to be rather the opposite in Finland. A specific analysis was also conducted in order to test the hypothesis of increasing differentials between insiders and outsiders in relation to the labour market. By and large, the findings did not support this hypothesis.

In sum, given the macroeconomic changes that have taken place, the results are most surprising for Finland; not only because of the improvements detected in many respects but also because of the striking lack of substantial increases in inequality. However, it is important to remember that the years covered in this study did not include only the recession years of the early 1990s; the economic boom of the mid–late 1980s is also included.

An exception to the above general remarks is the relative deterioration that occurred among the youngest age group. This can to a large extent be explained by the fact that young people by necessity are in a more vulnerable and uncertain position on the labour market. Otherwise, the findings in this respect support the perspective taken, for example, by Lahelma *et al.* (1997), that the rocketing rise of unemployment was felt in all segments of the society and therefore meant a sort of democratization of unemployment as a phenomenon.

It is hoped that this study has also demonstrated that changes in welfare and the social patterning of welfare are not very easily summed up in any aggregate measure, such as GDP, or even in a one-dimensional approach on the micro level, such as income.

Notes

1 Helpful comments on earlier drafts were made by Anders Barstad, Per Gillstöm, Erik Jørgen Hansen, Mikko Kautto, Olle Lundberg, Magnus Nermo, Niels Ploug and Hannu Uusitalo. The research was partly financed by a grant (F 572/95) from the Swedish Council for the Humanities and Social Sciences.
2 For discussions concerning the theoretical approach and the historical backgrounds of the Scandinavian welfare research, see, e.g. Allardt (1975); Erikson (1993); Erikson and Uusitalo (1987); Fritzell (1992); Johansson (1979); Tåhlin (1990).
3 Unfortunately, Denmark is not included in this comparison, since no corresponding data are available for Denmark in the 1990s.
4 Anonymous data from the Finnish surveys have been made available for analysis under the supervision of Stakes, Helsinki. Anonymous data from the Norwegian level of living surveys have been placed at my disposal from the Norwegian Social Science Data Services (NSD). The Swedish data, in anonymous form, were bought from Statistics Sweden. Neither the central statistical agencies nor NSD or Stakes are in any way responsible for the analyses or interpretations presented in this chapter.
5 A precise description of the variables is available from the author upon request.
6 The equivalence scale adopted is the square root of the number of persons in the household. This scale has frequently been used in recent income distribution studies. It is also the prime scale used in the recent OECD study on income distribution in OECD countries (Atkinson, Rainwater

and Smeeding 1995). This scale, for example, assumes that a four-person household needs to have twice the disposable income of a single-person household in order to have the same equivalent income.

7 For datatechnical reasons, the youngest age group in Finland are between 21 and 30 years of age.

8 More detailed results from the 120 regressions on which Tables 7.1 to Table 7.5 are based are available from the author upon request.

9 No doubt some changes are masked by the fact that this study includes data from only two cross-sections from each country. For example, as reported by Uusitalo (1997), average real disposable income in Finland actually fell during the latter years studied here. Obviously, the increase was greater in the years prior to the recession.

10 It is important to realise that many of the results presented below are not necessarily age effects in the strictest sense of the word, but also capture what may in reality be generational effects.

11 The decreasing age gradient in health status in Finland was confirmed in a more thorough analysis conducted by Lahelma, Rahkonen and Huuhka (1997).

12 The relatively positive situation for the oldest age group is striking in many respects. For example, according to the criteria set up for this study, the occurrence of economic difficulties was least common among those above 60 years old in both Norway and Sweden.

13 An exception here is the experiencing of severe economic difficulties in Sweden. It is important to stress, however, that the slight equalization between different age groups are those that are found when studying relative differences in terms of odds ratios. When a phenomenon has become more common, as is the case here, it is not self-evident that the conclusion reached would be the same if other relative, or absolute, differences were investigated. Thus, in this case, the proportion of respondents facing economic difficulties increased by about 3 percentage points (from 9.3 to 12.2 per cent) among the youngest age group, whereas it increased by a little more than 1 percentage point (from 1.8 to 3.1 per cent) among those aged 61 to 75. This, however, is equivalent to a decrease in relative odds, from about 5.7 to 4.3, for the youngest age group as compared to the oldest.

14 The choice of equivalence scale can, of course, have a major influence on the respective level of equivalent income (for a thorough analysis of this topic in general, see Buhmann *et al.* 1988). However, given that the average household size and structure within age groups are fairly constant over time, this choice does not have a substantial impact on the trends reported here. As a sensitivity test, the same analysis was repeated with one of the two extremes in the equivalence scale choices, that is to exclude this factor altogether. The result of this exercise was, in terms of trends, remarkably similar to the ones reported in Figure 7.1, thus supporting the above argument.

15 Interestingly enough, the same conclusion was reached when studying the changes in Sweden during the 1980s (Fritzell and Lundberg, 1994). Apparently, it is, at least in Sweden, a phenomenon that cannot fully be explained by the 1990s' recession. An obvious explanatory factor for part of the both absolute and relative betterment of the oldest age group in all

three countries is the fact that the pension system has, so to speak, matured.

16 The reason why the results indicate a significant relative decline for the youngest (and in fact also for those aged 31–45) in Finland might be connected to imperfect measurement of full-time employees (since earnings are measured the year prior to survey year) but could of course also reflect true changes.

17 This is also supported by the fact that if all individuals with positive earnings are included in the earnings analysis by age, the results are more in line with those reported for equivalent income (see Fritzell 1997).

18 In fact, though somewhat different measures were used, trends along this line were found in earlier analyses on Swedish data for the 1980s. Thus, while a slight increase of the gender gap in wage rates was detected, there was a simultaneous decrease in the annual individual income gap (cf. le Grand 1994; Fritzell and Lundberg 1994). Evidently these trends are not affected only by the recession of the 1990s.

19 Students have been excluded from this analysis since they can hardly be regarded as the prototype of any eventual underclass or as a marginalized group of the present or future.

20 The table does show a pattern in line with the hypothesis also with regard to social support in Finland. In this case, it has become less frequent to lack a close friend in all three 'classes', but the relative improvement is of lesser magnitude among 'others'.

8 Poverty and social exclusion in the Nordic countries

Björn Halleröd and Matti Heikkilä

Introduction

Most people can agree that the main objectives of the welfare state are to combat poverty and to diminish the risk of welfare problems and social exclusion among its citizens. Changes in poverty rates and in the incidence of social exclusion are, therefore, not only indicators of living conditions among individuals as such, but are also a sign of the relative success or failure of the welfare state. For example, sickness insurance is designed to ensure that illness or injury does not lead to poverty. Free or subsidized health care prevents the transformation of poverty into bad health. Unemployment benefits are supposed to protect the unemployed from poverty. Housing policy is aimed at preventing bad housing conditions among the poor. Thus, when there are cutbacks in the welfare state system one would expect that the occurrence of multiple welfare problems would increase; that is, we will see an increase in the process of social exclusion.

However, the welfare state is not on its own responsible for the occurrence of different forms of social problem. What it can do is to some degree mediate effects of macroeconomic changes on the individual level and breed an economic environment that can continue to produce economic growth. Thus, before judging the achievement of the welfare state one has to look at the basic differences in economic conditions and development.

This chapter is organized in the following way. The next section contains some remarks on general economic development, unemployment and poverty in the four Nordic countries. A brief theoretical discussion of the concepts of poverty and social exclusion is given after that, and data and operationalizations of the concepts are presented. The empirical part of the chapter will focus on the coexistence of welfare problems. The focus of attention will be on poverty and the objective is to analyse how poverty is related to other types of welfare problems. By comparing the mid-1980s and mid-1990s, the hypothesis about increasing social exclusion can be tested. The conclusions are discussed at the end of the chapter.

At this point we inform the reader that the empirical analysis of social exclusion covers only Finland, Norway and Sweden. Denmark is left out because of a lack of comparable data.

Economic development and income poverty in the Nordic countries

As has been pointed out in Chapter 2 in this book, general economic development in the Nordic countries has been different. Norway succeeded best in the beginning of the 1980s and 1990s while the growth rate was more modest in the mid-1980s. Denmark has experienced relatively stable growth from the beginning of the 1980s onwards. Sweden had the lowest growth rate during the first five years of the 1980s, improved slightly during the second phase of the decade and then turned downward during the 1990s. Finland showed the most fluctuating development, with impressive growth in the late 1980s, followed by negative growth during the period from 1991 to 1995.

The consequences of economic crisis have been most obviously reflected in unemployment rates (see Chapter 2, Table 2.9). Both Norway and Sweden were able to keep unemployment below the 4 per cent level during the whole of the 1980s, which in a global perspective was exceptional. In Finland the unemployment level during the relevant period was somewhat higher while Denmark, like most other European countries, experienced high unemployment early in the 1980s and the unemployment rate thereafter remained at a relatively high level. In accordance with the economic crises in Finland the unemployment rate rocketed to a level between 17 per cent and 19 per cent in a few years. Also Sweden was hit by a massive increase in unemployment, although the figures never reached the same staggering levels as in Finland. Both Finland and Sweden have in the last couple of years shown positive growth figures, but the unemployment rate has nevertheless remained high.

Economic poverty, defined as having an income that is less than 50 per cent of the mean income in the country, and the degree to which people are dependent on social assistance can both be seen as indicators of economic hardship. However, these indicators are not to be looked upon as alternatives to each other. Economic poverty is a

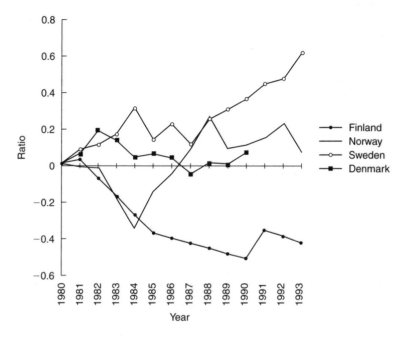

Figure 8.1 Economic poverty (< 50 per cent of mean income) ratio (1980 = 0)
in the Nordic countries
Source: Puide 1996.

relative indicator that basically is a function of the income distribution. Social assistance is to some degree also a relative indicator since
rules and legislation in practice are changed according to the development of the general life style and norms in a society. However, this
relative aspect of social assistance works with a certain degree of
inertia.

The figures on the economic poverty rates used here cover the
period from 1980 onwards and have been borrowed from Puide's
work (1996). However, comparing economic poverty rates between
countries is always a complicated task. Differences in definitions of
'income', 'household' and so on make it difficult to state which
country has the highest or lowest poverty rate even when comparing
relatively similar countries as is the case here. Therefore we have, to
avoid overinterpretation of differences in the poverty rate, calculated
a standardized ratio which compares the poverty rate in each country
with the situation in 1980. The incidence of economic poverty in the
Nordic countries from 1980 to 1993 is shown in Figure 8.1.

We can see that there has been an increase in economic poverty since the mid-1980s in Denmark, Norway and Sweden. In the 1990s the poverty rate in Sweden has continued to increase while it has decreased in Norway, a development that reflects the differences in macroeconomic performance between the countries. Finland deviates from the pattern; the poverty rate declined from the beginning of the 1980s to 1990. There was a moderate increase in 1991 but, thereafter the poverty rate again decreased. Hence, the impact of the deep economic crisis and rocketing unemployment in Finland on the poverty rate has been more or less negligible.

The pattern revealed when looking at recipients of social assistance (see Chapter 4, Figure 4.7) diverges from the picture given by economic poverty. Social assistance dependence increased in Finland, Norway and Sweden during the first part of the 1980s, it stabilized from 1985 to 1990 and then again increased during the 1990s. Denmark departed partly from this pattern, especially during the 1990s when there was a decrease in social assistance dependence.

The economic crisis in Finland and Sweden has manifested in an increased share of the population being dependent on social assistance. The positive economic development in Denmark is reflected in a decrease in social assistance dependency. The increase in Norway is harder to understand from the point of view of macroeconomic development.

It is difficult to draw a straightforward conclusion from the developments presented above. Sweden seems to be the least contradictory case. The weak growth rate of the early 1980s did correspond with relatively slow growth of purchasing power and an increase in poverty and in the number of recipients of social assistance. The growth rate increased somewhat and the situation stabilized during the later part of the decade. We can finally spot the economic crisis in the 1990s. The growth of purchasing power halted, unemployment increased and so did both the poverty rate and the proportion of the population that received social assistance. Denmark's case is also relatively easy to understand. Stable economic growth generated an increase in purchasing power. However, the positive economic development did not lead to a fall in the poverty rate and the social assistance rate has only started to fall in the last couple of years. It is tempting to interpret this development as an effect of the persistently high unemployment figures. Norway is a more difficult case that in the 1990s has seen a combination of a high growth rate and low unemployment with a stable poverty rate and an increasing social assistance rate, showing that there is no straightforward connection between macroeconomic growth and poverty alleviation. Finally, Finland stands out as the most contradictory case, at least in the 1990s. A persistent decline in poverty has been combined with negative economic growth, falling incomes, rocketing unemployment and a massive increase in the number of people receiving social assistance.

Social exclusion and poverty: theory

The discourse on social exclusion emerged in France during the 1960s and has since then spread across the rest of Europe. In the 1980s the concept was introduced by the European Commission and is now widely used by both social scientists and politicians. Today, combating social exclusion has been made an objective of the EU. How to interpret the concept is nevertheless unclear and the definition of social exclusion varies among countries, among different schools of thought and among different experts and researchers (Silver 1994). Social exclusion is in some cases used as a substitute for poverty, just another word for the same phenomenon. Persistent rumours say that the term 'poverty' has been replaced by 'social exclusion' since certain governments within the EU dislike the connotations inherent in the former concept. Others have tried to establish a distinction between poverty and social exclusion. Several arguments have been suggested for such a distinction. First, poverty is said to be a narrow concept dealing with problems that are directly related to economic resources, while social exclusion deals with a broad range of questions dealing with an individual's integration in society.

> notions such as social exclusion [. . .] focus primarily on relational issues; in other words, inadequate social participation, lack of social integration and lack of power. Social exclusion is the process of becoming detached from the organisations and communities of which the society is composed and from the rights and obligations that they embody.
>
> (Room 1995: 243)

Second, poverty is seen as a static phenomenon, dealing with people's economic situation at one point in time, while social exclusion represents a dynamic perspective focusing on the processes that lead to a situation of exclusion and, for that matter, poverty. Third, social exclusion is in some cases seen as an extreme form of poverty. The socially excluded are the worst off, the poorest among the poor (Abrahamson 1996).

If poverty and social exclusion are defined as two separate but interrelated concepts, one can also argue that there exists a causal relationship between them. What that causal relationship looks like is, however, unclear. Berghman (1995) argues, for example, that social exclusion is the process and poverty the outcome, while Walker (1995) claims that a long-lasting spell of poverty could lead to a state of social exclusion.

> It is clear, therefore, that the seeds of social exclusion are inherent within the very experience of poverty: increased social isolation, reduced morale, deviant behaviours and even the experience of ostracism that are linked more or less directly to the limited choice and restricted opportunities imposed by inadequate resources.
>
> (Walker 1995: 116)

To emphasise the ambiguity, Walker also argues that social exclusion and poverty can exist independently of each other and that social exclusion in some cases can result in poverty (Walker 1995: 128).

The view that poverty is narrow and static whereas social exclusion is broad and dynamic is from several perspectives an inadequate one. There is definitely a broad range of poverty research that focuses on the dynamics and the processes that create poverty (Nolan and Whelan 1996). Nevertheless, it is clear that the concept of poverty does not cover the same scope as social exclusion, but that does, on the other hand, mean that poverty as a concept is more stringently defined and has more depth (Nolan and Whelan 1996). The relationship between access to resources and outcome in terms of living conditions has also been explored, both theoretically and empirically, within the realm of poverty research (Townsend 1979; Callan *et al.* 1993; Mac Cárthaigh 1994; Halleröd 1995; Nolan and Whelan 1996). The notion of poverty also has a meaning in ordinary language. Most people know what we are talking about when we discuss poverty; social exclusion does not carry with it the same understanding.

This theoretical discussion will not be dealt with here any further. Instead the definition of social exclusion and poverty used here will be based on the first argument mentioned above. Hence, poverty will be defined and operationalized in a narrow and exclusively economic manner, that is, in the way it most often is defined and operationalized. Social exclusion will be defined and operationalized as an effect of accumulation of welfare deprivation that occurs in a broad range of areas. Defining social exclusion in this way seems to be in line with a common understanding of the concept of social exclusion, even though it very rarely is defined *and* operationalized at all. This way of dealing with social exclusion is also in line with parts of the Nordic research tradition based on the level of living standard (LLS) surveys. Erikson and Thålin's (1987) study, the 'Coexistence of Welfare Problems', is one example. Heikkilä's (1991), Halleröd's (1991) and Tham's (1994) analyses of deprivation and poverty are other examples.

Data and operationalization

The purpose of the analysis is, first, to study the incidence and accumulation of welfare problems in the three countries in the mid-1980s compared with in the mid-1990s. Second, the purpose is to analyse the risk of different sections of the population of suffering from accumulated deprivation. The analysis will be restricted to Finland, Norway and Sweden since, as mentioned above, a lack of comparable data makes it impossible to include Denmark. There are six different nationwide level of living surveys used for this purpose. These survey samples represent the total adult population in each country. However, in this study the sample has been restricted to cover the age span 20 to 64 years of age.[1] The main reason for this limitation of the sample is that we want to concentrate on the part of the population that is or at least is supposed to be active in the labour market. The surveys and the size of the working samples used in the analyses are shown below.

Basic information about the data on level of living survey is contained in Table 8.1. All of the data sets represent the Nordic tradition of level of living survey and to a large extent they cover the same areas. There are nevertheless several problems that have to be solved to make the analysis possible. First, even though the surveys in the three countries are following the same tradition, they are not co-ordinated in detail between the countries. This fact imposes some serious limitations on the study. Second, the Norwegian and Swedish surveys are fairly well co-ordinated over time. However, this is not the case with the Finnish surveys, a fact that adds additional limitations for the analysis.

Despite the problems of co-ordination, it is possible to define welfare problems in six areas for all three countries. These are:

Table 8.1 Information about Nordic level of living surveys

Country	Data source	Response rate	Total sample size	Working sample
Norway	Level of Living Survey 1987[a]	78.2	4,373	2,973
	Level of Living Survey 1995	75.4	3,630	2,933
Finland	Survey of Living Conditions 1986	86.9	12,057	9,168
	Survey of Living Conditions 1994	73.0	9,650	6,510
Sweden	Survey of Living Conditions 1986/8	78.4	11,818	8,616
	Survey of Living Conditions 1994/9	79.4	11,650	8,872

Sources: The Norwegian data set was originally collected by Statistic Norway and has been made available to us via Norwegian Social Science Data Service (NSD). The Finnish data were made available by Statistic Finland. The Swedish data were obtained from Statistic Sweden (SCB). All data sets were obtained in anonymous form. Neither Statistic Norway, NSD, Statistic Finland nor SCB is responsible for any of the analysis or interpretations in this chapter.

Note:
a   There is an extra sample of elderly people in the 1987 survey that explains the large difference between the total sample and the working sample.

1   Problems making ends meet in the household economy;
2   Low material standard;
3   Unemployment problems;
4   Poor health;
5   Social isolation; and
6   Exposure to violence.[2]

It should be mentioned that no assumptions about the causal relationship between different forms of welfare problems have been made at this stage. It is important to keep in mind that the exact operationalization can differ among the countries to some degree. *This means that it is incorrect to compare differences in the percentages among the countries.* The only exception to this rule is the category 'unemployment problems'. However, the operationalizations are identical for the two points in time looked at for each country. So, what can be compared is to what degree within a country the incidence of a certain problem decreased or increased from one year to another.

In the next step the six variables will be combined to form a simple index. The index will tell us to what degree people have more than one welfare problem at the same time. If a person has two or more problems, this will be taken as an indicator of social exclusion.

The incidence of poverty and social exclusion

Table 8.2 shows the percentages of the population that suffer economic poverty and different forms of welfare problems. In Norway there has been a significant increase in economic poverty. We can also observe that there has been an increase in unemployment problems and health problems. The situation looks otherwise stable and there was no significant change in the share of Norwegians that suffer from social exclusion.

In Finland there were significant changes in every area except violence. However, the pattern is not at all clear. Owing to the unfavourable economic developments in Finland one could expect a remarkable increase in economic poverty as well as in the incidence of welfare problems. On the other hand we have to keep in mind that in the two years of the cross-section – 1986 and 1994 – the GDP per capita remained steady. This common-sense expectation is only confirmed when looking at problems making ends meet, unemployment and health problems. There was also an increasing fraction of the

Table 8.2 The incidence of economic poverty and welfare problems in Norway, Finland and Sweden, mid-1980s and mid-1990s

	Norway 1987	Norway 1995	Finland 1986	Finland 1995	Sweden 1986/87	Sweden 1994/95
Economic poverty	5.7[a]	7.1[a]	5.8[a]	3.9[a]	4.3[a]	5.9[a]
Welfare problems:						
Problem making ends meet	5.7	6.7	6.3[a]	11.3[a]	7.5[a]	12.9[a]
Low material standard	9.6	9.3	21.1[a]	10.4[a]	13.1[a]	14.5[a]
Unemployment problem	6.1[a]	13.2[a]	12.0[a]	23.2[a]	7.8[a]	16.5[a]
Poor health	7.2[a]	9.4[a]	3.3[a]	4.8[a]	4	3.9
Social isolation	11.2	10.5	5.3[a]	4.5[a]	7.9	7.3
Exposure to violence	1.8	1.7	2.2	2.5	1.7[a]	2.7[a]
Social exclusion (2 or more welfare problems)	7.3	8.5	9.2[a]	11.9[a]	8.8[a]	13.4[a]

Note
a Changes between the years are significant at p < 0.05 level.

population that suffers from social exclusion. An interesting finding is the halving of the percentage of those living at a low material standard and the significant decrease in economic poverty.

The decrease in the Finnish low material standard group could possibly be explained by the fact that the indicators used to measure this area, especially in the case of Finland, are focused on housing. The housing standard in Finland improved rapidly during the booming economy of the late 1980s. Even though the Finnish economy was thrown into free fall in 1991, the welfare state prevented a situation where people would have been forced to sell their durable goods or their houses. In fact, what happened in the early 1990s was a remarkable increase in income transfers which then kept the relative poverty level unchanged (Heikkilä and Uusitalo 1997a). One can also assume that people suffering from economic hardship nevertheless would hesitate or find it impossible to sell their assets in a situation when demand and prices are falling. Instead they reduce their consumption of non-durable goods such as food, clothing and travel (Heikkilä *et al.* 1994). Thus, the explanation for the sharp decrease in the low material standard group could be that the variable used is able to reflect the economic improvement of the late 1980s, but was not affected by the crisis of the 1990s.

The figures that show a decrease in economic poverty are consistent with other estimates of economic poverty in Finland. One explanation offered for this development may be that the crisis in the Finnish economy hit almost every section of the population and initially led to a general decrease in income (Uusitalo 1997). So, in contrast with Sweden, the economic crisis in Finland was not accompanied by an increase in income inequality, which in turn, can at least partly serve as an explanation for the decrease in economic poverty measured in relative terms as is the case here.

The development in Sweden seems to have followed a straightforward path, consistent with the country's macroeconomic development. Economic poverty increased. There was an increase in all welfare problems that are directly related to labour market and economic well-being. The only areas where there was no significant increase are health and social isolation. Consistent with these results, we can also observe a large increase in the percentage of people suffering from social exclusion.

Table 8.3 shows the risk that a person who suffers from one specific welfare problem also suffers from at least one other problem. For example, 61.7 per cent of the Norwegians who had problems making

Table 8.3 The risk of having at least one additional welfare problem among people with welfare problem, percentages

	Norway 1987	Norway 1995	Finland 1986	Finland 1995	Sweden 1986/87	Sweden 1994/95
Problem making ends meet	61.7	61.8	62.6	67.3	64.6	68.1
Low material standard	40.9	48.2	32.3	50.2	49.0	61.8
Unemployment problem	53.4	43.6	47.9	40.3	44.6	45.8
Poor health	40.5	42.7	46.5	42.1	45.2	53.3
Social isolation	27.1	39.1	23.3	20.5	35.9	48.9
Exposure to violence	47.2	53.8	57.7	55.0	50.7	56.9

ends meet in 1987 also showed up in at least one of the other problem groups.

The pattern shown in Table 8.3 clearly reveals differences among the countries. The situation in Norway has been more or less stable. That is also the case in Finland, except among those in the low material standard group. The reason for this group being an outlier in the Finnish case may be that the group was much smaller in 1994 compared with 1986. It is possible, therefore, that those who in 1994 had a low material standard represented a more homogeneous and marginalized group compared to the very large group in 1986. Sweden again represents a more clear-cut example of increasing social exclusion. It is not only the case that the size of the problem groups has increased over time: the risk of having an additional welfare problem has also increased in each and every one of the defined problem groups.

Table 8.4 displays the correlations between welfare problems. The first thing to notice is that most of the correlations are significant and positive in all three countries. Thus, having one welfare problem generally increases the risk of having yet another welfare problem. However, there are some deviations from this 'rule'. In Finland social isolation is either negatively correlated, or not correlated at all, with other types of welfare problems.

Looking at the correlations country by country we can again observe that the situation in Norway seems to have been stable. Some correlations are weaker and some are stronger for 1995 compared to 1987, but the overall patterns are similar in both years and

Table 8.4 Correlation (Kendall's Tau_b) between different welfare problems in Norway, Finland and Sweden

Norway

Welfare problem	1987					1995				
	Unemployment	Making ends meet	Health problem	Social isolation	Material standard	Unemployment	Making ends meet	Health problem	Social isolation	Material standard
Making ends meet	0.163[b]					0.169[b]				
Health problem	0.071[b]	0.119[b]				−0.005	0.115[b]			
Social isolation	0.016	0.065[b]	0.050[b]			0.040[a]	0.068[b]	0.073[b]		
Material standard	0.091[b]	0.163[b]	0.059[b]	0.064[b]		0.096[b]	0.147[b]	0.051[b]	0.059[b]	
Violence	0.093[b]	0.088[b]	0.041[a]	−0.24	0.037	0.073[b]	0.070[b]	0.003	0.032	0.051[b]

Finland

Welfare problem	1986					1994				
	Unemployment	Making ends meet	Health problem	Social isolation	Material standard	Unemployment	Making ends meet	Health problem	Social isolation	Material standard
Making ends meet	0.223[b]					0.260[b]				
Health problem	−0.011	0.056[b]				−0.023	0.056[b]			
Social isolation	−0.037[b]	−0.037[b]	−0.036[b]			−0.081[b]	−0.047[b]	−0.039[b]		
Material standard	0.106[b]	0.096[b]	0.047[b]	−0.032[b]		0.081[b]	0.106[b]	0.055[a]	−0.032[a]	
Violence	0.063[b]	0.090[b]	0.0013	−0.023[a]	0.025[a]	0.042[b]	0.060[b]	0.028[a]	0.005	0.038[b]

Sweden

Welfare problem	1986/87					1994/95				
	Unemployment	Making ends meet	Health problem	Social isolation	Material standard	Unemployment	Making ends meet	Health problem	Social isolation	Material standard
Making ends meet	0.171[b]					0.197[b]				
Health problem	−0.004	0.064[b]				−0.021	0.070[b]			
Social isolation	0.001	0.041[b]	0.056[b]			0.011	0.077[b]	0.056[b]		
Material standard	0.124[b]	0.268[b]	0.050[b]	0.063[b]		0.145[b]	0.312[b]	0.056[b]	0.111[b]	
Violence	0.029[b]	0.082[b]	0.004	0.008	0.053[b]	0.055[b]	0.100[b]	0.007	0.005	0.093[b]

Note:
Correlation is significant at the: a = 0.05 level, b = 0.01 level (2-tailed).

there is no general direction to the changes. Also in Finland stability is the most dominant feature when comparing 1986 with 1984. Thus, the deep recession of the early 1990s has not led to an increased probability of accumulation of deprivation, and the significant increase in the number of people that suffer from two or more problems seems to be an effect of an increased number of people with welfare problems, not tighter connections between different problems.

Again, Sweden departs from the other two countries and the tendency is a strengthening of the correlations between welfare problems. Hence, the development in Sweden has not only been characterized by an increase in the number of people that report different welfare problems. The incidence of social exclusion increased in Sweden both as an effect of an increased number of people suffering from welfare problems and an increased connection between these problems.

Multivariate analysis

The multivariate analysis explored the risk among individuals in different sections of the population of being socially excluded. Six independent variables were used in the analysis and they were operationalized in the following way:

> *Equivalent income*: Income was measured in the national currency for each country. Disposable income was converted to equivalent income using the so-called OECD equivalence scale (the first adult = 1, each successive adult = 0.7 and children = 0.5).
>
> *Economic poverty*: Those who had an equivalent income under 50 per cent of the median in each country were regarded as poor. Poverty was therefore, in technical terms, a dummy variable that discriminates the households in the lowest segments of the income variable. The hypothesis is that poverty will increase the risk of being socially excluded. Such an effect would give justification to the use of this definition of poverty since it will clearly indicate a qualitative uniqueness of this category, a uniqueness that deviates from the linear effect of income distribution.
>
> *Socioeconomic class*: The populations were divided into nine categories based on their position in the labour market. The classification system, the so-called socioeconomic code, is very

similar to the well-known CASMIN system introduced by Erikson and Goldthorpe (1993).

1 Unskilled blue-collar worker
2 Skilled blue-collar worker
3 Lower white-collar worker
4 Middle-range white-collar worker
5 Upper white-collar worker (including free professions and managerial positions)
6 Self-employed
7 Farmers
8 Students
9 Others (including non-students who are not participating in the labour market)

Education: The populations were ranked according to highest completed level of education.

1 Only compulsory school
2 Comprehensive school I (less than three years)
3 Comprehensive school II (three years or more)
4 University less than three years
5 University three years or more

Household type:

1 Male single adult without children
2 Female single adult without children
3 Single parent, male and female
4 Couple without children
5 Couple with children

Age: This variable was entered into the analysis as a set of dummy variables in order to capture the possibilities of a non-linear relationship between age and social exclusion.

1 Age 20 to 24
2 Age 25 to 30
3 Age 31 to 40
4 Age 41 to 50
5 Age 51 to 64

Gender: Men were assigned value 0 and women assigned value 1. Hence, it is the effect of being a woman that is estimated in the model.

The analytical model

The analyses were organized according to the analytical model shown in Figure 8.2. The model should be interpreted as a 'soft causal model' aiming more at testing relationships than definite causal effects. The model was based on the assumptions that all variables affect social exclusion directly and that the weak part of the chain is the relationship between 'income and poverty' and 'social exclusion'. One could very well assume that the causal effects in some cases work the other way around; that is, social exclusion causes low income and poverty.

Age and gender are presumed to affect household, education, class, income and poverty. Household composition is mainly presumed to influence income. There will in fact also be a test of the associations between household, on the one hand, versus class and education, on the other. However, we do not assume any strong relationship and we are also aware of the fact that any definite assumption about the causal relationships between these three variables is dubious. Education is

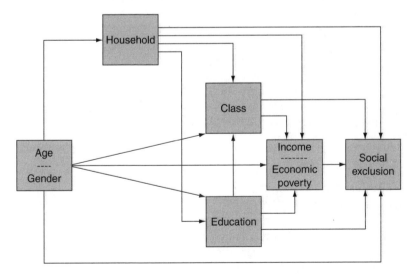

Figure 8.2 Analytical model

supposed to affect class, income and poverty. Finally, class is assumed to affect income and poverty.

The analyses were conducted in a series of logistic regression models.[3] The causal relationship was analysed according to the so-called effect change design strategy (Hellevik 1992). This means that the analysis was conducted in several steps, starting with the estimations of the bivariate effects. In the second step income and economic poverty were introduced as control variables for the other independent variables. Thus, all the independent variables were analysed one by one together with income and poverty. These analyses show to what degree the bivariate effects are mediated through the income/poverty variables. In the third step class was added as a control variable together with income. In the fourth step education was added as a control variable, and in the fifth step household type was also used as a control variable. Finally the total multivariate model was estimated.

The basic assumption was that the effects of the independent variables would decrease in every step of the analysis, suggesting an indirect relationship with deprivation. However, it is rather common that the effects increase as new control variables are introduced, indicating the occurrence of interaction effects. The interaction effects were estimated in an additional set of regression models. The results from these models are not shown here, but any significant estimate of interactions will be commented on in the text. Lastly, we tested to what degree differences over time within each country were significant. This was done by pooling the two data sets for each country and respecifying all the regression models by including an interaction term between time (year of survey recoded as 0 and 1) and each independent variable in the model.

In the following sections we will first try to interpret the broad causal pattern shown by the regression analysis and then compare the probability of social exclusion in different groups of the population.

Changes over time

In Tables 8.5, 8.6 and 8.7 we try to summarize and compare the situation in the 1980s with the situation in the 1990s: the focus is on changes over time in each country. The figures should be read as follows: the first column tells us if there have been any changes in the bivariate estimates between the years. Bold print was used if the difference between the years was statistically significant. If changes are indicated with normal print the result should be interpreted as

Table 8.5 Summary of changes over time in Finland

Indicator	Bivariate estimate	Full model estimate	Indirect effect via income and economic poverty	Indirect effect via class	Indirect effect via education	Indirect effect via household composition
Equivalent income poverty	Stable	Stable				
Economic poverty	Increased (negative)	Increased (negative)				
Class	Decreased	**Decreased***	Increased			
Education	**Increased***	**Increased***	**Stable***	**Stable***		
Household	Increased	**Increased***	Stable	No interaction	No interaction	
Age	**Increased***	**Increased***	**Increased***	**Stable***	**Stable***	**Stable***
Sex	Increased	Increased	Stable	Stable	Stable	Stable

Note
* Statistically significant.

being just a tendency. For example, in Table 8.5 we can see that the impact of education on social exclusion increased significantly in Finland. There is also a tendency telling us that household composition became more important. However, this is just a tendency that cannot be stated with statistical certainty. The second column is a summary of the results from the estimation of the full regression model. Again looking at Finland, we can see that the impact of education was still significantly larger in 1994 compared to 1986. We can also see, looking at columns three and four, that there is an indirect effect of education via income and class. Hence, people with different education levels had different incomes and different class positions, which partly explains why people with low education had a higher risk of being excluded than highly educated persons. However, these indirect effects did not change over time and they do not offer a full explanation as to why education has an impact on social exclusion.

If we continue to look at Finland's case we can see that the effect of income was stable at the same time as we can observe that the direct, negative effect of economic poverty increased over time. The direct effect of class decreased while the indirect effect via income increased. The increased effect of education is clear in Finland. The household type seems to have been somewhat more important in Finland in the 1990s compared to the 1980s. We can see that the effect of age became stronger over time and the gap between those over 50 years of age, who generally are better off, and the rest of the population increased. We can also observe an increased difference between Finnish men and women. The risk of exclusion was already higher in the mid-1980s among men than among women, a difference that had become greater in 1994 (although the change is not statistically significant).

In Finland there were a number of interaction effects between age and the other variables in the model. The interaction between age and household indicates that young single women and young couples without children were worse off than older people in the same household type in 1986. In 1994 there was still an interaction between age and couples without children, but the interaction between age and single women has been replaced by an interaction between age and single men.

We can, when it comes to age and education, observe an interaction that shows that older people with a short (< 3 years) university education had an increased risk of exclusion in 1986. It is hard to understand why this particular group had an increased exclusion risk and it is tempting to regard it as a one-time flux. (The estimated coefficient is rather big, but so is the standard error of the estimate and the effect did not reappear in 1994.) The interaction in 1994 points to a totally different group, namely young people with only a basic education. Here the interpretation is more straightforward and plausible. Young people without any or with only little work experience and with a low amount of human capital have been the losers in the early 1990s. Finally, looking at the interaction between age and class we can see that the combination of being young and a lower white-collar worker increased the risk of exclusion during both years.

Looking at Norway, the effects of income and economic poverty were basically unchanged, and low income increased the risk of being socially excluded. The direct effects of class weakened at the same time as one could see an increase in the indirect effect of class via income. The direct effect of education increased slightly over time while the indirect effect via class increased somewhat. The impact of household type decreased significantly between the years. Behind this change lies an improvement in the situation of couples with children. Finally, age and sex had an increasing effect, both directly and indirectly via income. There were no significant estimates of interactions effect in Norway (Table 8.6).

The effect of income was fairly stable also in Sweden and, as in Finland, we can observe an increased, negative effect of economic poverty. Sweden followed the other two countries regarding the weakening of class effect and the strengthening of the impact of education. The indirect effect of class via income became stronger. Education had a more substantial effect on exclusion via income in the 1990s. On this point, Sweden departs from the two other countries (Table 8.7).

Age became a more important factor in Sweden over time and it has been the young section of the population that has faced an increased risk of social exclusion. The direct effect of age on exclusion increased, and so did the indirect effects via household and income. In the 1980s the risk of exclusion was significantly higher among men compared to women. This difference disappeared in the 1990s.

There are also some interaction effects in the Swedish data. However, there is only one interaction that in a significant way affected the risk of exclusion and that is the interaction between class and age in 1994/95. The interaction clearly shows that young blue-collar and lower white-collar workers suffered from exclusion to a higher degree than their older counterparts. Finally, there were no general differences

Table 8.6 Summary of changes over time in Norway

Indicator	Bivariate estimate	Full model estimate	Indirect effect via income and economic poverty	Indirect effect via class	Indirect effect via education	Indirect effect via household composition
Equivalent income	Stable	Stable				
Economic poverty	Stable (negative)	Stable (negative)				
Class	Decreased	Decreased	Increased			
Education	Increased	Stable	Increased	Stable		
Household	**Decreased***	**Decreased***	**Stable***	**Stable***	**Stable***	
Age	Increased	Increased	Increased	Stable	Stable	Stable
Sex	Increase	Increased	Increased	Stable	Stable	Stable

Note
* Statistically significant.

Table 8.7 Summary of changes over time in Sweden

	Bivariate estimate	Full model estimate	Indirect effect via income and economic poverty	Indirect effect via class	Indirect effect via education	Indirect effect via household composition
Equivalent income	Stable	Stable				
Economic poverty	Increased (negative)	Increased (negative)				
Class	Stable	Decreased*	Increased			
Education	Increased*	Increased*	Increased*	Decreased*		
Household	Increased*	Stable	Increased*	No effect	Increased*	
Age	Increased*	Increased	Increased*	Stable*	Stable*	Increased*
Sex	Stable	Decreased*	Stable	Decreased	Stable	Decreased*

Note
* Statistically significant.

between men and women in Sweden that were not accounted for by the household variable.

Summarizing the changes over time there are at least some findings that are worth an extra note. First, the direct effect of class on social exclusion decreased over time in all three countries. At the same time the indirect effect of class via income has increased. Second, the direct effect of education has in all three countries increased. Third, young people have been more exposed to exclusion than others. This difference has increased over time, indicating growing cleavages between different generations. The effect of age via income also strengthened in all three countries. In both the Finnish and the Swedish data there were also interaction effects showing that young people in some cases were worse off than older people in otherwise similar situations. Thus, the main findings are: declining importance of class, increasing importance of education and widening of generation cleavages.

The probability of being socially excluded

In this section the probabilities of being socially excluded are calculated for different sections of the population. The calculations were based on the 'full model' logistic regression estimates. Probabilities for twelve different cases (or 'individuals') were calculated. The input value for these cases are shown in Table 8.8. In every step of the calculations some changes in the conditions were made. The changes from one step to another are marked with bold print. The results of the calculations are shown in Figure 8.3.

The estimated risk of social exclusion was, as expected, very low in the first case in all three countries and as we changed the conditions towards less favourable situations the probabilities increased. However, there were some differences between the countries. The risk of being excluded in Norway and Sweden was generally higher in the 1990s compared to the 1980s. In Norway the gap increased when case number 5 was estimated. The results show that the development in Norway resulted in a clear difference between skilled and unskilled blue-collar workers. The gap continued to widen when cases 6 and 7 were estimated, a result that shows that the impact of low income increased in Norway. In case 8 the analysis moved from estimating probabilities among couples to estimating probabilities among single adult households. The gap between the curves for Norway further increases here except for women in single adult households, but this group was, on the other hand, clearly an outlier in 1987. This

Table 8.8 Input values for probabilities calculations

Case no	Input value
1	Male, married but no children. High income earner,[1] upper white-collar worker. University degree, 55 years of age
2	Male, married with children. **Average income,**[2] **middle range white-collar worker.** Less than three years university education, 35 years of age
3	Male, married with children. Average income, **lower white-collar worker. Three years comprehensive school,** 35 years of age
4	Male, married with children. Average income, **skilled blue-collar worker. Two years comprehensive school,** 35 years of age
5	Male, married with children. Average income, **unskilled blue-collar worker. Compulsory school,** 35 years of age
6	Male, married with children. **Low income,**[3] unskilled blue-collar worker. Compulsory school, 35 years of age
7	Male, married with children. **Very low income,**[4] unskilled blue-collar workers. Compulsory school, 35 years of age
8	Male, **single adult. Below the poverty line**[5] **(effect of poverty estimated),** unskilled blue-collar worker. Compulsory school, **27 years of age**
9	**Female,** single adult. **Very low income,** unskilled blue-collar worker. Compulsory school, 27 years of age
10	**Male,** single adult. **Very low income,** unskilled blue-collar worker. Compulsory school, 27 years of age
11	Male, single adult. **Below the poverty line (effect of poverty NOT estimated),** unskilled blue-collar worker. Compulsory school, 27 years of age
12	**Female, single parent.** Below the poverty line (effect of poverty NOT estimated), unskilled blue-collar worker. Compulsory school, 27 years of age.

Notes
1 Belongs to the highest income decile.
2 Belongs to the fifth income decile.
3 Belongs to the second income decile.
4 Belongs to the lowest income decile.
5 Has an income below 50 per cent of the median income.

indicates a worsening of the situation for young single adults, male and female, with and without children.

The picture is somewhat different when looking at the case of Sweden. The increased effect of low class, education and low income that was revealed for Norway is not as clear for Sweden. Here we mainly find differences among young, single adult households. In Norway the highest risk of exclusion was found among single women.

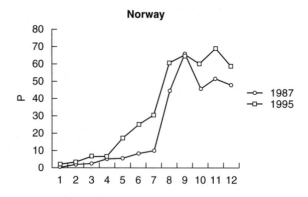

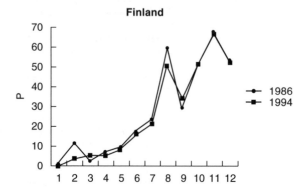

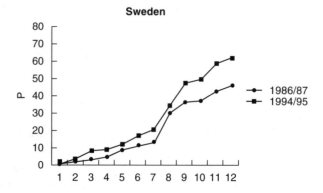

Figure 8.3 The probability of being socially excluded for different sections of
the population in Finland, Norway and Sweden in the mid-1980s
and mid-1990s

In Sweden the highest risk was found among single parents, a group that to a large degree is equivalent to single mothers.

Finland deviates from the two other countries mainly because of the small changes between the years studied. Thus, the distribution of the risk of being socially excluded, as measured here, seems to have remained more or less unchanged in Finland. This result is, of course, somewhat mysterious since Finland was the country to go through the most dramatic macroeconomic development of all three countries. However, it is worth emphasizing that these results are in line with what other researchers have found and they support the overall picture of Finland passing unexpectedly untouched through the economic recession of the 1990s.

The impact of economic poverty

The effect of economic poverty on the risk of being excluded was negative in every one of the regression models, although it was not always significant. This result is, at least at a first glance, puzzling since it indicates that people below the poverty line were somewhat better off than people with an income just above the poverty line. Looking at the charts in Figure 8.3 we can see that the exclusion risk in all three countries was higher for case number 11 compared to case 8. The only difference in input value between these cases was that the effect of economic poverty was estimated in number 8 but not in number 11. However, the most likely explanation for this result is not that low income in reality had a positive impact on people's standard of living, instead we have to acknowledge that income, *as far we were able to measure it*, was an inadequate indicator of standard of living. This seems especially to have been the case among those with the lowest income, i.e. those usually regarded as the poor. Under-reporting of income and access to non-monetary resources in some cases lead to a mismatch between the incomes that are registered and the economic resources that individuals actually possess. Thus, there are probably always a number of well-off people that are wrongly classified as poor. The probability that these people also will be defined as socially excluded is, of course, low and we will thereby get a negative estimate of economic poverty (when economic poverty is regressed together with income).

The differences between cases number 8 and 11 can be interpreted in the following way. In number 11 we assumed that the effect of income among the poor follows the general log-linear relationship found in the total population when we controlled for the peculiarity in the lowest segment of the income distribution. In case 8 we estimated exclusion risk among those that actually fell below the defined poverty line. We then included the measurement error in the estimate. So the argument here is that the true impact of low income is best shown by case 11, not by case 8.

A summary of the results

To sum up this part of the analysis we can conclude that both Norway and Sweden were broadly following the same pattern of social exclusion risk. The risk of exclusion was generally higher in the 1990s compared to the 1980s. This is especially true among those living in single adult households and among unskilled, less educated, and low income earners. The overall picture is that there seems to be the same sort of process working in both these countries. To discuss and analyse these processes in detail is way beyond the scope of this chapter. What the results indicate is that these processes have had a major impact on the level of social exclusion in Sweden because of unfavourable economic developments and social policy retrenchment. These difficulties have led to a larger number of people living in 'risk situations' where they are exposed to welfare problems and social exclusion. Norway has managed to avoid this development, not because they have been able to eliminate the risk factors, but because they have had economic development that has served to keep the number of people at exclusion risk at an unchanged, or decreasing, level. An economic downturn in Norway would therefore probably have the same effect as in Sweden.

The Finnish pattern is deviant. We do not see any clear-cut effects of the very deep economic crisis that hit the country in the beginning of the 1990s regarding the distribution of the probability of being excluded. Instead the results indicate different parts of the population have all been hit in a similar way by the economic recession, a conclusion that corresponds with other analysis of the effect of the economic crisis in Finland (Heikkilä and Uusitalo 1997b).

Conclusion

The Nordic countries are often looked upon as a group of nations with a lot in common. Even though this is partly true, it is also partly wrong. Differences between the Nordic countries are clearly visible when comparing their development during the 1980s and the first half of the 1990s. Denmark started out in the 1980s as the 'sick man' in the Nordic family. High unemployment, budget constraints and welfare cuts were a part of the Danish reality that did not, at least not with the same magnitude, affect the other three Nordic countries included in this study. However, Danish development during the 1990s has been positive, and when looking at the situation in the middle of the decade, Denmark has turned out to be a prosperous country with a strong economy and a per capita income that clearly exceeds those of both Finland and Sweden. The 1990s has been for the two latter countries a problematic period. Both Finland and Sweden experienced their deepest recession since the 1930s, and even though their economies have recovered, they are still in the aftermath of the crisis, manifested in welfare retrenchment, seemingly persistent high unemployment and, in comparison with their Nordic neighbours, a degradation of per capita income. Norway can be seen as an outlier in a more narrow Nordic perspective, as in the wider Western context. Since the beginning of the 1980s Norway has been the richest country in the Nordic family (when looking at GDP per capita), a position that has been reinforced during the 1990s.

The aim of this chapter has been to analyse poverty and social exclusion in the Nordic countries, comparing the situation in the mid-1980s with that in the mid-1990s. Because of limitations in data these analyses were limited to only three countries; Finland, Norway and Sweden. The focus of attention in the analysis was the incidence of social exclusion within each country, its distribution within the populations and changes over time in both incidence and distribution.

First, considering the differences in macroeconomic development we expected differences between the countries regarding changes over time in the incidence of different welfare problems as well as social exclusion. Comparing Norway and Sweden, this turned out to be true. The situation in Norway was stable, with no increase in welfare problems or in social exclusion, while in Sweden there was a clear increase in single welfare problems and social exclusion. However, this picture, indicating a straightforward relationship between macroeconomic performance and individual welfare was, at least partly, blurred by the addition of Finland's case. Even though the economic crisis in Finland was deeper than in Sweden, the development towards increased incidence of welfare problems and social exclusion was less clear-cut in Finland than in Sweden. In the future, the explanation for these differences has to be analysed more thoroughly regarding the ways the recession hit the populations and the ways the welfare states in these two countries managed to counterbalance the failures of the market.

The second part of the analysis concerned the risk of being socially excluded among different parts of the population. Here the analysis revealed some general patterns. People's class positions are traditionally seen as a main predictor of people's standard of living. However, the analysis done here indicates that class has lost some of its significance. Class was not as important in determining the risk of being socially excluded in the 1990s as it was in the 1980s. At the same time as class lost some of its impact, education gained importance. To be highly educated has become more important over time. This is a development that corresponds to and gives empirical support for the general discussion about the increasing importance of education. Another factor that seems to play a more important role is age. The risk of social exclusion is unevenly distributed among age categories both in the 1980s and 1990s and at both points in time the younger sections of the population suffer from an increased social exclusion risk. Still, the impact of age has increased and there are substantial differences between age groups in the mid-1990s indicating growing cleavages between different generations.

Looking at the broad pattern of the risk distribution we can see that for many groups the risk of social exclusion has increased over time in Norway and Sweden. This result is interesting since it indicates a similarity in the development in these two countries that has occurred despite the difference in macroeconomic achievements. Thus, the changes in the incidence of social exclusion are different in Norway and Sweden because of the differences in economic development. But the fundamental forces that create social exclusion seem to be very much the same in the two countries, a result that indicates that Norway will follow the same road of increasing social exclusion as Sweden if the Norwegian economy for one reason or another loses its pace. When looking at the risk of being socially excluded, Finland once again behaved in an unexpected way since the distribution of exclusion risk did not change in any visible sense between the mid-1980s and mid-1990s. Hence, it seems the deep economic recession in the beginning of the 1990s did not hit certain parts of the population harder than other parts. This result, and the fact that the increase over time in welfare problems and social exclusion was less marked in Finland compared with Sweden, blur the assumed relationship between macroeconomic achievements and individual welfare. But the results regarding Finland do, nonetheless, correspond to what other researchers have found when analysing the effects of the economic crisis in the 1990s. Different statistical sources tells us that the relative poverty rate did not increase, that the income distribution remained quite stable and that the internal structure of household consumption among low-income earners did not deviate essentially from the general consumption pattern (Uusitalo 1997; Sihvo 1997). On the basis of our own analysis and these other observations we have good reason for saying that the 1990 recession was a real test of the Finnish welfare state and the results we have indicate that the system worked as it should and as expected – i.e. it prevented large masses of people from falling into poverty and from suffering other material miseries when the market income fell, mainly due to quickly rising unemployment (Heikkilä and Uusitalo 1997a: 179–91).

The problem is that there also exists a second picture of the Finnish reality that is reflected by a social assistance dependency rate that has risen more than twofold over the five years from 1989 to 1994 while at the same time the duration of this dependency has become prolonged. Over-indebtedness is a problem in many households and there is clear evidence that both the need and actual use of unofficial help, i.e. NGO-based activity, have increased. This has been said to indicate that the formal system cannot respond to all the new material and immaterial problems of people. The problem is, of course, to understand how these two divergent pictures can exist simultaneously. It might be argued that our analysis of social exclusion is not sensitive enough to capture the impact of the economic crisis in Finland. However, we should not overlook the fact that our findings on Finland fit other findings based on income and expenditure data. We also have to understand why we can trace the effect of the economic crisis on social exclusion in a very clear way in Sweden but not in Finland. There is clearly a need for further research regarding these matters.

There is finally one point that we want to stress. The analysis of exclusion risk shows that the risk of exclusion actually decreases among the part of the population that has an income below the economic poverty line, i.e., a disposable income under 50 per cent of the median income. What this result implies is that it is worse to have an income just above the poverty line compared to an income below the poverty line. The explanation for this phenomenon that has been put forward here is that the income variable lacks reliability, especially among households classified as low income. This has an important policy implication when it comes to targeting social transfers. One reason for moving from a universal transfer system to a selective targeting transfer system is to improve the efficiency of the system. Only those in need should get transfers, the rest can easily do without support from the welfare state. However, the problem of identifying the poor via their disposable income pinpoints the weakness in this reasoning. Targeting will, to a not negligible degree, direct transfers to parts of the population that are not in need and it will to a certain degree miss parts of the population that are in need. A majority of those defined as socially excluded in this study will, for example, not be affected at all by transfers directed at those parts of the population that fall below the poverty line.

Notes

1 In Sweden people aged eighteen years or older are regarded as a household of their own, even if they still live with their parents. This manner of defining a household departs from both that of Norway and Finland (as well as most other countries). The Swedish definition of a household tends to lead to an overestimate of the incidence of economic poverty among young people. The most obvious category in this respect is young students living with their parents. The assumption that they are a household of their own and that they don't share any resources with their parents is not viable. Therefore students who live together with their parents have been excluded from the Swedish data set.
2 The exact description of the operationalization of these indicators can be obtained from the authors.
3 The results from these analyses (logistic regression estimates) can be obtained from the authors.

9 The distribution of income in the Nordic countries

Changes and causes

Björn Gustafsson, Rolf Aaberge, Ådne Cappelen, Peder J. Pedersen, Nina Smith and Hannu Uusitalo

Introduction

The Nordic welfare states are in many analyses characterized by their emphasis on equality, referring not only to the principles of their social policies but also to distribution of income and other living conditions. In the last two decades or so our knowledge of the distribution of well-being has improved considerably. This is particularly true as regards income distribution. The Luxembourg Income Study (LIS), which, in particular, has harmonized household level data across countries, has meant great progress in the study of economic inequalities. A relatively recent study using this data and published by the OECD showed that in the latter part of the 1980s Finland, Norway and Sweden were the countries with the smallest inequality in equivalent disposable income (Atkinson *et al.* 1995). Another recent study, using mainly data from the European Community Household Panel from 1994 and from the Nordic Level of Living Surveys, reveals the same pattern: Finland, Norway, Sweden and Denmark have more equal distributions of income than the other European Union countries (Vogel 1997: 79).

This chapter focuses on the development of income distribution in the Nordic countries, particularly during the 1980s and 1990s, and aims to describe income distribution trends. We use national data sets, which are not exactly comparable between the countries, but the trends can, within the limits specified in the relevant context, be adequately compared. The second task is to analyse the causes of the changes, if any. Here we focus particularly on the impact of unemployment and on social and tax policies. Our method is to survey the relevant literature, filling some holes in our knowledge by reporting new results. This means, for example, that for Norway we present a new time-series.

The chapter is laid out as follows: in the next section we address general methodological issues and then go on to present time series of income distributions for each country. After that we ask if there is a direct relation between the unemployment rate and income inequality. The role of changes in the composition of the population on inequality and changed income for various subgroups is addressed subsequently and then we trace changes in inequality to various components making up disposable income. The results are summarized in the final section.

Methodological issues

There seems to be wide agreement that comparisons of inequality should preferably focus on welfare and that income is just one of the arguments of the welfare function. The problem is that there is no consensus on which other aspects to consider, nor on how to weight various arguments of the welfare function. Therefore, when trying to monitor the development of inequality regarding welfare, analysts are most often left with evaluating the development of inequality in the distribution of disposable income.

There are several issues in the measurement of disposable income which can be discussed. Some sources of income are more difficult to define and measure than others. The former include income from capital and business as well as imputed income from owner-occupied housing. All measures of income refer to a specific time interval, most often one year. There is also the issue of how to define the income-receiving unit. Finally, sample selection and the method of collecting data can vary. There are thus many reasons why comparability of income distribution data is limited between countries. However, for a given country there is often rather a large continuity in how all the above-mentioned issues are treated, making comparisons over time less problematic.

From a welfare perspective it is essential to consider the fact that individuals live in households having a certain household disposable income. However, the individual welfare implications of a given household income are quite different depending on how many persons are living on it. This consideration motivates attempts to control for the size of the household (and sometimes also characteristics of the persons). Most often this is done by using an equivalence scale.

Unfortunately, there is no consensus on which equivalence scale to use or on the method of arriving at a scale. As empirical equivalence scales differ widely it seems potentially dangerous to arrive at a time series by combining studies which have used different equivalence scales.

The view that welfare measurements should use the individual as a unit of analysis is rather widespread today. This means that when computing Lorenz-curves and inequality indices individuals are weighted equally, not in inverse proportion to the size of the household they live in, which is the case if households are used as unit of analysis. This approach means that each member of a household is assumed to have the same income. Although questionable, this assumption seems to be reasonable from various perspectives. Present policies in modern societies attempt only to a very limited extent to affect the distribution of consumption within the household. Statistics showing how much each family member is consuming are not easily available. A large part of consumption within a household (for example, housing) has a considerable collective element.

The time-series of the distribution of income for the four countries which we report in the next section are relatively comparable across countries on a conceptual level. A problem is that when one inspects more closely how data are collected in the various Nordic countries several differences are apparent (Zamanian 1993). For example, a household is not defined in the same manner in all countries and the same applies to disposable income. Therefore comparability across the Nordic countries at one point in time is limited, but the evolution over time can be compared with greater accuracy.

How have income distributions changed in the Nordic countries?

Consistent time series covering a long span of years do not exist for Denmark. As regards the 1970s, Egmose (1985) found a strong decrease in the Gini-coefficient for the distribution of taxable income between individuals. Some estimates are available for the 1980s (see Table 9.1). Tentative conclusions from this somewhat confusing picture are: the decline in inequality regarding disposable income seemed to continue in the first half of the 1980s; but different series point in different directions as regards the development since the mid-1980s.

Uusitalo (1989) presented a time series on the distribution of equivalent income for Finland using the household budget surveys carried out in 1966, 1971, 1976, 1981 and 1985. The time series show

Table 9.1 Gini-coefficients for the distribution of disposable income in Denmark, 1981–94

Year	Disposable income per adult, married couples, 25–59, CLS data	Disposable income per adult, Aaberge et al. (1996) period I, 25–59	Disposable income per adult, Aaberge et al. (1996) period II, 25–59	LIS data square root equivalence scale, person weighted	Finansministeriet (1995) average income per adult in household	Danish Economic Council (1996), square root equivalence scale
1981	0.222	0.220				
1982	0.217	0.217				
1983	0.211	0.215			0.210	
1984	0.210	0.219				
1985	0.209	0.221				
1986	0.206	0.221	0.228		0.209	
1987	0.201	0.224	0.229	0.257		
1988	0.205	0.232	0.239			0.220
1989	0.202	0.234	0.240		0.208	
1990	0.206	0.245	0.247			
1991						
1992				0.240	0.213	0.220
1993					0.210	
1994					0.201	

a dramatic decrease in inequality during the first part of the period studied. This time series has also been used for a comparison with Sweden where large parallels were found during the first part of the period investigated (Gustafsson and Uusitalo 1990). Jäntti and Ritakallio (1997) analysed the same survey for 1981, 1985 and added 1990. They report surprisingly small changes during the 1980s. In later work Uusitalo updated his original time series using income distribution statistics up to 1995 (Uusitalo 1997).

While income inequality is found to have been increasing in many industrialized countries during the 1980s (Gottschalk and Smeeding 1997), Finland seems to be a clear exception (see Figure 9.1). Although the Finnish economy experienced a deep recession in the first part of the 1990s, the distribution of income changed very little. The Gini-coefficient changed only marginally during the one and a half decades elapsing between the beginning of the 1980s and 1995.

Although there are time series published for Norway, they are not without problems.[1] Therefore we present two new time series estimated from microdata. We use the Income Distribution Survey of Statistics Norway which is based on filled-in and approved tax reports and various administrative registers of social transfers. The survey provides detailed information about reported incomes, legal deductions, taxes paid and transfers received. A household includes all persons living in the same dwelling and having common board.

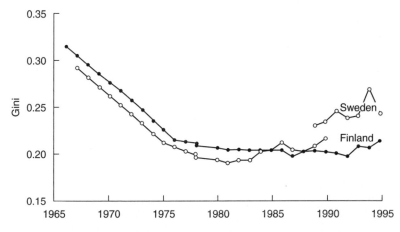

Figure 9.1 Gini-coefficient for disposable equivalent income in Finland 1966–95 and in Sweden 1967–95

Sources: Gustaffson and Uusitalo (1990); Uusitalo (1989, 1997); Gustaffson and Palmer (1997); Statistics Sweden (1997b).

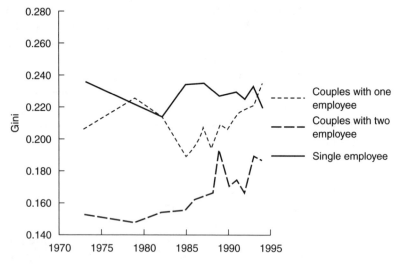

Figure 9.2 Inequality in distributions of disposable income for single
employees and couples with one and two employees in Norway.
Gini-coefficients, 1973–94
Source: Statistics of Norway (Annual data).

Figure 9.2 reports Gini-coefficients for equivalent income in the
period 1973 to 1994 for the three family types: couples with one
employed, couples with two employed and single employed persons.[2]
Inequality within each of the three categories reduced from the first
period of measurement to the second (1979). Changes thereafter are
more irregular and varied for different family types. The series for
single employees and couples with two employed both point upward
during the 1980s, while this is not the case for the third series.

For the period 1985 to 1994 we can report results annually for the
entire population using two different equivalent scales. Figure 9.3
shows an upward trend in Norwegian inequality starting at the second half of the 1980s and with a noticeable spike in 1989.

Most work on the Swedish distribution of income has used the
Household Income Survey which is done annually. Gustafsson
(1987a), Jansson (1990), Jansson and Sandqvist (1993) as well as
Gustafsson and Palmer (1997) have all worked with the concept of
equivalent disposable income per person. Due to the large tax reform
in 1990/91 which broadened the tax base, more income was recorded
in the survey which is the reason for the discontinuity in the time
series.[3]

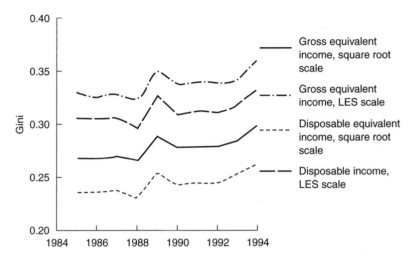

Figure 9.3 Inequality in distributions of gross and disposable equivalent
income in Norway, 1985–94
Source: Statistics of Norway (Annual data).

The time series of Gustafsson and Palmer (1997), based on HINK
1975 to 1991 and linked to estimates for 1992–95 based on the same
source reported by Statistics Sweden (1997b), are reported in Figure
9.1. In the figure we also show estimates from the Level of Living
Survey 1967 (reported in Gustafsson and Uusitalo 1990) as well as
the development for Finland discussed above. For the first period
there are strong parallels with the development in Finland, but thereafter trends differ. In Sweden inequality increased profoundly from
1983.[4] The development during the 1990s needs more comment:
there was a large increase from 1993 to 1994 followed by an equally
large drop in 1995 (back to the same level as in 1991). Available
information indicates that this spike to a very large extent can be
attributed to realized capital gains driven by changes in the tax
code.[5]

On the basis of this somewhat scattered description, the following
picture of the development of income inequalities in the Nordic
countries during the 1980s and 1990s can be presented. All evidence
points in the direction of decreased inequality up to the beginning
of the 1980s. Thereafter the trend is different in these countries. In
Norway and Sweden there are clear signs of increases in income
inequality while changes in Finland appear rather modest. The

development in Denmark is more difficult to judge because available evidence points in different directions.

These differences in trends are not very easily explained. What follows is a survey of the possible role of some explanatory factors.

The impact of unemployment on income distribution

There is empirical literature in which changes in the distribution of income are linked to macroeconomic development. For example, a number of authors have followed Blinder and Esaki (1978) who estimated regression models with the income share of each quintile as dependent variables and measures of unemployment and inflation as independent variables. Results from such studies for the US and UK (for example Blank and Blinder 1986; Nolan 1986) indicate that high unemployment has had an unfavourable effect on the income share of the lower quintiles. The effects of inflation are less clear.

Among the Nordic countries the Blinder and Esaki framework has been used in studies for Sweden (Gustafsson 1987b; Björklund 1991, 1992; Gustafsson and Palmer 1997). While some weak signs of the impact of unemployment on income inequality have been revealed in earlier studies, such results do not appear in studies covering the period up to the recent deep recession.

A new study by Gustafsson and Johansson (1997) also cast doubt on the existence of a strong relationship between unemployment rates and inequality. In the study, data covering 16 OECD countries from 1966 to 1994 were analysed. The results suggest that many factors affect how inequality in equivalent disposable income measured by the Gini-coefficient develops: factors are both strictly economic, such as the sector composition of the economy, or outside a strictly defined market-sphere (the proportion of the labour force that are members of a trade union and the size of the public sector), as well as demographic. However, a relation between the unemployment rate and inequality could not be found.

Simple comparisons of the time series for unemployment and income inequality in Denmark and Finland also cast doubts concerning a relationship between the unemployment rate and inequality. It is remarkable that while the Danish unemployment rate increased after the first oil price shock, available evidence presented in the preceding section does not show increases in inequality. It is even more remarkable that inequality went up in Sweden during the 1980s when the country had full employment.

Our conclusion is that unemployment rates cannot account for changes in income distribution in the Nordic countries during the period after 1980. One obvious reason why increases in the unemployment rate do not have consequences for income inequality in the Nordic countries is the existence of counterbalancing processes. Most unemployed people receive unemployment benefits. This is not the full story, since not all unemployed people receive unemployment benefits and compensation rates are less than 100 per cent.

The role of unemployment can be further elaborated by looking at Aaberge *et al.*'s study (1997). It focused on persons living in households whose head was between 30 and 54 years of age. Factor income was disaggregated into the three components: earnings, self-employment income and capital income. In addition there were two components of public sector transfers: unemployment benefits and tax-free transfers plus income taxes. This analysis used concentration-coefficients of income components. The Gini-coefficient of equivalent disposable income is equal to the weighted sum of concentration-coefficients with weights equal to the average share of each income component in disposable equivalent income. Thus each income component contributes to total inequality by its average size multiplied by its concentration-coefficient.

Table 9.2 summarizes the main conclusions of Aaberger *et al.*'s analysis. Years in the table have been chosen to represent years of low and years of high unemployment, respectively. First we see how various components affect inequality at one point in time. All factor income components have positive concentration-coefficients, with the exception of capital income for Denmark in 1986. This means that they tend to increase disposable income inequality. In Denmark and Norway self-employment income has high concentration-coefficients and in the table there are many instances of high capital-income concentration-coefficients. Unemployment benefits as well as other public sector transfers have negative concentration-coefficients, meaning that they reduce inequality, as do direct taxes.

Looking at changes over time, differences between countries are clearly visible for the component earnings. Increased unemployment has led to earnings contributing more to inequality by larger concentration-coefficients in Norway and Sweden, while the opposite is the case for Denmark and Finland. It seems that the direct effects of increased unemployment have been different in the four Nordic countries. Also working towards increased inequality when unemployment increased is smaller contributions of the income tax system for Finland, Norway and Sweden while this is not the case for Denmark. From the table it can also be seen that in all countries

Table 9.2 Income component contributions to the Gini-coefficient of disposable income for years of 'low' and 'high' unemployment

	Denmark 1986 'low'	Denmark 1990 'high'	Denmark LIS-1987 'low'	Denmark LIS-1992 'high'	Finland 1989 'low'	Finland 1993 'high'	Norway 1986 'low'	Norway 1993 'high'	Sweden 1989 'low'	Sweden 1993 'high'
Earnings										
Share in disposable income	1.243	1.299	1.328	1.290	1.016	0.900	1.001	0.935	1.257	1.181
Concentration-coefficient	0.242	0.255	0.229	0.241	0.300	0.307	0.206	0.251	0.231	0.277
Contribution to Gini	**0.300**	**0.331**	**0.304**	**0.311**	**0.305**	**0.276**	**0.206**	**0.235**	**0.291**	**0.327**
Self-employment income										
Share in disposable income	0.126	0.100	0.082	0.075	0.137	0.099	0.178	0.148	0.038	0.031
Concentration-coefficient	0.571	0.605	0.596	0.791	0.359	0.328	0.518	0.548	0.048	0.190
Contribution to Gini	**0.072**	**0.060**	**0.049**	**0.059**	**0.049**	**0.032**	**0.092**	**0.081**	**0.002**	**0.006**
Capital income										
Share in disposable income	0.027	0.014	0.040	0.025	0.058	0.113	0.055	0.079	0.109	0.062
Concentration-coefficient	-0.174	0.976	0.442	0.345	0.385	0.415	0.346	0.628	0.648	0.580
Contribution to Gini	**0.005**	**0.013**	**0.017**	**0.009**	**0.022**	**0.047**	**0.019**	**0.050**	**0.071**	**0.036**
Unemployment benefits										
Share in disposable income	0.057	0.073	0.050	0.074	0.019	0.081	0.006	0.026	0.009	0.047
Concentration-coefficient	-0.175	-0.232	-0.166	-0.164	-0.230	-0.241	-0.140	-0.088	-0.240	-0.153
Contribution to Gini	**-0.010**	**-0.017**	**-0.008**	**-0.012**	**-0.004**	**-0.019**	**-0.001**	**-0.002**	**-0.002**	**-0.007**
Tax-free transfers										
Share in disposable income	0.022	0.041	0.035	0.077	0.153	0.172	0.086	0.120	0.055	0.066
Concentration-coefficient	-0.442	-0.283	-0.136	-0.235	-0.140	-0.030	-0.166	-0.210	-0.251	-0.313
Contribution to Gini	**-0.010**	**-0.011**	**-0.005**	**-0.018**	**-0.021**	**-0.005**	**-0.014**	**-0.025**	**-0.014**	**-0.021**
Taxes										
Share in disposable income	-0.474	-0.526	-0.534	-0.541	-0.384	-0.365	-0.325	-0.308	-0.468	-0.387
Concentration-coefficient	0.238	0.260	0.258	0.258	0.371	0.350	0.268	0.326	0.281	0.306
Contribution to Gini	**-0.113**	**-0.137**	**-0.138**	**-0.139**	**-0.142**	**-0.128**	**-0.086**	**-0.100**	**-0.132**	**-0.119**
Gini	**0.245**	**0.240**	**0.220**	**0.209**	**0.208**	**0.204**	**0.215**	**0.238**	**0.215**	**0.223**

unemployment benefits have counterbalanced inequality increases.[6] However, the counterbalancing effect of unemployment benefits is typically not as large as the counterbalancing effect of tax-free transfers.

Can changes in income distribution be due to changes in the composition of the population?

Consider a population made up of two categories of persons having different mean income. Using an additively decomposable inequality index, inequality in the total population is then the weighted sum of inequality within each category and a term named 'between group inequality'. The latter expresses the extent of inequality in cases there was no inequality within each category, while the mean incomes of the two categories were kept constant. Changes in total inequality can in turn be attributed to terms expressing (a) changes in mean income for the categories, (b) changes in the number of persons belonging to the categories and (c) changes in inequality within each category.

This framework has recently been used to shed light on reasons for changes in income inequality at the household level in several countries, for example Jenkins (1995) for the United Kingdom, Tsakloglou (1997) for Greece and Jäntti (1997) for Canada, the Netherlands, Sweden, the United Kingdom and the United States. Uusitalo (1989) has studied the impact of changes in socioeconomic structure and household structure on equivalent disposable income distribution in Finland between 1966 and 1981. He found that the changes in socioeconomic structure (decrease in the proportion of farmers, increase in the proportion of white-collar groups and in the economically inactive) had only a small equalizing impact on income distribution. Similarly, changes in household structure had no great impact. The equalization of income distribution in Finland between 1966 and 1981 cannot be explained by changes in the population structure.

A similar analysis was done for Sweden by Gustafsson and Palmer (1997), who studied the period of decreased inequality from 1975 to 1983 as well as the period of increased inequality between 1983 and 1991 by disaggregating the population along six different socioeconomic and sociodemographic categories (age of the person, degree of employment of household, household composition, socioeconomic classification of household head, region of residence, citizenship of household head). Also this research revealed that only a small proportion of changes in total inequality can be attributed to changed composition of the population. Some part of changes in total inequality can be attributed to changed mean incomes for the various categories. For example, about one fourth of the decrease in inequality in equivalent income in Sweden between 1975 and 1983 can be attributed to decreased differences in mean income between individuals in households with different degrees of employment.

We are left with the result that most of the changes in income inequality are due to changes that have taken place in various population groups. In most cases, changes in income distribution within population groups go in the same direction as the changes in overall inequality, although their quantity might vary. For example, the explanatory power of some variables describing the household may decrease or increase. Uusitalo (1989) shows that in Finland the relative equivalent income of persons in white-collar households fell rapidly between 1971 and 1976, reducing the explanatory capacity of socioeconomic position. A remarkable result for Sweden is that while the average equivalent real income of the Swedish population was 28 per cent higher in 1991 than in 1975, the average equivalent real income of persons aged 18 to 24 years was the same at the beginning as at the end of the period (Gustafsson and Palmer 1997). There is also a clear pattern in how the deep recession in Sweden during the 1990s has hit people of different ages. The median equivalent income of people below 50 years of age decreased by at least 10 per cent from 1990 to 1995, while decreases for those aged 50 to 64 were smaller and the median equivalent income for persons above 65 years of age actually increased (Statistics Sweden 1997b).

It should also be said that the relative unimportance of demographic changes for the distribution of equivalent household income hides the dramatic changes when individuals, not households, are the income-receiving unit. Female labour force participation rates have increased in all the Nordic countries during the 1980s, and as a consequence a part of the gap in annual income between women and men has disappeared. At the same time inequality in the personal annual income of women has decreased dramatically. For example, for Denmark based on the longitudinal data at CLS (the Centre for Labour Market and Social Research), Pedersen and Smith (1995) reported that the Gini-coefficient for women aged 25 to 59 decreased from 0.379 in 1981 to 0.288 in 1990 while the corresponding numbers for men were 0.294 and 0.304.

Are the changes in income distribution explained by the changes that have taken place in the components of disposable household income?

Household income is made up of many components. There are rewards for factors of production among which those for labour make up the largest proportion. There are payments from the public sector in the form of social insurance benefits and other transfer payments. The public sector also modifies household income through income taxation. Therefore, the changes in the distribution of disposable income can be accounted for by the changes in its constituents.

To analyse these questions we first look at the development of wage inequality among full-time and full-year workers in the four Nordic countries. Second, we decompose equivalent disposable income into three components: factor income; public sector transfers; and income taxes, which makes it possible to investigate the role played by each component in the development of income distribution. This we can do only for Finland and Sweden.

Figures 9.4a–d show how earnings dispersion among full-time and full-year workers has developed from the end of the 1970s to the beginning of the 1990s. Figures 9.4a and 9.4b show how much greater the earnings share of the ninth decile is compared to that of the fifth decile, while Figure 9.4c and 9.4d display the same relation between the fifth and the first (lowest) earnings deciles. It is evident that in comparison to the increase in earnings inequality in the United Kingdom

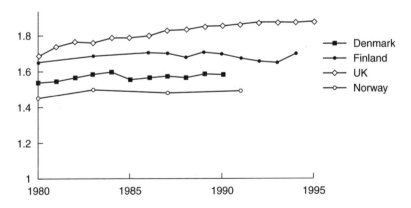

Figure 9.4a Trends in earnings dispersion in Denmark, Finland, UK and Norway, 1980–95 (D9/D5)
Source: OECD (1996a).

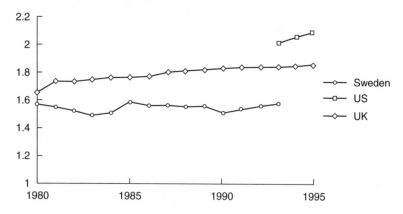

Figure 9.4b Trends in earnings dispersion in Sweden, US and UK, 1980–95 (D9/D5)
Source: OECD (1996a).

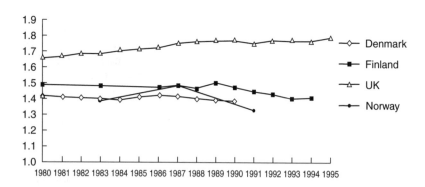

Figure 9.4c Trends in earnings dispersion in Denmark, Finland, UK and Norway, 1980–95 (D5/D1)
Source: OECD (1996a).

and the United States, changes in earnings inequality in the Nordic countries have been small, and partly they have developed differently in the upper and lower parts of the earnings distribution. Increased inequality in earnings for full-time and full-year employed workers seems to be one, but not the only, reason why inequality in equivalent income has changed (see for example Gustafsson and Palmer, 1997).

Now we turn to the second question posed earlier and look at what changes in which of the various components of disposable income

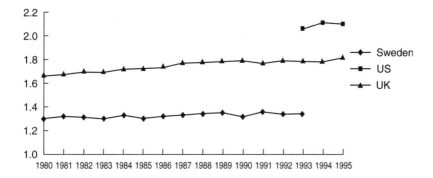

Figure 9.4d Trends in earnings dispersion in Sweden, US and UK, 1980–95
(D5/D1)
Source: OECD (1996a).

can account for the changes in income distribution. One way to answer this is by simulating income distribution, making the assumption that transfers and taxes (both or one in turn) are set equal to zero while factor incomes are unaffected. This is of course unrealistic, but might nevertheless be informative. Here we report results from three different simulations done in similar ways for Finland and Sweden covering the entire population in both countries and the development from the end of the 1960s up to the beginning of the 1990s (Sweden) or to the middle of the 1990s (Finland). This exercise was done by putting together earlier results by Gustafsson and Uusitalo (1990), Uusitalo (1997) and Gustafsson and Palmer (1997).

Figure 9.5 describes time series for inequality in equivalent factor income for these countries. The Gini-coefficients are much larger compared to those based on disposable income. This means that the combined effect of transfers and taxes reduces income inequality.

In Sweden, there. has been an almost continuous trend towards increased inequality in equivalent factor income. In Finland the trend was towards decreasing inequality between 1966 and 1976 and increasing inequality from the early 1980s onwards. Many factors contribute to these developments. In both countries there is a long-term trend towards an increasing proportion of the population being retired (and therefore with no factor income or with only very small factor income) due to the ageing of the population. Another trend is that people enter the labour market at a later age due to lengthening of education (which means that an increasing proportion of young adults

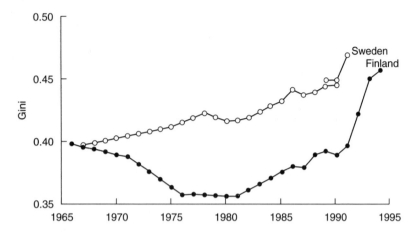

Figure 9.5 Gini-coefficient for equivalent factor income in Finland 1966–94
and in Sweden 1967–91
Sources: Gustafsson and Uusitalo (1990); Uusitalo (1997); Gustafsson and Palmer (1997).

have no or only small factor incomes). In the 1990s, larger proportions
of the population are unemployed in both countries.

In any case it is obvious that the changes in factor income distribution do not account for the changes in disposable income distribution. The trends were the same in Finland from the mid-1960s to
the early 1980s, but after that they diverged. In Sweden, the trends
were different from the 1960s to the early 1980s, after which they have
moved in similar directions. In both countries, however, the changes
in factor income distribution have been more sizeable than those in
disposable income distribution.

Figure 9.6 shows the redistributive effect of transfers. The curves
are derived from simulations of inequality in equivalent factor
income and equivalent gross income (defined as the sum of factor
income and transfers).[7] The redistributive effects of transfers
increased dramatically in both countries from a period starting in
the mid-1960s. Thus the growth of the welfare state must have been a
very important factor in declining inequality in these countries.
However, there are differences between Finland and Sweden. At the
beginning of the period the redistributive effect increased more rapidly
in Sweden, which is consistent with a faster growing public sector
during those years. While the redistributive effect did not change
much in Sweden from the beginning of the 1980s, it continued to

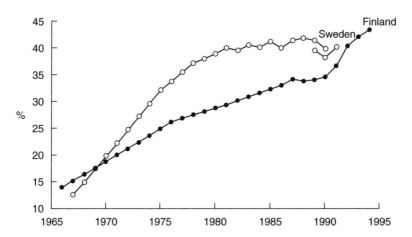

Figure 9.6 Redistributive effect of transfers in Finland 1966–94 and in
Sweden 1967–91
Sources: Gustafsson and Uusitalo (1990); Uusitalo (1997); Gustafsson and Palmer (1997).

increase in Finland, and with a more steeply upward slope during the
deep economic recession, despite cuts in many welfare programmes.

Finally, we compare inequality in equivalent gross income and
inequality in equivalent disposable income and thereby receive a
conception of the redistributive effects of income taxes. Figure 9.7
shows similarities in the beginning of the period for Finland and
Sweden: the redistributive effect increased rapidly in both countries.
This development is understandable because taxes as a GDP share
increased. From the early 1980s onwards the countries differ: the
changes in the redistributive effect of taxes were small in Finland
but in Sweden we find a clear decreasing trend.

Sweden experienced tax-reforms leading to greater inequality during the first half of the 1980s, and particularly when the 1990–91 tax
reform was institutionalized. Several studies have evaluated the distributional consequences of the latter, all showing decreased redistribution effects (Schwarz and Gustafsson 1991; Klevmarken and
Olovsson 1994; Björklund *et al.* 1995). However, this was counterbalanced by increased transfers, making the entire reform package
relatively neutral (Schwarz and Gustafsson 1991; Björklund *et al.*
1995).

Our conclusion is the following: the development of factor income
distributions has naturally had an impact on the changes in disposable income distribution, just because factor income is an important

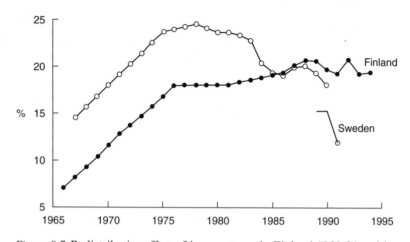

Figure 9.7 Redistributive effect of income taxes in Finland 1966–94 and in
  Sweden 1967–91
Sources: Gustafsson and Uusitalo (1990); Uusitalo (1997); Gustafsson and Palmer (1997).

part, although for most of the period studied here a declining part, of
disposable income. Since the redistributive role of income transfers
and taxes has generally become more important, their impact on the
development of disposable income distribution has been decisive.
Their increasing role accounts for the maintenance or increase in
disposable income equality, despite the trends in factor income distribution which have been working for increased inequality since the
1980s in both countries.

Conclusion

The first task of this chapter was to describe how inequality in
equivalent household income has developed in the four Nordic countries. All evidence points in the direction of decreased inequality up to
the beginning of the 1980s. Thereafter trends differ. In Norway and
Sweden there are clear signs of increases in income inequality while
changes in Finland appear rather modest. Some signs of increased
inequalities have been visible during the latest years, when Finland
has been recovering from the deep recession. The development in
Denmark after the 1980s is left open, since available evidence is
somewhat conflicting.

  Our second task was to analyse the causes of these changes. We
first examined the role of unemployment and found, partly contrary

to some existing literature, that there is no immediate and systematic impact of unemployment on disposable income inequality. As regards the impact of the composition of the population in terms of its socioeconomic position and age, our conclusion is that the changed population structures are not responsible for the changes in disposable income inequality. This does not mean that there have been no changes in the relative income position of different population groups. On the contrary, it has been shown that, for example, aged persons have gained in relative position while young adults have lost; a result that is confirmed also by a recent study on the development and structure of poverty in the Nordic countries (Puide 1996). Also other changes in the relative income positions of, for example, various socioeconomic groups have taken place.

The trends in disposable income distribution can be understood largely in terms of how the various components of disposable incomes, factor incomes, transfers received by households and income taxes paid by them have developed, although our analysis here was based on a comparison of Finland and Sweden only. In Sweden, the trend in factor income inequality has been upwards since the mid-1960s, while in Finland this type of development started only at the beginning of the 1980s. In both countries the redistributive impact of income transfers has grown almost constantly, but the speed has varied: in Sweden this was fast from the 1960s to 1980, while in Finland the early years of the 1990s, i.e. the deep recession years, witnessed a steep increase. The stories of the redistributive impact of income taxes are also partly different. In both countries it grew until the mid-1970s, after which it has been declining in Sweden, while it grew in Finland until the late 1980s. An analysis based on the households headed by workers in their prime age supports these conclusions also for Denmark and Norway.

The general conclusion of this exercise is that the changes in the welfare state, both in its provision of benefits and its collection of resources for this purpose through income taxes have been crucial determinants of disposable income distribution.

Notes

1 For example, Epland (1992) quoted by Atkinson (1996) refers to household income per household. There is also a time series by Ringen (1991) which, however, differs from what is reported by Statistics Norway as discussed by Atkinson *et al.* (1995). The literature also covers Ström *et al.* (1993), Aaberge *et al.* (1996) and Aaberge *et al.* (1997).
2 Thus the non-employed are not covered.

3 Another source of data for Sweden is the Level of Living Survey which was first done in 1967 (see Spånt 1981; Åberg *et al.* 1984; Fritzell 1991). One advantage of this survey is that the first measurement was taken considerably earlier than the first Household Income Survey. The disadvantage of these data is limited possibilities of measuring household income accurately each year.

4 These results are in line with what has been reported from the same survey but using different concepts by Statistics Sweden (1997a) and the Ministry of Finance, Sweden (1996). The increase is more profound than reported in the studies by Björklund and Freeman (1995) who, however, excluded persons 18 and 19 years old as well as those 65 and older.

5 This might very well also be the case for Norway, which implemented a tax-reform in 1992. The most recent increase in inequality in Norway might thus be temporary due to recording of capital gains in 1993 and 1994.

6 Looking at the numbers in brackets one sees that this is the outcome of larger sums paid to households, not of unemployment-compensation being more negatively related to disposable income.

7 The redistributive effect of public sector transfers is defined as one minus the ratio of the inequality index for gross equivalent income to the inequality index for equivalent factor income (multiplied by 100). The redistributive effect of income taxes is defined as one minus the ratio of the inequality index for equivalent disposable income to the inequality index for equivalent gross income (multiplied by 100).

10 The legitimacy of the Nordic welfare states

Trends, variations and cleavages

Jørgen Goul Andersen, Per Arnt Pettersen, Stefan Svallfors and Hannu Uusitalo

Problems and hypotheses

As the previous chapters of this book have demonstrated, the Nordic welfare states have had both common and different experiences during the last 15 years. In Denmark, the restructuring of the welfare state had already started in the 1980s. Norway had economic problems in the late 1980s, but because of the country's oil economy these were minor ones compared to those which Finland and Sweden experienced in the early 1990s. As a reaction to the fiscal problems of the state, Finland and Sweden have made changes to social benefits in order to save costs. In all countries, however, the discourse concerning social policy has moved from emphasizing the pitfalls of social security in securing the welfare of the citizens to underscoring the concern about the costs and incentive effects of social security and taxation.

How are these economic and social policy changes related to a constituency's support for welfare policies? Is there evidence showing that these policies have followed public opinion or, rather, is it the other way round? Is there evidence that the Danish population wanted to change social policies in the early 1980s? Did the economic crisis in Finland and Sweden change public opinion to back the cuts in social benefits? Has the support for the welfare state been most stable in Norway, where the economic and social policy changes have been less pronounced than in the other countries?

These being our comparative questions, it is also important to refer to broader sociological discussions concerning the tendencies in support for the welfare state. Roughly up to the early 1980s, the history of the Nordic welfare states was one of expansion, both in level and scope – sometimes conceptualized as 'decommodification' that makes people's living conditions increasingly independent of their market position (Esping-Andersen 1990), sometimes conceptualized as 'regulation of risk' (Svallfors 1996; Øverbye 1995). These perspectives mean that the expansion of the welfare state has mainly been backed by groups with weak market positions – notably the working class and the labour movement – although other social forces have also been involved (Baldwin 1990).

Some sociological analyses claim that support for the welfare state is declining in the long run. One of the reasons is that the growth of middle-class life styles, alongside increasing individualism (Gundelach and Riis 1992), tends to erode the welfare state's popularity (Wilensky 1975). Against this view we can put the institutional perspective (see Goul Andersen 1993; Svallfors 1996), according to which such arguments are far more applicable to residual welfare states than to the Nordic ones where nearly everybody is a potential welfare user or client. This blurs the calculation of self-interest, and probably reduces reasoning in terms of narrow self-interest. Ironically, this institutional perspective implies that the countries with the highest tax rates, such as Western European countries and the Nordic countries in particular, are the least susceptible to tax protest (Esping-Andersen 1996a).

Legitimacy problems may arise from other concerns. A relatively common discourse in the Nordic countries emphasizes the negative effects of high taxes, social security arrangements and high minimum wages on economic incentives and hence employment and growth. This may create negative attitudes towards the welfare state among the public. This makes particularly appealing the comparison of developments in the 1980s and the 1990s in the Nordic countries, where economic and social policy developments have been somewhat different and where there has been different timing of economic problems and of economic and social policy reactions. Finland and Sweden have experienced dramatic economic problems and social benefits have decreased. Denmark has had a very long period of high unemployment, while Norway has managed to avoid large-scale unemployment throughout the period. Are the temporal patterns of opinion changes in these countries related to such economic and policy changes?

We should distinguish between medium- or short-term changes (changes taking place in a few years) and long-term trends that occur over decades. Short-term changes may include economic crisis effects but they may also derive from political mobilization. It is tempting to suggest that unless such mobilizations lead to more profound institutional change, welfare state support is likely to return to 'normal' levels relatively soon. From this perspective, it becomes especially interesting to examine the reactions in severe recession periods as in Denmark in the early 1980s and in Sweden and Finland in the 1990s.

When analysing opinions concerning particular benefits, there are diverging hypotheses as well. 'Samaritan' wisdom might suggest that people are most likely to support spending for the 'poor' or the most 'needy'. In contrast, a rational choice perspective would lead us to expect that the support for different benefits depends on the size of their (potential) constituencies. These views lead to differing hypotheses concerning universal and means-tested benefits. In addition, public opinion is not undivided. Different population groups have different views on the welfare state, and therefore it is also of interest to examine these differences in a comparative perspective.

As already mentioned, the labour movement was a main although not the only driving force behind the building of the welfare state. It represented the interests of people with smaller market resources and more exposure to the risks connected with market dependency. This emphasizes the importance of class, and of class-related factors such as education and income as a producer of structural cleavages for the support of the welfare state. This leads one to ask whether class continues to be important for attitudes towards welfare, and if so, whether this impact is similar in the Nordic countries. For example, the comparative histories of the making of the welfare states suggest that in Sweden class politics has been more important than, for example, in Norway, where the welfare state has emerged from a greater consensus among the major political forces.

The Nordic welfare states have been known as woman-friendly welfare states. There is a sort of symbiotic relationship between welfare arrangements, women's increasing integration in the labour market and what may perhaps be labelled the achievement of full citizenship among Scandinavian women (Hernes 1988; Karvonen and Selle 1995) – although the causal relationships are not necessarily simple (Jensen 1996). It is obvious to suggest that the welfare state enjoys greater support among women than among men. To the extent that this is the case, there are three standard explanations, however (Goul Andersen 1994): gender values, gender interests and class interests. From the structure of preferences it may be possible to distinguish between the two first mentioned: do we find the strongest gender differences on issues that pertain to gender interests or on issues where gender values are involved? From the analysis of social variations we may distinguish between the class interest hypothesis and the two others: do gender effects disappear when we control for the different class/sector position of men and women?

Age effects are of course also interesting – not least in comparisons between the countries – although it may be difficult to decide whether we meet generation, life-cycle or period effects. In particular, it is interesting to see if the support of the welfare state is lower among the younger age groups, as this may signal the beginning of a long-term decline. If we find such a result in all countries, it is tempting to infer a generation effect even from cross-sectional data.

But there are other social differences as well, some of which relate to potential new social cleavages between the public and the private sector, or between the gainfully employed and the publicly supported. In some of the countries, divisions between public and private employees have become highly significant, in fact quite dramatic, in relation to party choice and the party system (Borre and Goul Andersen 1997; Goul Andersen and Bjørklund 1997). It is extremely relevant to ask whether welfare state support is maintained only because of the increasing number of people depending on the public sector for their main income (as this group encompass more than 60 per cent of the adult population in some of the Nordic countries).

The differing levels of endorsement of the welfare state in different income layers may reflect interests as taxpayers. Is this association especially pronounced in Denmark which has the most visible income-tax system? And are class differences mainly explained by income inequality and different interests as taxpayers, or do they remain significant even when we control for income, indicating that identities or way-of-life factors rather than inequality constitute the decisive link between class and attitudes?

These being our topics and hypotheses, we start by analysing temporal changes in opinions concerning the welfare state. We have data from the 1960s or mid-1970s to the 1990s which allow us to display long-term trends and short-term fluctuations in opinions and to discuss, although not to assess with certainty, their causes. The welfare state consists of a large variety of programmes, the support for which may vary, as indicated above. Therefore, our third section focuses on the support for various welfare programmes. We ask whether the Nordic populations have similar popularity rankings of various benefits and we also examine the support for welfare measures in comparison to other activities of the state. The fourth section compares the variation in opinions of different population groups. It asks whether opinion differences are similar or different in the Nordic countries. In the last section, the conclusions to which the analysis gives rise are discussed.

Decline, stability or increase? Trends in welfare state opinions

As already noted, there are two contradictory views of the long-term development of welfare state legitimacy (Svallfors 1996: 47–8). Partly as a result of welfare policy, the level of education and living standard rises which in turn promotes individualistic values. Such values might undermine the willingness of the growing and well-to-do middle class to finance benefits. Furthermore, geographical and social mobility may weaken those social structures which maintain social solidarity and thereby may splinter the common interest base which is necessary for welfare policy. This perspective argues that support for the welfare state is withering away (see also Pettersen 1995: 199).

An opposite view claims that the welfare state has become an essential constituent of people's performance in everyday life (Rose 1989). This has created strong groups who have interests in the welfare state (Korpi 1983). The mere existence of the welfare state reproduces its support. The claim is that the support for the welfare state does not show a declining trend, but is rather stable. Institutionalization works against the eroding factors.

Interpretations of comparative empirical studies on welfare state opinions have given credit to both perspectives. Stein Ringen (1987) came to the conclusion that there is a downward trend in the support for the welfare state in many countries. Some analysts point out that the evidence is more in favour of stability (Svallfors 1996; Page and Shapiro 1984).

Within the general long-term trends, short-term fluctuations, ups and downs in the public endorsement of the welfare state may exist. One particular cause of 'downs' is economic crisis and the concomitant problems in public economy, which have been particularly prevalent in Finland and Sweden (Sihvo and Uusitalo 1995). Another cause of reduced support is connected to right-wing political movements, which had importance particularly in Denmark but also in Norway in the 1970s (Pettersen 1995: 202).

This section aims at comparing changes – both long- and short-term – in support for the welfare state in the Nordic countries. We have tried to construct time series as far back in time as possible, reaching to the 1960s in Denmark, Norway and Sweden, and to the mid-1970s in Finland, and to include the most recent data as well, so that the developments in the 1990s, which are of particular interest for this book, can be revealed. The Appendix includes a brief description of our data sets and references to publications including further details. Our national surveys have used different questions and also the study designs have varied. Therefore, we are not in a position to compare the *levels* of support in the Nordic countries. We believe, however, that *trends* can be compared, since each national data set relies on the same survey questions each year. It should be emphasized that in this chapter we only present data which describe general support for the welfare state, but in the background we have data describing the trends in other aspects of social policy. This background data is not shown here, but we have used it as a check point concerning the conclusions that can be made on the basis of the data presented here.

Denmark experienced a sudden 'welfare backlash' in 1973 when Mogens Glistrup's newly formed antitax Progress Party gained 15.9 per cent of the votes and 28 seats in Parliament. At the time of conducting the first comprehensive Danish election survey in 1971, there were no signs of such backlash and that is why the survey did not include any questions on welfare. However, from a comparative Nordic survey, we have a single item that may be traced back to 1969 (Figure 10.1a). Not surprisingly, it confirms the conventional impression that there was widespread support for the welfare state in the 1960s. After Glistrup's triumph, which was accompanied by a dramatic decrease in support for the welfare state, support gradually recovered, and in the booming mid-1980s it even exceeded the level of the 1960s. In the latter part of the 1980s support declined, a trend which has continued slowly also in the 1990s. However, the support is now somewhat higher than it was 20 years ago.

The Danish case seems to give little confirmation of the view that there is a general long-term trend in the welfare state's popularity. There are fluctuations, however. The welfare backlash in 1973 was, first and foremost, a reaction to the extremely rapid growth of the public sector which peaked under the bourgeois majority government during the 1968–71 period (Glans 1986; Goul Andersen and Bjørklund 1997). Although some observers, notably Wilensky (1975), interpreted this as an effect of long-term social change (more precisely, economic prosperity and the expansion of the 'middle mass'), it was clearly a short-term reaction. The expansion of the

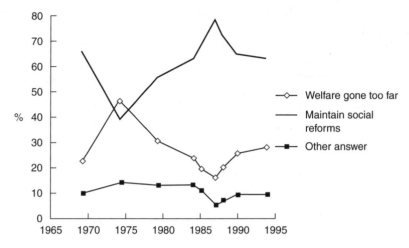

Figure 10.1a Support for the welfare state in Denmark, 1969–94
Sources: The data 1969 and 1974 are based on surveys conducted by Ingemar Glans, University of Aarhus. The 1985 data were collected for the study on Class Structure and New Social Cleavages, conducted by Jørgen Goul Andersen and Jens Hoff. The other data are derived from the surveys of the Danish Election Programme, conducted by Ole Borre, Jørgen Goul Andersen *et al.* All samples are nation-wide representative samples. N = approximately 2,000 in 1974, 1979, 1994; N = approximately 1,000 in 1984, 1987, 1990; N = approximately 700 in 1969, 1988. Interviewing was conducted by AIM in 1987/88 (panel), otherwise by Danish Gallup. For details about the Danish Election Surveys, see Borre and Goul Andersen 1997.

Note
The surveyed samples were asked: 'First a question about government spending on social programs. A says: Social reforms have gone too far in this country. More than now, people should manage without social support and support from government. B says: Those social reforms that have been made in our country should be maintained at least to the same extent as now. Do you agree mostly with A or B?'

public sector continued at an only slightly lowered speed in the 1970s, but support for the welfare state nevertheless recovered during the latter half of the 1970s. Besides, questions concerning cutbacks reveal that even in 1973 voters generally abstained from demanding savings on the most basic welfare issues, i.e. on public spending for health and pensions (Goul Andersen 1988: 152).

We would expect that economic crisis awareness would tend to limit the demand for increased spending. This is reflected in the *de facto* acceptance of the harsh retrenchment policies of the bourgeois government of 1982–83 (Petersen *et al.* 1987; Goul Andersen 1995; see also Goul Andersen 1988: 164). Unfortunately, there is a break in our time series between 1979 and 1984. From 1980 to 1982,

Denmark experienced its most severe economic crisis in the postwar period, and the crisis awareness among ordinary people was higher than at any other time (Petersen *et al.* 1996; Goul Andersen 1994). We do, however, have one indication that welfare attitudes may have followed this crisis awareness: in the 1981 election survey, the question used in Figure 10.1a was presented in an abridged version. The respondents were simply asked whether they would agree with the first item, in other words that 'Social reforms have gone too far in this country . . .'. It turned out that a majority agreed, which means that the distribution was almost the same as in 1973. Even if we acknowledge that there may be a persuasion effect in the omission of the other response alternative from the question wording, there seems to be little doubt that welfare support dropped in response to the economic crisis. But it also seems to have been a contingent reaction; it did not change the basic values that reproduce welfare state legitimacy in 'normal' times. In 1996, a vivid political debate over the uncontrollable increases in transfer expenditures and the burden of support in the future seems to have sparked off a similar reaction, even though people's willingness to sacrifice tax relief for improved public services increased at the same time (Goul Andersen 1997).

In Finland, as well, there are fluctuations without any long-term trend in support for the welfare state. In 1975, public approval of the welfare state was at a high level, but declined in the following ten years. From 1985 to 1990 support increased again close to the 1975 level. Although there is a break in the time series reported in Figure 10.1b, other poll questions support the conclusion that from 1990 to 1994 we witness quite a considerable drop in the willingness of the Finns to provide more tax money for social security. In 1995 and 1996 this declining trend turned into increased support.

These downturns in the 1970s and 1990s have been interpreted in economic terms. Finland met with a severe economic crisis in the 1970s and more especially again in the first years of the 1990s. The public economy was presented with great fiscal constraints and the interpretations of major decision-makers emphasized the need to curtail public expenditure. The Finns took a more reserved attitude towards the welfare state (Sihvo and Uusitalo 1995: 251–62).

As in Denmark, one can also see an underlying stability in these temporal changes. Even in a deep recession, only a small minority of the Finns expressed a preference for cuts in social benefits. Temporal changes have been between those who want more welfare state and those who are satisfied with the present situation. In this sense, a

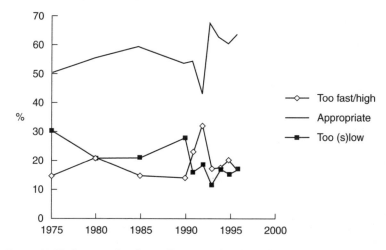

Figure 10.1b Support for the welfare state in Finland, 1975–96
Sources: The Finnish data are collected by Finnish Gallup in connection with their annual Omnibus interviews. The number of interviews is approximately 1,000 in each year, representing the Finnish population over 15 years of age (excluding Åland Islands). For further details, see Allardt, Sihvo and Uusitalo (1992: 25–6).

Note
The surveyed samples were asked: 'The development of social security in recent years has been too fast, appropriate or too slow?' (1975–92); 'What do you think about the current level of social security in Finland? Is it too high, appropriate or too slow?' (1993–6).

claim can be made that in the eyes of the Finnish population, the welfare state has always been legitimate in that it is regarded as worthy of tax money, either current amounts or more.

No successive surveys on attitudes towards the welfare state have been performed in Norway, but since the election in 1965 the Norwegian Electoral Programme has included a question on how much people support the social security system. The results are displayed in Figure 10.1c.

The results show that Norwegian willingness to develop the welfare state was high in 1965, when the Norwegian welfare state was at its peak of expansion. The proposal for an integrated national pension scheme had been introduced, and the People's Pension Act was passed by Parliament in 1967 with the support of all parties. Obviously popular support for the reform was prominent with less than 10 per cent in opposition. The next datum is for the year 1973. Between these years the People's Pension Act had been amended

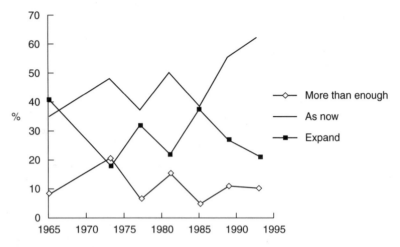

Figure 10.1c Support for the welfare state in Norway, 1965–94
Sources: The Norwegian data were collected by the Central Bureau of Statistics for the Norwegian Election programme for the years 1977 to 1993. Earlier data were collected by Norwegian Gallup. Data for 1996 were collected by the Central Bureau of Statistics for the research project, 'The pleasures and burdens of the welfare state'. Each data set is based on a representative sample of the voting age population in Norway.

Note
The surveyed samples were asked: 'Many people think that by now we have more than enough social security benefits, and we should attempt to limit them in the future, while others claim that we should maintain our social benefit programmes and if necessary extend them. . . . What is your opinion?'

several times to include new categories of recipients inside various programmes. The popular mood had changed from endorsement of expansion of the welfare state to satisfaction with the existing schemes. The increase to 33 per cent in favour of expansion in 1977 is again explained by reforms that were supported. In 1977 the Norwegian sickness insurance was reformed to compensate wage earners' incomes 100 per cent from the first day of sickness.

The next drop in support occurred when the conservatives had their victory in the election of 1981, but the proportion preferring expansion increased to the second highest level at the subsequent election in 1985, when the Labour party brought welfare state issues on to their election campaign agenda. After that peak, support for expansion has declined.

As in Denmark and Finland, the diminishing support in Norway for welfare state expansion has not produced welfare state opposition. Those who want to dismantle the welfare state have accounted only about 10 per cent of the population since the mid-1970s. What has increased is the proportion of those who perceive the welfare state programmes as satisfactory: no need for expansion; but no passion for reduction either. So basically the population of Norway (and the other Nordic countries as well) has moved from a position of preference for welfare state expansion towards a position of welfare state contentment.

Data from Sweden, as displayed in Figure 10.1d, show that the general attitude towards welfare state expansion became more sceptical in the 1960s and early 1970s. After that period, however, there have been no clear signs of either declining or increasing approval. The data show a 'trendless fluctuation', which is clearly connected to the political debate about welfare policies (Svallfors 1996: 60–1).

We find that Swedish opinion towards welfare state expansion became more sceptical in the early 1980s, but swung back in a more positive direction in the mid- and late 1980s. In the early 1990s there was again a decline in support for welfare state expansion, but just as in the 1980s this decline was soon followed by a

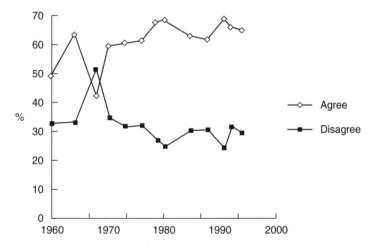

Figure 10.1d Support for the welfare state in Sweden, 1960–95
Sources: The Swedish data come, with one exception (1992), from the Swedish election studies. They sampled about 3,000–4,000 respondents each time, representing eligible voters aged 18–80 years. The non-response rate varies from approximately 20 to 30 per cent. For a description of 1992 data, see Appendix.

Note
The surveyed samples were asked: 'Have social reforms gone so far in this country that government should reduce rather than increase social support and benefits in the future?'

return of support. These pendulum-like swings in the welfare opinion at the general level are clearly reflected also in attitudinal indicators other than the single one we have used here (Svallfors 1996: 50–1). In contrast to Finland, the severe economic problems in the 1990s in Sweden have not led to a decline in welfare state support.

The conclusions of our comparative analysis of the trends in support for the welfare state seem relatively straightforward. None of our data from the Nordic countries gives credit to the view that there is a long-term decline in general support. However, the support for welfare state expansion was at its highest in the 1960s and in early 1970s before the backlash in Denmark and Norway, i.e. in the period when social protection schemes were in the making. Since then, the popular mood has moved towards approval of the maintenance of these schemes. The proportion of those who would like to see curtailments in benefits and services has remained low in all countries. In this sense, support for the welfare state continues to be at a high level in all Nordic countries, a result which is confirmed by another study focusing on welfare state attitudes in Denmark, Norway and Sweden in the early 1990s (Nordlund 1997: 233–46).

Variations in approval for the welfare state also relate to economic and political situations which are often historically constituted. In Denmark and Norway, there was a simultaneous drop in welfare state popularity with the success of 'tax revolt' parties in the early 1970s. In Finland, in particular, severe economic problems made people more reserved, while in Sweden, where economic problems were almost as great as in Finland, we do not see this kind of decline.

Some welfare state programmes are more popular than others

The Nordic welfare states have a large number of welfare programmes, the purposes of which vary substantially. There are many forms of income transfers and social and health services to provide help in various life situations. The Nordic model of the welfare state has also many responsibilities in the areas of housing and education. In addition, there is a nightwatch state, the one that takes care of defence, law and order and infrastructure.

To analyse the legitimacy of the welfare state requires that the multifaceted nature of programmes and schemes be taken into account. Obviously, some programmes are more popular than others. The variations are due to the differing principles on which the programmes are founded, which groups of citizens are covered and whether the question is about income transfers or services. In this section we ask whether the popularity rankings of the state activities are similar in the Nordic countries.

The popularity of welfare state programmes can be measured in several ways. We investigate the support for programmes in two ways: we look at the proportion of the population who would like to see more resources used in the policy area in question and the proportion of people who would like to see less. Results are reprinted in Table 10.1.

The public health system is pretty much the 'queen' of the welfare state in all four nations. In all countries health services receive most support for more government spending. There is variation between the countries, but if we look at the proportions of those wanting to spend less, the differences are small. For old-age pensions the picture is rather similar. Very few prefer a reduction, but there is some variation with regard to the proportion who want more money spent on pensions. The most prominent difference between the nations is that, among the Finns, there is less demand for more spending on both health services and pensions. This probably indicates the severe economic crisis of the 1990s in Finland, which has made people cautious. In contrast is Norway, where the economic situation has given opportunity for demands to increase money for health services and old-age pensions. It is interesting to note that in the national elections in 1997 these issues were very prominent in Norway.

Child care comes third in the popularity ranking, although we have data for Denmark and Norway only. As regards child allowances we find that the preferences in Finland, Norway and Sweden are very similar, with around 30 per cent wanting more spending. In Denmark the proportion is considerably smaller. An interesting difference can be found between Finland and the other countries. In these three countries, health care and pensions are far more popular than measures for children, while in Finland the rankings are the same but the gaps are much smaller. In other words, the priorities of the Danes, Norwegians and Swedes clearly favour health care and pensions, while in Finland the priorities are more disposed to include child benefits as well.

Data on sickness insurance exist only for Finland and Norway. The Norwegians have a much lower proportion of people demanding expansion, probably because sickness insurance already compensates for 100 per cent of income loss from the first day of sickness.

Less popular welfare state programmes include unemployment

Table 10.1 Support for various welfare state programmes in Denmark, Finland, Norway and Sweden. Percentages supporting more, or less, government money spending on programmes. Answers indicating 'current amount' and 'don't know' have been omitted

	Denmark 1994		Finland 1996		Norway 1992		Sweden 1992/1996	
	More	Less	More	Less	More	Less	More	Less
Health service/Hospitals	74	1	44	4	88	1	77	1
Public pension/Old age pension	52	0	35	5	63	1	57	3
Child care/Day care centres	38	6	—	—	47	11	—	—
Child allowance	13	13	31	6	31	4	32	14
Sickness insurance	—	—	31	6	16	7	—	—
Unemployment benefits	12	12	28	21	12	21	43	15
Social assistance	11	22	25	13	18	19	13	26
Housing allowance	—	—	24	15	—	—	13	38

Notes
The question in Denmark: 'Now, I'd like to ask about your view on public expenditure for various purposes. For each purpose, please tell me if you think the public sector spends too much money, an appropriate amount, or too little for this purpose.' Source: The Danish Election Survey 1994.
The question in Finland: 'The following is a list of cash benefits financed mainly by taxes. Please say in each case whether more tax money, the same amount as now, or less tax money should be used to finance these benefits.' The data source are described in Figure 10.1b.
The question in Norway: 'Consider the government use of money for different purposes, should the government use more money, about as much as today or less money on (the different items following)?'
The question in Sweden: 'Taxes are used for different purposes. Do you think that the amount of tax money used for the following purposes should be increased, remain the same or be decreased?' This question goes for the items of – child allowance (support for families with children) – social assistance – housing allowances. The questions relating to support for health services, old age pensions and unemployment benefits are from the ISSP 1996 survey. In this survey the question is (quoted from the 1990 survey): 'Listed below are various areas of government spending. Please show whether you would like to see more or less government spending in each area.'

benefits, social assistance and housing allowances. A much smaller proportion prefers increased spending in all four nations, and a significant percentage actually want to decrease spending. The popularity rankings of these benefits are relatively similar from one Nordic country to the next, but some interesting differences can be observed. The dislike of social assistance and housing allowances seems to be most distinct in Sweden, while the Swedes are most favourable towards unemployment benefits, the popularity of which is greater than that of child allowances. The Norwegians are least sympathetic towards unemployment benefits. The Danes and the Finns are in an intermediate position. Even for these least popular programmes, we never find a majority who want reductions.

In conclusion, in the Nordic countries we find relatively similar popularity patterns among social benefits. The first and most obvious difference between the 'very popular' programmes and the 'not so popular' programmes is linked to universalism and targeting/means-testing. Universal programmes are more popular than selective programmes. However, there are variations in popularity also among the universal programmes. Health services and hospitals, together with old-age pensions, generally enjoy wider support than child allowances, although the difference is not substantial in Finland. Programmes targeted at children seem to fall into an intermediate position. Child allowances are universal in that every family with children receives support. Less universal programmes (unemployment benefits) and means-tested programmes (social assistance and housing allowances) are less popular. These are benefits which many people see as going to others, and probably many are afraid that fraud is frequent here. These results are not only characteristic of the Nordic countries, but are found in other countries as well, for example in Great Britain and in the USA (Coughlin 1979; Pöntinen and Uusitalo 1986; Taylor-Gooby 1989; Svallfors 1996; Pettersen 1995, 1997).

Table 10.2 shows the priorities people have on a broader range of issues. As far as the data go, the patterns are rather similar in each country. The two most popular programmes, education and law enforcement, are old activities of the government, and concern every citizen. Environment protection seems to be in an intermediate position. Two of the least popular sectors are defence and culture. Only Finland and Norway have data concerning the giving of support to industry, and the countries differ considerably. In Norway public support for industry subsidy is much higher than in Finland.

Table 10.2 Support for various non-welfare state sectors in Denmark, Finland, Norway and Sweden. Percentages supporting more, or less, government money spending on sectors. Answers indicating 'current amount' and 'don't know' are omitted in the table.

	Denmark 1994		Finland 1996		Norway 1996		Sweden 1992/1996	
	More	Less	Not at all	Cuts could be made	More	Less	More	Less
Education	44	2	80	18	50	4	59	3
Law enforcement	53	2	72	26	61	4	47	6
Employment support	21	20	60	34	86	5	61	7
Environment protection	48	6	48	49	42	7	53	4
Defence	4	39	29	68	10	48	14	50
Culture and arts	6	40	13	84	8	58	15	44
Support for industry	–	–	13	78	59	18	–	–

Notes

For Denmark the same source and the same wording as Table 10.1

The question in Finland: 'I am now going to list certain items in the state and local budget. If the state and local authorities need to cut their expenditures, which items could they economise considerably, which to some extent and which not at all?' The data are described in Figure 10.1b.

The question in Norway: 'Below you will find a list of initiatives which the government may use to stimulate the economy. Are you for or against these initiatives?'

– support for projects to create new jobs
– support industry in decline to save jobs

The following questions are asked both in Norway and Sweden: 'On the list below you will find various areas of public expenditures. Should the government spend more or less on each of these areas? Remember that if you answer "much more", there might be an increase in taxes to pay for the increase.'

– environment
– police and judicial system
– education
– defence
– arts and culture

The data is based on International Social Survey Program 1996.

The question for employment support in Sweden is from the Welfare Survey of 1992.

Structural cleavages and support for the welfare state

In this section we analyse the linkages between people's socio-demographic characteristics and their attitudes towards welfare policies in the Nordic countries. Support for the welfare state has often been connected to position in the market, especially in the labour market (Matheson 1993; Svallfors 1991, 1995). Those less endowed with market resources, and more exposed to the risks connected with market dependency would, *ceteris paribus*, be more prone to support welfare state intervention in order to redistribute resources and risks. Those less favoured by the play of market forces may also more easily develop norms and values favouring redistribution and equality. This highlights the importance of class, and of 'class-related' factors such as education and income. We would expect that blue-collar workers, and those with low education and income, would be more in favour of government redistribution than upper white-collar employees and those with high education.

Our class variable distinguishes between blue-collar workers, lower and higher white-collar employees and the self-employed. In Norway and Sweden, retired and other people outside the labour force have been classified according to their last occupation, if any. In Denmark and Finland, only present occupation is available, and students and retired respondents have been entered in the analysis as separate categories. The income variable distinguishes between levels of individual incomes. The education variable distinguishes between those who have only primary education as their highest formal education level, those who have some sort of secondary education and those who have a university degree. Assessing a more fine-grained and yet roughly comparable classification proved impossible.

Some have argued that the privileged role of class and class-related cleavages in relation to welfare policies is complemented or even superseded by other structural cleavages in contemporary capitalism. The first one is obviously gender. This argument is based, first, on the fact that women are more dependent on the welfare state, both as employees, as family members relieved of heavy and unpaid care work and as recipients of benefits from the state. Women often have a more precarious market position than men, leaving them either dependent on a male bread-winner or more dependent on the state than men are (Hernes 1987a, 1987b; Borchorst and Siim 1987). Second, the specific experiences of women may make them more inclined to embrace a 'rationality of caring' in which concern, consideration and devotion to others are more prominent (Waerness 1987). The institutionalization of caring services brings into the public realm what was previously a private matter, thus transforming a 'moral economy of domesticity' into support for state welfare (Piven 1985).

Issues of gender are tightly wedded to the question of public and private sector location. Divisions between public and private sector employees can, just like gender divisions, be separated into those emanating from the self-interest of those employed by the public sector and those emerging from specific socialization experiences in the public sector compared to the private one. Those employed by the public sector have an obvious interest in guarding their employment, wages and working conditions (Dunleavy 1980; Zetterberg 1985), at the same time as their working conditions may create bonds of sympathy and solidarity between public sector employees, and their clients, patients and other 'welfare dependants' (Lafferty 1988). According to many analysts, this suggests possibilities for 'paternalistic' alliances between welfare clients and higher level administrators in the public sector (Kolberg and Pettersen 1981; Zetterberg 1985; Dunleavy 1986; Cloward and Piven 1986; Joppke 1987). Following from the debate on new social cleavages, our analysis compares men to women, and public sector employees to those working in the private sector. Furthermore, we separate the unemployed as a category more or less completely dependent on public benefits, temporarily (or even permanently) excluded as they are from the labour market.

Another variable is age, which is neither a class-related nor a 'new' social cleavage. Age may be taken to represent either an indication of position in the life-cycle, where the young and the old are most exposed to precarious situations in terms of market conditions, or as an indicator of belonging to a specific cohort or generation. In the latter case, arguments have been put forward (Inglehart 1990) according to which the young would be more sceptical towards the welfare state in various respects.

The above-mentioned variables place a person in the social structure in objective terms. Party preference is an interesting variable since it taps the social and political views of the individual, part of which may include his/her views about the welfare state. Political parties mould perceptions and attitudes, but party sympathy can also be affected by attitudes towards the welfare state. We should therefore not compare the links between party sympathy and attitudes with those we find between various other variables and attitudes. It may nevertheless be interesting to see to what extent attitudes towards the welfare state constitute a watershed between the political left and right in the Nordic countries. In the analysis, we will compare attitudes towards the welfare state between different categories of party sympathizers, but enter this variable in a second model in order not to confound relations between various structural variables and attitudes towards the welfare state.

Many of the variables had some problems of comparability, due to differences in categorizations and coding between the countries. Small differences should therefore not be interpreted, but rather we should concentrate on the broader patterns.

In the tables below, we compare how opinions are structured in the case of six different aspects or programmes. First, we enter the general question on 'social reforms', which has been posed in all the Nordic countries (see pages 239–46), in order to study how such a general view about the welfare state is structured. Second, we analyse how opinions towards spending on universal and encompassing programmes such as pensions, health care and child allowances are influenced by structural variables. These programmes are similar in their universality, but different in how they affect people at various stages in the life-cycle. Finally, we include two more programmes which are tightly connected to risks and resources in the labour market: social assistance and unemployment benefits, the first of which also is means-tested and thus highly selective.

The responses to the question on social reforms is simply dichotomized between those who are in favour of further social reforms (1) and those who are against them (0). The responses to the other items are trichotomized between spending more (2), keeping the level of spending intact (1) and decreasing spending (0).

In Tables 10A.1 to 10A.4 in the Appendix, correlations between the variables and attitudes towards welfare policies are displayed in the form of Eta and Beta coefficients, computed with multiple classification analysis (MCA). MCA provides a number of useful measures. The Eta and Beta coefficients give estimates of the amount of variance which the independent variables contribute, without controlling for other variables (Eta) and with controlling for other variables in the equation (Beta). Apart from this, MCA also supplies empirical and adjusted means for the categories of the independent variables, which give estimates of the direction and magnitude of categorical differences. These figures are not displayed in the tables, but interesting patterns and country differences are discussed in the text.

We find both similarities and differences between the Nordic countries. Patterns between various groups are similar between the countries, and with a few exceptions, in the expected direction.

Women, public sector employees, workers, people with low income or less education, and the unemployed are more supportive of welfare state spending than other groups are. Older people are generally more prone to support spending on pensions and health care, and less prone to support spending for families with children than the young are. One interesting exception is that in Denmark, once other variables are controlled for, the old are less prone to support spending on pensions than the young are.

As discussed in the introductory section, age differences could be an outcome of generation, life-cycle or period effects. Because age differences go in different directions in the case of different benefits, we are tempted to interpret this in terms of life-cycle effects. Old people have more interest in pensions and health care than the young just because of their age, and the same is true for the support of young people for family policy benefits.

Views on welfare state spending also constitute a clear dividing line between supporters of the political left and right. Conservative and right-wing populist party sympathizers are less prone to support welfare spending than supporters of the left.

The magnitude of these differences does, however, vary greatly between the countries. Without going into too much detail, which the minor discrepancies in variables should stop us from doing, a few obvious differences between the Nordic countries should be pointed out. When we compare the impact of the variables, and the amount of explained variance, we find that the level of disagreement between population groups on welfare state spending seems to be highest in Sweden, followed by Finland and Denmark, with Norwegian population groups displaying the most consensus on welfare spending. This is, first, owing to the larger differences between various class, education and income categories in Sweden than elsewhere, while such differences are very small in Norway. It seems as if class, and 'class-related' factors such as income and education, have a greater impact in Sweden than in the other countries, and that Norway displays more 'class consensus' than the other countries.

Second, divisions between the political left and right are particularly pronounced in Sweden, and are particularly small in Norway. Denmark displays almost the same pattern as Sweden, and Finland falls somewhere between Denmark and Norway. Again, the Norwegian pattern is much more 'consensual' than the Swedish or Danish one.

As far as gender is concerned, our analysis shows that gender differences are reduced when we control for other variables. However, significant direct gender effects remain in all four countries as regards opinions on pensions and health care, and as regards unemployment benefits in three cases out of four. These findings would suggest an interpretation following the argument that care issues are more important for women than they are for men. However, this is not supported by the fact that gender effects are insignificant as regards support for families with children (except in Denmark).

Now that we have pointed out some interesting categorical and country differences, we should also emphasize some expected differences that more or less failed to materialize. Differences between public and private sector employees were mostly small and insignificant. We find no support that this dividing line is an important new one. Even less is the impact of unemployment. With the exception about views on spending on unemployment benefits, where the livelihood of the unemployed is most obviously at stake, there are very small differences to be found between the unemployed and the others.

Conclusion

This chapter has compared the trends in public support for the welfare state, the popularity of various welfare programmes and the factors which are related to such support. Our main findings are the following.

Against some expectations, we do not find any declining long-term trend in support for the welfare state. There are fluctuations, but it would require considerable imagination to see long-term trends in our data. Developments in different countries do not display similar trends, but they may still be explained by similar factors. The support for welfare state expansion was at its highest in the 1960s and in the early 1970s, i.e. in the period when social protection schemes were in the making. Since then, the popular mood has moved towards approval of the maintenance of these schemes. The proportion of those who would like to see curtailments in benefits and services has remained low in all countries. In this sense, support for the welfare state continues to be at a high level in all Nordic countries.

As regards the more short-term developments in the 1980s and 1990s, the patterns are different. In Denmark, one can observe slightly declining support in recent years. In Finland, the willingness to finance the welfare state declined dramatically in the unforeseen economic recession of the early 1990s, while in Sweden popular support has stayed quite stable. In Norway, popular opinion has moved from wanting more welfare to maintaining the current levels in the 1980s and 1990s.

There are fluctuations which can be interpreted in the context of political and economic situations. In Denmark and Norway, the emergence of antitax parties was a concomitant feature to the decline in the support for the welfare state, but the causal directions probably go in both ways. Economic crises have had negative effects on the public's endorsement of the welfare state in Finland, but this does not seem to be true in Sweden in the early 1990s. It is therefore likely that economic problems as such are not a cause in themselves, but rather it is how they are interpreted, what kind of economic policy measures are suggested and how unanimous various opinion makers are in their diagnoses.

When we examined the priorities the Nordic populations have concerning the welfare state, we found relatively similar patterns. Universal welfare schemes are in all countries more popular than selective ones. Health care and health-related income transfers and old-age pensions are the most popular welfare programmes. Family policy benefits and services are in an intermediate position. At the bottom are selective and often stigmatizing programmes like social assistance, unemployment benefits and also housing benefits. There are some national variations, but these are the main patterns.

When comparing the prioritization of non-welfare policies of the state, we again find relatively similar patterns. In all countries, education has much support, as has law enforcement, while defence and culture are less often seen as areas which need expansion.

As regards explanatory factors, the similarity is again rather striking. Patterns between various groups are similar between the countries, and with a few exceptions, in the expected direction. Women, blue-collar workers, people with low income or education and the unemployed are more supportive of welfare state spending than other groups are. Older people are generally more prone to support spending on pensions and health care, and less prone to support spending for families with children than the young are.

However, the magnitude of impacts varies in an interesting way. When we compare the amount of explained variance, we find that the level of disagreement between groups on welfare state spending seems to be highest in Sweden, followed by Finland and Denmark, with Norway displaying the most consensus on welfare spending. This is, first, owing to the larger differences between various class, education and income categories in Sweden than elsewhere, while such differences were found to be very small in Norway. It seems as if class, and 'class-related' factors such as income and education, have a larger impact in Sweden than in the other countries, and that Norway displays more 'class consensus' than the other countries.

Second, divisions between the political left and right are particularly pronounced in Sweden, and are particularly small in Norway. Denmark displays almost the same pattern as Sweden, and Finland falls somewhere between Denmark and Norway. Again, the Norwegian pattern is much more 'consensual' than what is found in Sweden and Denmark.

We should also emphasize some expected differences that more or less failed to materialize. Differences between public and private sector employees were mostly small and insignificant. We found no support that this dividing line is an important new one. Even less is the impact of unemployment. With the exception of views on spending on unemployment benefits, where the livelihood of the unemployed is most obviously at stake, there are very small differences to be found between the unemployed and the others.

Appendix

Table 10.A1 Structural cleavages and attitudes towards welfare policies in Denmark (1994). Multiple classification analysis

	Social reforms			Pensions			Health care			Child allowances			Social assistance			Unemployment benefits		
	Eta	Beta	Beta	Eta	Beta	Beta	Eta	Beta	Beta	Eta	Beta	Beta	Eta	Beta	Beta	Eta	Beta	Beta
Gender	0.04	0.01	0.08[b]	0.09	0.08[b]	0.08[b]	0.16	0.12[a]	0.12[a]	0.09	0.07[c]	0.07[c]	0.07	0.03	0.02	0.08	0.05[a]	0.06[a]
Sector	0.10	0.06	0.00	0.00	0.00	0.01	0.02	0.04	0.04	0.05	0.01	0.01	0.10	0.08[b]	0.04	0.08	0.07[a]	0.04
Class	0.19	0.11[c]	0.16[a]	0.16	0.16[a]	0.14[b]	0.17	0.09	0.08	0.20	0.11[c]	0.08[c]	0.14	0.14[c]	0.10	0.22	0.15[c]	0.11[a]
Education	0.05	0.05	0.09[c]	0.11	0.09[c]	0.07	0.11	0.11[a]	0.11[a]	0.05	0.05	0.06	0.04	0.03	0.03	0.10	0.10[a]	0.09
Income	0.11	0.09[c]	0.04	0.06	0.04	0.04	0.18	0.11[a]	0.10[b]	0.11	0.07	0.06	0.09	0.04	0.02	0.12	0.05	0.05
Age	0.15	0.11[c]	0.07[a]	0.07	0.17[a]	0.15[c]	0.06	0.09[c]	0.13[a]	0.18	0.17[a]	0.16[b]	0.15	0.21[a]	0.15[b]	0.14	0.15[c]	0.10
Unemployment	0.09	0.06[c]	0.02	0.06	0.02	0.01	0.08	0.05[c]	0.04	0.07	0.03	0.01	0.07	0.07[c]	0.04	0.17	0.16[c]	0.12[c]
Party sympathy	0.36		0.33[a]	0.20		0.17[a]	0.21		0.17[a]	0.21		0.17[a]	0.31		0.29[a]	0.32		0.26[c]
R2 (%)	5.0		14.8	4.7		7.7	7.0		10.6	6.2		9.3	4.6		12.5	9.3		15.7

Significance: [a] = 0.001 level [b] = 0.01 level [c] = 0.05 level.
Specification of categories: See notes below.

Denmark
Sector: Public employee vs. all others (including people outside the labour force).
Class: Present occupation (except for temporarily absent), six categories: workers, lower white-collar, higher white-collar, self-employed, students, pensioners.
Education: Basic school (7–9 years), secondary school (10–12 years), university.
Income: Yearly income before tax for the respondent. Four categories: <120 000 DKK; 120–199 000, 200–299 000, 299 000 >.
Age: Five categories (18–29; 30–39; 40–49; 50–59; 60+).
Unemployed: Unemployed vs. all others (including people outside the labour force).
Party choice (six categories): Left wing party; Social democrats; Centre (radical liberals, centre democrats, Christian democrats); Right (liberals, conservatives); Progress party; Independent candidates.

Table 10.A2 Structural cleavages and attitudes towards welfare policies in Finland (1996). Multiple classification analysis

	Social reforms			Pensions			Health care			Child allowances			Social assistance			Unemployment benefits		
	Eta	Beta	Beta	Eta	Beta	Beta	Eta	Beta	Beta	Eta	Beta	Beta	Eta	Beta	Beta	Eta	Beta	Beta
Gender	0.06	0.05[c]	0.03	0.06	0.04[a]	0.03	0.07	0.07[b]	0.05	0.03	0.02	0.02	0.03	0.03	0.03	0.08	0.06[c]	0.06[b]
Sector		—		0.01	0.03	0.03	0.01	0.05	0.05	0.00	0.04	0.04	0.04	0.04	0.04	0.03	0.04	0.03
Class	0.24	0.18[a]	0.14[a]	0.19	0.20[a]	0.20[a]	0.15	0.15[a]	0.14[a]	0.10	0.09[b]	0.09[b]	0.19	0.15[a]	0.15[a]	0.26	0.21[c]	0.20[c]
Education	0.18	0.09[a]	0.07[a]	0.10	0.10[a]	0.09[a]	0.11	0.08[a]	0.07[a]	0.09	0.07[c]	0.06[c]	0.16	0.11[a]	0.10[a]	0.22	0.14[c]	0.12[c]
Income	0.21	0.17[a]	0.16[a]	0.15	0.12[b]	0.11[b]	0.12	0.08	0.07	0.11	0.09	0.10	0.18	0.11	0.11[c]	0.14	0.14[c]	0.14[c]
Age	0.07	0.09	0.10	0.12	0.18[a]	0.18[a]	0.05	0.06	0.05	0.20	0.23[a]	0.23[a]	0.08	0.13[c]	0.12[c]	0.11	0.16[c]	0.15[c]
Unemployment		—		0.07	0.06	0.06	0.08	0.01	0.01	0.11	0.04	0.05	0.15	0.07[c]	0.07	0.10	0.10[b]	0.10[b]
Party sympathy	0.32		0.27[a]	0.11		0.08	0.12		0.08	0.07		0.05	0.13		0.08	0.15		0.15[c]
R2 (%)		9.3	16.3		7.5	7.9		4.4	4.9		6.7	7.1		7.9	8.7		14.8	17.0

Significance: [a] = 0.001 level [b] = 0.01 level [c] = 0.05 level.
Specification of categories: See notes below.

Finland

Two data-sets were used in the multivariate analysis. The first one was collected by the Finnish Gallup and is described in Figure 10.1b. The wording of the question: 'What do you think about the current level of social security in Finland? Is it too high, appropriate or too low?' 'Don't know' answers were treated as missing.

The second data set was collected by Statistics Finland in November and December 1996 (N = 1548). Telephone interviewing was used, except for with people over 74 years of age, who were interviewed face to face. The data represent the Finnish population over 15 years of age. These data were utilized when analysing opinions on financing of five different social policy programmes. The wording of the question was as follows: 'The following is a list of cash benefits. Please say in each case whether more tax money, the same amount as now or less tax money should be used to finance these benefits.' 'Don't know' answers were treated as missing.

Age (five categories): (15–24, 25–34, 35–49, 50–65, over 65).
Education (three categories): primary, secondary, university.
Class: Present occupation (six categories): worker; upper white-collar; lower white-collar; self-employed (including farmers and entrepreneurs); student; pensioner.
Sector of employment: public and private.
Unemployment: Unemployed vs. all others (including people outside the labour force).
Income: Monthly income before tax for the respondent. For the first item (four categories): below 7500 FIM; between 7501-15000; 15001 and over; Income not known. For the other items (five categories): < 8,000 FIM; 8,001–16,000; 16,001–20,000; 20,000+; Income not known.
Political party: (Seven categories): Social Democrats; National Coalition; Centre Party; Left League; Green League; Other parties; No party affiliation.

Table 10.A3 Structural cleavages and attitudes towards welfare policies in Norway (1996). Multiple classification analysis

	Social reforms			Pensions			Health care			Child allowances			Social assistance			Unemployment benefits		
	Eta	Beta	Beta	Eta	Beta	Beta	Eta	Beta	Beta	Eta	Beta	Beta	Eta	Beta	Beta	Eta	Beta	Beta
Gender	0.09	0.04	0.04	0.10	0.10[a]	0.10[a]	0.11	0.10[a]	0.09[b]	0.04	0.02	0.00	0.04	0.01	0.04	0.00	0.02	0.03
Sector	0.05	0.04	0.02	0.04	0.05	0.05	0.04	0.05[c]	0.07[c]	0.01	0.01	0.03	0.03	0.01	0.01	0.03	0.03	0.04
Class	0.10	0.06[c]	0.03	0.09	0.06	0.06	0.08	0.04	0.05	0.11	0.08[b]	0.08[c]	0.05	0.06	0.07	0.09	0.08	0.06
Education	0.10	0.07[c]	0.08[c]	0.17	0.14[a]	0.15[a]	0.13	0.11[a]	0.09[b]	0.07	0.02	0.01	0.05	0.01	0.03	0.08	0.05	0.04
Income	0.16	0.11[b]	0.10[b]	0.13	0.08	0.08	0.13	0.06	0.09[c]	0.10	0.10[b]	0.12[b]	0.14	0.13[b]	0.13[b]	0.11	0.10[a]	0.09
Age	0.08	0.05	0.05	0.05	0.09[c]	0.08	0.08	0.06	0.08	0.22	0.22[a]	0.22[a]	0.08	0.06	0.07	0.09	0.05	0.06
Unemployment	0.04	0.04	0.02	0.01	0.02	0.00	0.01	0.00	0.00	0.01	0.03	0.03	0.02	0.01	0.01	0.07	0.05[a]	0.04
Party sympathy	0.14		0.11[b]	0.07		0.11[b]	0.09		0.09[c]	0.07		0.04	0.17		0.15[a]	0.16		0.15[c]
R2 (%)		4.0	5.3		5.3	7.0		4.2	5.9		6.9	7.3		2.5	5.3		2.9	4.6

Significance: [a] = 0.001 level [b] = 0.01 level [c] = 0.05 level.
Specification of categories: See notes below

Norway
Data collected by the Central Bureau of Statistics for the research project 'The pleasures and burdens of the welfare state'. The data represent the voting-age population in Norway.
Sector: Public employee vs. all others (including people outside the labour force).
Class: Present or last occupation (four categories): workers, lower white-collar, higher white-collar, self-employed.
Education (three categories): primary school, secondary education, university
Income: Yearly income before tax for the respondent (five categories): < 99,999 NOK; 100,000–149,999; 150,000–199,999; 200,000–249,999; > 250,000
Age (six categories): (18–20; 20–29; 30–39; 40–49; 50–64; 65+).
Unemployed: Unemployed vs. all others (including people outside the labour force).
Party sympathy (Six categories): Left Socialist; Social Democrats; Liberals; Christian People's Party, Centre Party; Conservatives; Progress Party; No party sympathies.

Table 10.A4 Structural cleavages and attitudes towards welfare policies in Sweden (1992/1996). Multiple classification analysis

	Social reforms (1992)			Pensions (1996)			Health care (1996)			Support for families with children (1992)			Social assistance (1992)			Unemployment benefits (1996)		
	Eta	Beta	Beta	Eta	Beta	Beta	Eta	Beta	Beta	Eta	Beta	Beta	Eta	Beta	Beta	Eta	Beta	Beta
Gender	0.06	0.01	0.00	0.20	0.12[a]	0.12[a]	0.17	0.12[a]	0.14[a]	0.07	0.01	0.01	0.02	0.01	0.02	0.16	0.07[a]	0.10[b]
Sector	0.08	0.05	0.03	0.10	0.02	0.01	0.13	0.08[c]	0.07[c]	0.12	0.12[a]	0.10[a]	0.06	0.05	0.05	0.14	0.08[b]	0.05
Class	0.12	0.08	0.04	0.26	0.10[c]	0.09	0.25	0.11[b]	0.09[c]	0.13	0.03	0.03	0.13	0.07	0.04	0.32	0.18[c]	0.13[c]
Education	0.05	0.08[c]	0.09[c]	0.24	0.14[b]	0.12[c]	0.24	0.25[a]	0.23[a]	0.04	0.09[c]	0.06	0.17	0.10[c]	0.10[c]	0.22	0.18[c]	0.13[b]
Income	0.12	0.07	0.08	0.33	0.24[a]	0.21[a]	0.26	0.15[a]	0.12[b]	0.14	0.05	0.05	0.14	0.08	0.08[b]	0.30	0.15[c]	0.12[b]
Age	0.17	0.15[a]	0.15[a]	0.11	0.15[a]	0.13[b]	0.05	0.08	0.06	0.24	0.25[a]	0.26[a]	0.19	0.16[c]	0.15[a]	0.17	0.15[c]	0.12[b]
Unemployment	0.09	0.07[c]	0.05	0.03	0.01	0.01	0.07	0.06	0.05	0.09	0.05	0.03	0.08	0.08[b]	0.06[c]	0.17	0.15[c]	0.13[c]
Party sympathy	0.33		0.32[a]	0.23		0.32[a]	0.24		0.14[a]	0.27		0.24[a]	0.29		0.27[a]	0.41		0.30[c]
R2 (%)		5.8	15.2		17.3	19.0		15.4	16.7		9.2	14.7		7.3	13.5		21.0	28.4

Significance: [a] = 0.001 level [b] = 0.01 level [c] = 0.05 level.
Specification of categories: See notes below.

Sweden
Two data-sets are used in the analysis. The first is a national survey from 1992 (February–May), asking about opinions towards welfare policies and taxation. The response rate is 76.0% of the net sample of 1992 respondents representing the Swedish population aged 18–74. The second data set is from the survey 'Role of Government', conducted within the International Social Survey Program in February–May 1996. The response rate is 68.3 % of the net sample of 1992 respondents representing the Swedish population aged 18–76. Both data were compiled by Statistics Sweden. The question wordings are found in Tables 10.1 and 10.2.

Sector: Public employee vs. all others (including people outside the labour force).
Class: Present or last occupation. (Four categories): Workers, Lower level non-manuals, Higher level non-manuals, Self-employed.
Education (three categories): primary school, secondary education, university
Income: Monthly income before tax for the respondent. (five categories): < 8,000 SEK; 8–12,000; 12–16,000; 16–20,000; 20,000+.
Age (six categories): (18–20; 20–29; 30–39; 40–49; 50–64; 65+).
Unemployment: Unemployed vs. all others (including people outside the labour force)
Party sympathy (five categories): Left Party; Social democrats; Middle (Centre Party, Liberals, Green Party, Christian Democratic Party); Right (Conservatives, in 1992 also New Democracy); No party sympathies.

11 Conclusion

The Nordic model stands stable but on shaky ground

Matti Heikkilä, Bjørn Hvinden, Mikko Kautto, Staffan Marklund and Niels Ploug

The question

These comparative studies started from a common interest to see what – if anything – had happened to the Nordic welfare state model after the early 1980s. Empirically, the background for this interest was threefold. All the Nordic countries had passed through turbulent periods in their macroeconomic development and levels of unemployment, although in different magnitudes and forms. At the same time the countries seemed to differ with respect to the pathways they had chosen in coping with these challenges. Consequently, there was good reason to believe that differing economic development and policy adjustments would have resulted in different outcomes in terms of people's well-being. As regards comparative welfare state research, our starting points were the recent discussions about the nature of changes in the welfare state and typologies. Moreover, some time had passed since the last comparative analysis of the whole spectrum of welfare state activities, focused on the Nordic countries.

The joint work started from this line of reasoning by developing a conceptual model and an analytical framework (see Chapter 1) which was used as a device to determine the collection of information. Here we made a distinction between four areas of interest. First, our interest was on *preconditions* of welfare policies, such as economic conditions, politics and demography. Second, we wanted to address possible shifts in or restructuring of *welfare measures*. Third, we were interested in the *outcomes* in terms of the observable welfare of citizens. Finally, the issue of welfare state *legitimacy* was addressed separately from the other categories. Changing attitudes towards welfare were thus seen both as prerequisites and outcomes of changing welfare state performance.

Developments in separate categories and the possible linkages between these categories have been the focus of the book. The empirical ambition has been to obtain answers to whether there have been system changes in the respective countries and how the actual welfare of the population has changed in the period between 1980 and 1995 in the four countries, Denmark, Finland, Norway and Sweden.

We started the book by presenting the major changes in the preconditions for the Nordic welfare states. Unsatisfactory macroeconomic development and consequent problems of unemployment became a major concern, although on different levels, for all Nordic countries. The process of European integration, resulting in Finland and Sweden becoming new EU members and Norway becoming part of the European Economic Area, added new dimensions for needs to adjust. In politics, social democracy was not in as strong a position as in the early 1980s, and with regard to social needs, demographic development added to the problem of unemployment, resulting in a growing dependent population.

As we remarked in the introductory chapter, modern welfare states have to respond in an adequate way to four major challenges – growing dependency ratios, new forms of organization of work, gender equality and finally the issue of social inclusion and exclusion. All these factors were seen as key determinants of the welfare policies adopted in the Nordic states. The special focuses when examining the restructuring of welfare arrangements were cash benefits, social and health services and various activation policies and measures. In the outcome section the interest was in possible changes in inequality of living conditions, poverty and social exclusion and income distribution.

Changing preconditions

In Chapter 2, Marklund and Nordlund analysed the macroeconomic and political development in the four Nordic nations from the early 1980s to the mid-1990s. The research question here was whether there have occurred such major changes that allow or push forward a restructuring process in the Nordic welfare states. Here – in contrast to the other chapters – we wanted to make comparisons not only between the Nordic countries but also between the Nordic group and other industrial countries and to put the Nordic model in an OECD context. It is a well-known fact that differences between the countries in their economic strategies and outcomes were clearly visible during the 1980s and early 1990s. Denmark had started out in the late 1970s as the 'sick man' of the Nordic family. High unemployment, budget constraints and lack of development of the welfare state were then a part of the Danish reality. There were no such problems in the other three Nordic countries at that point in time. Danish development has been positive during the first half of the 1990s and the country has emerged as a prosperous one with a strong economy and a per capita income exceeding that of Finland and Sweden.

For Finland and Sweden, the early 1990s proved to be a difficult period. Both countries experienced their deepest recessions since the 1930s with large increases in unemployment figures and troubled public economies. Although the economies of both countries had recovered by the mid-1990s, an essential and seemingly persistent hallmark of crisis – the high level of unemployment – still existed. Although social spending measured as the share of GDP increased during the years of deepest economic problems, the Finnish and Swedish governments introduced substantial cuts that affected almost all social policies.

Norway had from the beginning of the 1980s emerged as the richest Nordic country and this position was reinforced during the 1990s. This development is to a high degree linked to the country's good use of oil resources in the North Sea. But even Norway experienced a substantial increase in unemployment in the early 1990s and there have been national concerns about the long-term effects of the country's expansive economy.

Nevertheless, and despite dramatic developments in the macro-economies of and marked differences between the Nordic nations, Marklund and Nordlund's analysis suggested quite moderate effects when the Nordic countries were compared to other OECD countries in the light of macroeconomic indicators. The Nordic countries were still prosperous by international comparison. Some convergence in terms of overall labour-market participation rates between the Nordic countries and the rest of the OECD had taken place. The female labour market participation in the Nordic countries was still highest in the Europe of the mid-1990s. The welfare states of the Nordic countries were also distinctly larger in relative terms and they were still high spenders on social welfare compared to other industrial countries. No trend towards convergence between the Nordic group and the rest of the OECD in terms of spending on social transfers could be seen.

The main result from the analysis of political developments in the Nordic nations was that social democratic parties had lost influence while conservative parties had gained support. Increasing volatility among voters, the rise of new voter alignments and the rise of new parties made the parliamentary situation more complicated. Social democrats had to co-operate with parties from the Centre and/or the Right in various cabinet coalitions and alliances or seek support from these parties in the parliaments. This process could be seen either in terms of a strengthening of political forces through co-operation, or it could be seen as a sign of a general decline in political power in relationship to other social forces. However, these processes seem not to be unique to the Nordic nations.

In Chapter 3 Kautto analysed demographic developments in terms of the changing needs to be met by the welfare states. At the macro-level, the demographic development has been fairly similar in all four Nordic countries. This has resulted in increasing 'social needs' arising from such factors as the ageing of the population and increasing numbers of single parents and single households. When this analysis of demographic development was complemented with a look at phenomena such as postponed entrance into the labour market, early exit from the labour market and unemployment, we had a more finely nuanced picture of the 'burden of support'. Although ageing is a fact in all four countries, in Denmark and Norway this trend has been counterbalanced by a growth in the number of employed people. Thus, the economic dependency ratios have become less favourable in Finland and Sweden, but remained stable in Denmark and Norway.

Changes in demographies and in the composition of work forces are having clear consequences for available resources and spending. Moreover, anticipated demographic changes in the next century have also influenced present-day policies, for instance through perceived need to modify existing old-age pension schemes. Thus, in all four countries the perception has been that growing demands on the welfare state are about the sustainability of income protection systems and providing social care and health care services to increasing numbers of old people in need. Family developments and the overall consequences of demographic development on redistribution between generations or between different family types have not caused as much concern as the impact of ageing populations.

A key conclusion about changing preconditions could be that the Nordic countries still formed a distinct group of nations in terms of welfare policies in the mid-1990s. Only limited convergence with the rest of the OECD countries could be observed. But on the other hand, combining the facts of increased macroeconomic vulnerability and growing needs due to social and demographic pressures that have taken place in the Nordic countries, there appeared to be potential for more fundamental restructuring of the welfare state.

Minor changes in cash benefits, services and activation

Chapters 4 to 6 examined the modifications in the key outputs of the welfare state. In our analysis these outputs included cash benefits, services and measures to link welfare to work. The key issue that was addressed here was whether we could observe any notable structural modification or systemic changes in welfare state arrangements as a consequence of changing economic, political and social preconditions. As noted earlier, there was a clear potential for more fundamental changes during the period under examination. But did this potential materialize?

In the analysis of changes in cash benefits between 1980 and 1993 Ploug demonstrated that although cuts were made in all four countries and in most benefits, these cuts had not been dramatic. All the usual methods had been adopted when cutting benefits – tightening the conditions of entitlement, lowering the compensation levels, shortening the periods of payment, etc. There did not seem not to be any clear or common pattern in the changes that had been implemented, nor were there any distinct national differences. Most of the cuts and the systemic changes had been undertaken in unemployment benefit schemes, simply because the fastest increase in spending had occurred here alongside the recession and growing labour market problems. However, in the mid-1990s, the cash benefit system was still relatively generous in all Nordic countries compared with other countries. It offered universal coverage for all citizens but was somewhat less generous than in the 1970s and 1980s. The introduction of more work linkage and work incentives to cash benefits have been discussed but not many actual measures have been introduced or enforced. On the other hand, there has been a move towards more 'active' labour market measures.

As regards social and health services, Lehto, Moss and Rostgaard (Chapter 5) showed that the essential principles of the Nordic service model were still alive in the Nordic countries of the 1990s. The principles referred to included universalism, high quality, tax financing and public provision. On the other hand, the chapter indicated that universalism and supply of services had to some extent been circumscribed by introducing higher user fees, budget constraints and professional discretion. As was the case with cash benefits, there were clear differences in development between the different services. In the case of child care, the Nordic principles were especially strong and even gaining ground. All in all, the Nordic model was very alive in the area of services and the differences between the individual countries had decreased.

Drøpping, Hvinden and Vik (Chapter 6) examined the 'new' activation policies at the interface between work and welfare. They illustrated how 'active' labour market policies were a possible response to external and internal pressures on the Nordic welfare states. This was clearly reflected in the policy rhetoric in the Nordic countries. There were, however, significant differences between countries. Denmark was the country that most clearly had made a shift towards active measures; it had also adopted a broader understanding of activation than the other countries. All Nordic countries had spent more on active measures compared with income transfers to the unemployed, but on account of the simultaneous increase in unemployment compensation the rate between costs for active and passive measures remained fairly stable. While the activation debate indicated a shift in the 1990s' policies, it was hard to find firm evidence of the efficiency of these measures.

As a summary and conclusion of this section on policy responses, it may be stated that the obvious potential for restructuring coming from macroeconomic as well as demographic and political pressures had not been manifested in the form of fundamental changes in benefit or service provisions. Most forms of cash benefits had been reduced but not in a dramatic fashion. The existing safety net still offered universal coverage in the mid-1990s. When it came to services, all the known Nordic hallmarks were still present: universalism, high quality, tax funding and public provision. There are good reasons to repeat the conclusions of Alber (1988) and Marklund (1988) about the lack of evidence of a major welfare backlash or instability in the 1970s and 1980s. Even during the much more severe pressures of the 1990s, the Nordic countries seemed to be very resistant to dramatic changes. However, gradual and small changes combined with growing burdens of dependency and changed economic and political conditions have created a still existing potential for welfare reform. Time will show whether this potential will be realized.

Differing and unexpected outcomes

In examining the measurable well-being of Nordic citizens the interest was twofold. On the one hand, variations in income and well-being could be seen as an outcome factor, dependent on changes in welfare state policies. Thus, radical cutbacks in unemployment compensation or family benefits should logically be reflected in the material welfare of jobless people and families with children, respectively. On the other hand, turbulent macroeconomic developments could be regarded as predictors of the incidence of various welfare problems in the population. Thus an individual was potentially affected both by changes in the risk of needing support and by changes in the welfare system itself. Hence the research question was how the changes in the preconditions and/or in the Nordic welfare systems had affected the well-being of the population. This was studied with respect to living conditions, income differentials, poverty and social exclusion (Chapters 7 to 9).

In analysing changes in the distribution of living conditions, Fritzell (Chapter 7) adopted economic turbulence as his starting point. He assumed that at least in Finland and Sweden one would expect a notable deterioration in living conditions from the mid-1980s to the mid-1990s due to the severe recession in these countries after 1991. This expectation was not substantiated: in fact clear improvement in real earnings, disposable equivalent income and social support was found in the three countries studied, that is, Finland, Norway and Sweden. Against all common sense, the most positive development in the distribution of living conditions between the 1980s and 1990s had taken place in Finland. There was no substantial increase in inequality in Finland. The most notable weakening of living conditions in this period took place in Sweden, but also to some degree in Norway. These findings were both interesting and problematic.

In all three countries the young had more welfare problems than middle-aged people. Changes in living conditions between men and women and between social classes had been more modest. The relative deterioration in the living conditions of the young in the Nordic countries could mostly be explained by their increased vulnerability in the labour market. To some degree, increased intergenerational differences could also be seen as an indicator of less generous welfare state compensation for young people. In sum, the findings on changes in living conditions demonstrated that macroeconomic aggregate measures like GDP or one microeconomic measure like income cannot indicate or even predict the variation and social patterning of the welfare of individuals.

Recent macroeconomic changes were one of the background factors also for Halleröd and Heikkilä in their analysis of poverty and social exclusion (Chapter 8). Trends in relative economic poverty and in dependency on social assistance were used to examine social exclusion. Social exclusion was defined in terms of an accumulation of several single welfare problems.

Economic poverty increased from the mid-1980s in Denmark, Norway and Sweden but surprisingly not in Finland. On the other hand, the number of people who received social assistance payments increased radically in Finland, moderately in Norway and Sweden, but not in Denmark. The Finnish case could be used to argue that social assistance might be a better indicator of economic problems than the relative poverty measure. When analysing social exclusion in each country, Sweden appeared not only to have growing economic poverty but also a rising incidence of a number of other welfare problems from the mid-1980s to the mid-1990s. The same general trend occurred in Norway, although the development was less pronounced. And again, Finland experienced not only decreasing relative poverty but also stable incidence of other welfare problems – with the exception of unemployment, of course. These findings were not in line with the expectations stemming from macroeconomic development and reduced welfare spending. So, in Norway and Sweden the risk of social exclusion followed the expected pattern, but in Finland this was not the case.

The risk of becoming socially excluded was generally speaking higher in the mid-1990s than ten years earlier in all three countries examined (comparable data from Denmark were not available). Regarding the determinants of risk of social exclusion, class position lost its power to predict to a certain extent, whereas educational level gained importance. Age seemed also to be increasingly important, in the sense that the younger sections of the population suffered from increased risk. This finding was in line with Fritzell's findings.

Gustafsson *et al.* studied the income distribution in all the Nordic countries for a period from the late 1960s onwards (Chapter 9). The long-term trend in the distribution of equivalent household income had been a clear decrease in inequality until the early 1980s. This was mainly due to the maturation of pension schemes and the expansion of public transfers. After the early 1980s the trends differed between countries. In Norway and Sweden, there were clear signs of increased income inequality. Finland remained at the same level of inequality. Differing measures did not allow for assessment of the direction of development in Denmark.

It proved difficult to find clear factors to explain changes in income differences within and between nations. There was evidence to conclude that income inequality was not clearly related to the unemployment levels experienced by the Nordic countries. There was also support for the conclusion that the aged have gained and the young have lost over time in all four nations. This could be seen as an indicator of changed effects of social transfers.

What might then be concluded from the analysis of welfare outcomes? First, one may say that welfare outcomes turned out to be more complicated and more difficult to explain than they appeared from the outset. Second, it seemed that macrolevel changes better explained the variations in income and welfare than they did policy responses. These results indicate only that welfare performance during these years in the Nordic countries was a combination of a number of intricate forces that make simple interpretations impossible and call for both more detailed studies and a deflation on what one could reasonably expect in terms of change during a period of 15 years.

Broad support for welfare state measures

In examining the legitimacy of the welfare state, Goul Andersen *et al.* focused on three major questions – trends in support for the welfare state, popularity of various programmes and factors explaining population support (Chapter 10). As to the trends, no long-term decline in support for the welfare state was found. Support for the expansion of welfare policies was at its highest level in the 1960s and 1970s. Since then, the popular mood has been in favour of maintaining the existing schemes. Thus, in general, popular attitudes have been in line with policy changes.

Interestingly, in the short term, economic problems had negative effects on the support for welfare schemes in Finland but not in Sweden. As regards the popularity of different schemes, a similar pattern was found in all countries. As expected, universal welfare schemes, health care and health-related income transfers and old-age pensions have been most popular. Family policy schemes have occupied an intermediate position in terms of popular support. At the bottom of priorities were targeted programmes like social assistance.

Differences among various social groups in their support for the welfare state did not change much over time. Women, public sector employees, workers, low-income earners, unemployed people and those having the lowest educational levels have tended to support the welfare state most strongly. This is in line with the hypothesis of self-interest – those groups have also been more dependent on the welfare state, either in terms of being recipients of benefits and services or of being employees. The level of disagreement about the welfare state among various population groups was highest in Sweden because the class factor was most important there. Similarly, differences between the political right and left were also strongest in Sweden. The level of consensus was highest in Norway.

In conclusion, it seems as if the welfare state remained popular throughout the period. Differences in views between nations and between social groups have changed to only a limited degree.

Discussion

The main results concerning the development of the Nordic welfare states and the well-being of the population reported in this book indicate somewhat unexpected and surprisingly moderate changes. Changes in the structure and generosity of the welfare state measures as well as in most of the outcome indicators were smaller than expected. The analyses in this book give no evidence for 'retrenchment' or 'dismantling'. For the defenders of the welfare state the results are most agreeable: despite the 'colder climate', the Nordic welfare states seemed to stand relatively strong and they were supported by a clear majority of the population in the mid-1990s. The effects of the restructuring of the Danish welfare system in the early 1980s and the effects of the deep economic recession after the early 1990s, which mostly affected Finland and Sweden, were very moderate according to the kinds of indicators used here. All of the traditional hallmarks of the Nordic model (see Chapter 1) appeared to be very much alive.

This general conclusion requires some serious reservations. First, long-term changes both within systems and in welfare outcomes might not have manifested themselves and become observable in our data yet, as these have only covered a period of 10–15 years. In the moderate time span we have adopted, long-term trends may have been underestimated. Second, regarding the 'semimoderate' effects on individual welfare such as living conditions, poverty and exclusion, our data have admittedly been far from perfect. People on the margins of society are often hit more adversely by economic and labour market shocks and by cuts in benefits and services, and as a rule they are underrepresented in broad population surveys. Third, and perhaps most importantly, although average changes have relatively speaking and on an aggregate level been modest, changes on the individual level may still have been dramatic. A single family may well have been the victim of both increased risks in several respects and of reduced compensations in a number of welfare programmes.

Referring to the framework adopted for this study, we will finally comment on some of the key findings and interpretations stemming from the previous chapters. Macroeconomic and political changes have been seen as essential preconditions of welfare state policies as well as determinants of welfare outcomes. Worsening economic circumstances and more non-social democratic governance seemed to create almost optimal prerequisites for changes in policies in a more fundamental or systemic sense. But as we have demonstrated, such changes were very limited. This might be interpreted in different ways. One might say that the Nordic ways of organizing welfare production and distribution adapted fairly well to changing circumstances. They were internally stable, basically efficient and resistant to sudden changes. Another possibility would be to conclude that more dramatic economic, demographic or social changes would be needed to alter the Nordic model markedly. A third option might be to say that the Nordic model is so firmly rooted in the institutions and in the culture and everyday life of people that (party) politics do not affect it. This interpretation would be backed by the evidence of strong popular support for the major welfare state programmes.

There was more variation in outcomes – that is, in the changes in income and other parts of individual welfare – than that found in the structures of benefits and services. Outcomes seemed to be mainly affected by macroeconomic factors, at least this was assumed at the stage of setting hypotheses. This assumption was especially relevant, if not completely supported, in the examination of poverty, exclusion and inequality of living conditions. The general link between macroeconomic decline and increase in welfare problems at the individual level seemed to hold to some degree in Sweden and Norway (Denmark was excluded from the analysis for data reasons) but not in Finland.

The seemingly odd case of Finland has been accounted for in previous chapters. During the steep downfall of the economy this country increased the income transfers quite dramatically and was able to replace, although not fully, the lost market income of households. The result was that the relative share of the total income package of households coming from the transfers increased in five years from one-fifth to one-third. Thanks to this relative increase in transfers and the fact that all income groups were financially hit, income inequality did not increase. This explains the stable development of relative poverty over the recession period.

One important result was the weakening of the relative position of young adults *vis-à-vis* the stable or improved position of the elderly. This increasing generation gap was observed both in terms of overall risk of social exclusion and in terms of disposable income. Although this can partly be explained by the fact that the young had a weaker position in the labour market and were more affected by unemployment, it could also be seen as a sign of the inability of the welfare state to guarantee the living conditions of the younger generations. Thus, it could be interpreted in terms of the welfare states' lack of reorientation or adjustment to new conditions. In this respect the high level of institutional stability should perhaps be regarded as problematic.

Returning to our conceptual model, one may argue that the analyses have shown that politics did not explain much. The composition and political emphasis of the governments appeared not to have changed the direction of welfare policies essentially. On the other hand, nor did economics have the expected strong effect. General economic factors and increased vulnerability due to increased unemployment seemed to influence the living conditions of people more directly than did changes in the welfare machinery. But for large majorities of the populations and on crude indicators of welfare state performance, no signs of a welfare crisis caused by the recession could be detected. This raises the question of how we are to understand the relationship between general economic circumstances, welfare state support among the population and the political process. To answer this question more theoretical and empirical work is needed.

References

Aaberge, R., Björklund, A., Jäntti, M., Palme, M., Pedersen, P. J., Smith, N. and Wennemo, T. (1996) *Income Inequality and Income Mobility in the Scandinavian Countries Compared to the United States*, Discussion Paper No. 168, Statistics Norway, Oslo.

Aaberge, R., Björklund, A., Jäntti, M., Pedersen, P. J., Smith, N. and Wennemo, T. (1997) *Unemployment Shocks and Income Distribution: How Did the Nordic Countries Fare During Their Crises?*, Discussion Paper No. 201, Statistics Norway, Oslo.

Aardal, B. (1994) 'The 1994 Storting Election: Volatile Voters Opposing the European Union', *Scandinavian Political Studies* 17: 171–80.

Åberg, R., Selén, J. and Than, H. (1984) 'Ekonomiska resurser' (Economic Resources), in R. Erikson and R. Åberg (eds) *Välfärd i förändring*, Arlöv: Prisma.

Abrahamson, P. (1996) 'Social Exclusion in Europe: Old Wine in New Bottles?', *Druzboslovne razprave* XI (19–20): 119–36.

Agell, J. (1996) 'Why Sweden's Welfare State Needed Reform', *The Economic Journal* 106 (November), 1760–71.

Ahola, A., Djerf, K., Heiskanen, M. and Vikki, K. (1995) *Elinolotutkimus 1994*, Aineiston keruu. Tilastokeskus, Elinolot. Muistio 1995: 2, Helsinki.

Aktuell nordisk statistik (1996) Nordisk arbejdsmarkedsstatistik, I. Kvartal 1993–4. Kvartal 1995 og årene 1985–1995. Nordisk statistisk sekretariat, *Aktuell nordisk statistik*, nr. 35, September, Copenhagen.

Alban, A. and Christiansen, T. (eds) (1995) *The Nordic Lights: New Initiatives in Health Care Systems*, Odense: Odense University Press.

Alber, J. (1988) 'Is There a Crisis of the Welfare State? Cross-National Evidence from Europe, North America and Japan', *European Sociological Review*, 4(3): 181–207.

Aldrich, J. H. and Nelson, F. D. (1984) *Linear Probability, Logit and Probit Models*, Beverly Hills: Sage.

Alestalo, M. (1994) 'Finland: The Welfare State at the Crossroads', in N. Ploug and J. Kvist (eds) *Recent Trends in Cash Benefits in Europe*, Copenhagen: The Danish National Institute of Social Research.

Alestalo, M., Bislev, S. and Furåker, B. (1991) 'Welfare State Employment in Scandinavia', in J. E. Kolberg (ed.) *The Welfare State as Employer*, Armonk: M. E. Sharpe.

Allardt, E. (1975) *Att ha, att älska, att vara. Om välfärd i Norden.* Lund: Argos.

Allardt, M., Sihvo, T. and Uusitalo, H. (1992) *Mitä mieltä hyvinvointivaltiosta. Suomalaisten sosiaaliturvamielipiteet 1975–1991*, Helsinki: Sosiaali- ja Terveyshallitus, Tutkimuksia 17.

Andersen, A. and Laake, P. (1983) 'A Causal Model for Physician Utilization: Analysis of Norwegian Data', *Medical Care* 21 (3): 266–78.

Anttonen, A. and Sipilä, J. (1996) 'European Social Services: Is it Possible to Identify Models?', *Journal of European Social Policy* 6 (2): 87–100.

Arbeidsdirektoratet (1995–97) *Månedsstatistikk om arbeidsmarkedet,* Oslo: Arbeidsdirektoratet.

Atkinson, A. (1996) 'Seeking to Explain the Distribution of Income', in J. Hills (ed.) *New Inequalities: The Changing Distribution of Income and Wealth in the United Kingdom,* Cambridge: Cambridge University Press.

Atkinson, A., Rainwater, L. and Smeeding, T. M. (1995) *Income Distribution in OECD Countries: Evidence from the Luxembourg Income Study,* Social Policy Studies No. 18 Paris: OECD.

Baldwin, P. (1990) *The Politics of Social Solidarity,* Cambridge: Cambridge University Press.

Barstad, A. (1996) 'Flere aleneboende, men færre venneløse', *Samfunnsspeilet* 10: 24–9.

Benner, M. (1997) *The Politics of Growth and Economic Regulation in Sweden 1930–1994,* Lund: Arkiv.

Berghman, J. (1995) 'Social Exclusion in Europe: Policy Context and Analytic Framework', in G. Room (ed.) *Beyond the Threshold,* Southampton: The Polity Press.

Bille, L. (1992) 'Politisk kronik, 1. halvår 1992', *Økonomi & Politik* 65 (3): 50–9.

Bille, L. (1993) 'Politisk kronik, 2. halvår 1992', *Økonomi & Politik* 66 (3): 62–71.

Björklund, A. (1991) 'Unemployment and Income Distribution: Time Series Evidence from Sweden', *Scandinavian Journal of Economics* 93: 457–65.

Björklund, A. (1992) 'Långsiktiga perspektiv på inkomstfördelningen' (Long-run perspectives on the distribution of income), in *Inkomstfördelningens utveckling,* Bilaga 8 till LU 92, Stockholm.

Björklund, A. and Freeman, R. (1995) *Generating Equality and Eliminating Poverty – The Swedish Way,* Occasional Paper No. 60.2, Stockholm: Studieförbundet Näringsliv och Samhälle.

Björklund, A., Palme, M. and Svensson, I. (1995) 'Tax Reforms and Income Distribution: An Assessment Using Different Income Concepts', *Swedish Economic Policy Review* 2: 229–65.

Bjørn, N. H. (1996) 'The Apprenticeship System – Supply and Demand', in

E. Wadensjö (ed.) *The Nordic Labour Markets in the 1990s*, Part 2, Amsterdam: North-Holland.

Bjørn, N. H. *et al.* (1996) 'Strategies – the System of Transition from School to Work. A Comparison of the Nordic Countries', in E. Wadensjö (ed.) *The Nordic Labour Markets in the 1990s*, Part 2, Amsterdam: North-Holland

Blank, R. M. and Blinder, A. S. (1986) 'Macroeconomics, Income Distribution and Poverty', in S. Danziger and D. H. Weinberg (eds) *Fighting Poverty: What Works and What Does Not*, Cambridge, MA: Harvard University Press.

Blinder, A. S. and Esaki, H. Y. (1978) 'Macroeconomics Activity and Income Distribution in the Postwar United States', *Review of Economics and Statistics* 72: 414–23.

Borchorst, A. and Siim, B. (1987) 'Women and the Advanced Welfare State – A New Kind of Patriarchal Power?', in A. Showstack Sassoon (ed.) *Women and the State*, London: Hutchinson.

Borre, O. and Goul Andersen, J. (1997) *Voting and Political Attitudes in Denmark,* Aarhus: Aarhus University Press.

Brittan, S. (1977) *The Economic Consequences of Democracy*, London: Temple Smith.

Buhmann, B., Rainwater, L., Schmaus, G. and Smeeding, T.M. (1988) 'Equivalence Scales, Well-Being, Inequality, and Poverty: Sensitivity Estimates across Ten Countries using the Luxembourg Income Study (LIS) Database', *Review of Income and Wealth* 34: 115–42.

Burtless, G. (1989) 'Work Programs in Welfare and the Difference They Make', in R. M. Coughlin (ed.) *Reforming Welfare: Lessons, Limits, and Choices,* Albuquerque: University of New Mexico.

Callan, T., Nolan, B. and Whelan, C. T. (1993) 'Resources, Deprivation and the Measurement of Poverty', *Journal of Social Policy* 22 (2): 141–72.

Castles, F. G. and Mitchell, D. (1990) *Three Worlds of Welfare Capitalism or Four?*, Graduate Program in Public Policy, Discussion Paper 21, The Australian University, Canberra.

Castles, F. G. (ed.) (1993) *Families of Nations: Patterns of Public Policy in Western Democracies*, Aldershot: Dartmouth.

Christensen, U. *et al.* (1996) *Ventetid til operation,* Copenhagen: DSI and DIKE.

Cloward, R. A. and Piven, F. F. (1986) 'The Welfare State in an Age of Industrial Decline', *Smith College Studies in Social Work*, 56: 132–55.

Coughlin, R. M. (1979) 'Social Policy and Ideology: Public Opinion in Eight Rich Nations', *Comparative Social Research*: 3–40.

Daatland, S. (red) (1997) *De siste årene. Eldreomsorgen i Skandinavia 1960–95,* NOVA-rapport 22/97, Norsk insitutt for forskning om oppvekst velferd och aldring, Oslo.

Dahl, E. and Birkelund, G. E. (1996) 'Sysselsettning, klasse og helse 1980–1995', paper presented at the Nordic Workshop on Health Inequalities in Stockholm, November 1996, Oslo: FAFO.

Dahrendorf, R. (1987) *The Modern Social Conflict. An Essay on the Politics of Liberty*, London: Weidenfeld and Nicholson.

Danish Economic Council (1996) *The Danish Economy*, Autumn 1996, Copenhagen.

Danish Ministry of Health (1995) *Bekendgørelse om forsøgsordning på sygehusområdet*, Bekendgørelse af 8. marts 1995, Copenhagen: Shultz Forlag.

De Swaan, A. (1990) *In Care of the State*, Cambridge: Polity Press.

Dunleavy, P. (1980) 'The Political Implications of Sectional Cleavages and the Growth of State Employment', *Political Studies* 28: 364–83 and 527–49.

Dunleavy, P. (1986) 'The Growth of Sectional Cleavages and Stabilization of State Expenditures', *Society and Space* 4: 129–44.

Eardley, T., Bradshaw, J., Ditch, J., Gough, I. and Whiteford, P. (1996) *Social Assistance in OECD Countries: Synthesis Report*, Department of Social Security and OECD, Research Report No. 46, London: HMSO.

Egmose, S. (1985) 'Udviklingen i den personlige indkomstfordeling,' in S. Egmose, L. Egmose, G. V. Mogensen and H. Aage (eds) *Uligheden, politikerne og befolkningen. Sammenligningsundersögelsen* 2 (The Development in the Personal Distribution of Incomes, *Inequality, the Politicians and the Population*), The Danish National Institute of Social Research, Publication No. 139, Copenhagen.

Epland, J. (1992) 'Inntektsfordelingen i 1980-årene', *Økonomiske Analyser*, nr. 2, Statistisk sentralbyrå.

Erikson, R. (1993) 'Descriptions of Inequality: The Swedish Approach to Welfare Research', in M. C. Nussbaum and A. Sen (eds) *The Quality of Life*, Oxford: Clarendon Press.

Erikson, R. and Goldthorpe, J. (1993) *The Constant Flux: A Study of Class Mobility in Industrial Societies*, Oxford: Clarendon Press.

Erikson, R., Hansen, E. J., Ringen, S. and Uusitalo, H. (eds) (1987) *The Scandinavian Model: Welfare States and Welfare Research*, Armonk: M. E. Sharpe.

Erikson, R. and Thålin, M. (1987). 'Coexistence of Welfare Problems', in R. Erikson and R. Åberg (eds) *Welfare in Transition*, Oxford: Clarendon Press.

Erikson, R. and Uusitalo, H. (1987) 'The Scandinavian Approach to Welfare Research', in R. Erikson, E. J. Hansen, S. Ringen and H. Uusitalo (eds) *The Scandinavian Model: Welfare States and Welfare Research*, Armonk: M. E. Sharpe.

Esping-Andersen, G. (1985) *Politics against Markets*, Princeton: Princeton University Press.

Esping-Andersen, G. (1987) 'Citizenship and Socialism: De-commodification and Solidarity in the Welfare State', in M. Rein, G. Esping-Andersen and L. Rainwater (eds) *Stagnation and Renewal of Social Policy: The Rise and Fall of Policy Regimes*, Armonk: M. E. Sharpe.

Esping-Andersen, G. (1990): *The Three Worlds of Welfare Capitalism*, Cambridge: Polity Press.

Esping-Andersen, G. (1996a) 'After the Golden Age? Welfare State Dilemmas in a Global Economy', in G. Esping-Andersen (ed.) *Welfare States in Transition, National Adaptations in Global Economies*: London: Sage/ Unrisd.

Esping-Andersen, G. (ed.) (1996b) *Welfare States in Transition: National Adaptations in Global Economies*, London: Sage/Unrisd.

Esping-Andersen, G. and Korpi, W. (1987) 'From Poor Relief to Institutional Welfare States: The Development of Scandinavian Social Policy', in R. Erikson, E. J. Hansen, S. Ringen and H. Uusitalo (eds) *The Scandinavian Model: Welfare States and Welfare Research*, Armonk: M. E. Sharpe.

European Commission (1995) *The Demographic Situation in the European Union. 1994 report* DGV, COM (94)595, Luxemburg: Office for Official Publications of the European Communities.

European Commission Network on Childcare (1996) *A Review of Services for Young Children in the European Union 1990–1995*, Brussels: DGV.

European Observatory on National Family Policies (1995) *Developments in National Family Policies in 1994*, York: University of York.

Eurostat (1996) *Income Distribution and Poverty in the European Union*, Statistics in Focus, Luxemburg: Office for Official Publications of the European Communities.

Ferlie, E., Ashburner, L., Fitzgerald, L. and Pettigrew, A. (1996) *The New Public Management in Action*, Oxford: Oxford University Press.

Finansministeriet (1995) *Budgetredegørelsen*, Copenhagen.

Flora, P. (ed.) (1986) *Growth to Limits: The Western European Welfare States Since World War II, vol 1: Sweden, Norway, Finland, Denmark*. Berlin: de Gruyter.

Ford, M. (1993) *Attføring til arbeid? En oppfølgingsundersøkelse av forsøk på yrkesmessig attføring*, Oslo: INAS.

Forss, M. (1997) 'Om våra framtida pensioner', *EST* 3/97: 187–99.

Fritzell, J. (1991) *Icke av marknaden allena: Inkomstfördelningen i Sverige* (Not soley by the market: income distribution in Sweden), Stockholm: Almquist & Wiksell International.

Fritzell, J. (1992) *The Swedish Level of Living Approach to the Study of Welfare and Inequality*, Study of Social and Economic Inequality, Series No. 7, Sydney: Social Policy Research Centre and Centre for Applied Economic Research.

Fritzell, J. (1997) 'Distributional Changes of Economic Welfare in the Nordic Countries', paper presented at the ISA-RC 19 meeting in Copenhagen, August 1997, Stockholm: Swedish Institute for Social Research.

Fritzell, J. and Lundberg, O. (1994) 'Välfärdsförändringar', in J. Fritzell and O. Lundberg (eds) *Vardagens villkor. Levnadsförhållanden i Sverige under tre decennier*, Stockholm: Brombergs.

Fylkesnes, K. (1993) 'Determinants of Health Care Utilization – Visit and Referrals', *Scandinavian Journal of Social Medicine* 21 (1): 40–50.

Garrett, G. (1995) 'Capital Mobility, Trade and the Domestic Politics of Economic Policy', *International Organization* 49 (4): 657–87.

Garrett, G. and Mitchell, D. (1995) 'Globalization and the Welfare State: income transfers in the industrial democracies 1965–1990', paper presented to conference on Comparative Research on Welfare State Reforms, Pavia, September.

George, V. and Miller, S. (1996) 'The Welfare Circle towards 2000. General Trends', in V. George and S. Miller (eds) *Social Policy towards 2000: Squaring the Welfare Circle*, London: Routledge 1994. Reprint 1996.

George, V. and Taylor-Gooby, P. (eds) (1996) *European Welfare Policy: Squaring the Welfare Circle*, Basingstoke: Macmillan.

Glans, I. (1986), 'Fremskridtspartiet-småborgerlig revolt, högerreaktion eller generell protest?', in J. Elklit and O. Tonsgaard (eds) *Valg og vælgeradfærd,* Århus: Politica.

Gottschalk, P. and Smeeding, T. (1997) 'Cross-National Comparisons of Levels and Trends in Inequality', *Journal of Economic Literature* XXXV: 633–87.

Gough, I. (1979) *The Political Economy of the Welfare State*, London: Macmillan.

Goul Andersen, J. (1988) 'Vælgernes holdninger til den offentlige udgiftspolitik', in K-H. Bentzon (ed.) *Fra vækst til omstilling,* Copenhagen: Nyt fra Samfundsvidenskaberne.

Goul Andersen, J. (1993) 'Sources of Welfare State Support in Denmark: Self-Interest or Way of Life?', in E. J. Hansen, S. Ringen, H. Uusitalo and R. Erikson (eds) *Welfare Trends in the Scandinavian Countries*, New York: M. E. Sharpe.

Goul Andersen, J. (1994) 'Samfundsøkonomi, interesser og politisk adfærd', in E. Petersen *et al., Livskvalitet og holdninger i det variable nichesamfund*. Psykologisk Institut, Aarhus Universitet, i komm. hos Aarhus Universitetsforlag.

Goul Andersen, J. (1995) *(Hvorfor) vinder regeringen ikke på den økonomiske fremgang? Policy vurderinger, policy effects og andre forklaringer*, Arbejdspapir No. 2 fra Det danske valgprojekt, Institut for Statskundskab, Aarhus Universitet.

Goul Andersen, J. (1997) 'Krisebevidsthed og velfærdsholdninger i en højkonjunktur', in G. Graversen (ed.) *Et arbejdsliv. Festskrift tilegenet Professor dr.Phil Eggert Petersen*, Aarhus: Department of Psychology, University of Aarhus.

Goul Andersen, J. and Bjørklund, T. (1997) 'Radical Right-Wing Populism in Scandinavia: From Tax Revolt to Neo-Liberalism and Xenophobia', in P. Hainsworth (ed.) *The Politics of the Extreme Right: From the Margins to the Mainstream,* London: Pinter/Cassell (in press).

Grytten, O. H. (1995) 'Dagens og mellomkrigstidens arbeidsledighet i Norge i et vesteuropeisk perspektiv', *Tidsskrift for samfunnsforskning* 36 (2): 198–230.

Gundelach, P. and Riis O. (1992) *Danskernes værdier,* Copenhagen: Forlaget Sociologi.

Gustafsson, B. (1987a) *Ett decennium av stagnerande realinkomster* (A Decade of Stagnating Real Income), Stockholm: Statistiska Centralbyrån, Levnadsförhållanden, Rapport 54.

Gustafsson, B. (1987b) *Den offentliga sektorn – fördelningsaspekter* (The Public Sector – Distributional Aspects), Bilaga 20 till LU 87, Stockholm.

Gustafsson, B. and Johansson, M. (1997) 'In Search of a Smoking Gun – What Makes Income Inequality Vary Over Time and Across Countries?' Revised version of paper presented at the Tenth Anniversary Meeting of the European Society of Population Economics, Uppsala, Sweden, June 1996.

Gustafsson, B. and Palmer, E. (1997) 'Changes in Swedish Inequality: A Study of Equivalent Income 1975–1991', in P. Gottschalk, B. Gustafsson and E. Palmer (eds) *The Changed Distribution of Well-Being: International Aspects,* Cambridge: Cambridge University Press.

Gustafsson, B., Tasiran, A. and Nyman, H. (1997) 'Single Parent Families and Social Security – The Case of Sweden', in P. R. de Jong and and T. R. Marmor (eds) *Social Policy and the Labour Market. Volume Two.* International Studies on Social Security, Aldershot: Ashgate.

Gustafsson, B. and Uusitalo, H. (1990) 'Income Distribution and Redistribution During Two Decades', in I. Persson (ed.) *Generating Equality in the Welfare State,* Oslo: Norwegian University Press.

Habermas, J. (1975) *Legitimation Crisis,* London: Heinemann.

Hadenius, S. (1996) *Svensk politik under 1900-talet – konflikt och samförstånd,* Stockholm: Tiden Athena.

Halleröd, B. (1991) *Den svenska fattigdomen: en studie av fattigdom och socialbidragstagande,* Lund: Arkiv.

Halleröd, B. (1995) 'The Truly Poor: Indirect and Direct Measurement of Consensual Poverty in Sweden', *Journal of European Social Policy* 5 (2): 111–29.

Hallvarsson, M. (1994) *Välfärd och levnadsvillkor i Västeuropa.* Bilaga 9 till EG-konsekvensutredningen, samhällsekonomi; EG-konsekvensutredningen, social välfärd och jämställdhet, Stockholm.

Halvorsen, R. (1996) *Grunnbok i helse – og sosialpolitikk,* Oslo: Tano.

Hansen, E. Boll and Platz, M. (1995) *80–100-åriges levevilkår,* Copenhagen: Amterne og Kommunernnes Forskningsinstitut and Socialforskningsinstituttet.

Hatland, A. and Skevik, A. (1996) 'Changes in the Family', paper presented at the European Institute of Social Security's international colloquium 'The New Social Risks', at the University of Nantes, 3–5 October 1996.

Hedengren, G. (1994) *Vad händer inom barnomsorgen?,* VälfärdsBulletinen, No. 6.

Hedström, P. and Ringen, S. (1990) 'Age and Income in Contemporary Society', in T. Smeeding, M. O'Higgins and L. Rainwater (eds) *Poverty,*

282   *References*

Inequality and Income Distribution in Comparative Perspective, London: Harvester Wheatsheaf.

Heikkilä, M. (1991) 'Poverty and Accumulation of Welfare Deficit', in J. Lehto (ed.) *Deprivation, Social Welfare and Expertise*, Research Report No. 7, Helsinki: National Agency for Welfare and Health.

Heikkilä, M., Hänninen, S., Karjalainen, J., Kontula, O. and Koskela, K. (1994) *Nälkä* (Hunger), STM, Stakes, Raportteja (Reports) 153.

Heikkilä, M. and Uusitalo, H. (1997a) 'Postscript: Summary and Interpretations,' in M. Heikkilä and H. Uusitalo (eds) *The Cost of Cuts: Studies on Cutbacks in Social Security and their Effects in the Finland of the 1990s*, Helsinki: Stakes.

Heikkilä, M. and Uusitalo, H. (eds) (1997b) *The Cost of Cuts: Studies on Cutbacks in Social Security and their Effects in the Finland of the 1990s*. Helsinki: Stakes.

Hellevik, O. (1992) *Introduction to Causal Analysis*, Oslo: Scandinavian University Press.

Henrekson, M. (1996) 'Sweden's Relative Economic Performance: Lagging behind or Staying on Top?', *The Economic Journal* 106 (November): 1747–59.

Hernes, H. (1987a) *Welfare State and Woman Power*. Oslo: Universitetsforlaget.

Hernes, H. (1987b) 'Women and the Welfare State: the Transition from Private to Public Dependence', in A. Showstack Sassoon (ed.) *Women and the State*, London: Hutchinson.

Hernes, H. (1988) 'Scandinavian Citizenship', *Acta Sociologica* 31 (3): 199–215.

Hernes, T. (1995) 'Employment and Rehabilitation of People with Disabilities', in S. Bengtsson *Employment of Persons with Disabilities*, Copenhagen: Socialforskningsinstituttet.

Hoem, B. (1996) 'Some features of recent demographic trends in Sweden'. paper presented to the 30th Arbeitstagung der Deutschen Gesellschaft für Bevölkerungswissenschaft, Walferdange, Luxemburg, 11 April 1996. Stockholm Research Reports in Demography, No. 104, April 1996.

Hougaard Jensen, S. E. and Nielsen, S. B. (1995) 'Demographic Transition and Old Age Provision in Denmark', in C. Lundh (ed.) *Demography, Economy and Welfare. Scandinavian Population Studies, Vol. 10*, Lund Studies in Economic History 1, Lund: Lund University Press.

Hvinden, B. (1994) *Divided Against Itself*, Oslo: Scandinavian University Press.

Inglehart, R. (1990) *Cultural Shift in Advanced Industrial Society*, Princeton: Princeton University Press.

Janoski, T. (1994) 'Direct State Intervention in the Labour Market', in T. Janoski and A. M. Hicks (eds) *The Comparative Political Economy of the Welfare State*, Cambridge: Cambridge University Press.

Jansson J.-M. (1992) *Från splittring till samverkan – Parlamentarismen i Finland*, Söderström & C:O Förlags AB, Stockholm.

Jansson, K. (1990) *Inkomst och förmögenhetsfördelningen 1967–1987* (The

Distribution of Income and Wealth 1967–1987), Stockholm: Bilaga 19 till LU 90.

Jansson, K. and Sandkqvist, A. (1993) *Inkomstfördelningen under 1980–talet* (Income Distribution During the 1980s), Stockholm: Bilaga 19 till LU 92.

Jäntti, M. (1997) 'Inequality in Five Countries in the 1980s: The Role of Demographic Shifts, Market and Government Policies', *Economica* 64: 415–40.

Jäntti, M. and Ritakallio, V.-M. (1997) 'Income Inequality and Poverty in Finland in the 1980s', in P. Gottschalk, B. Gustafsson and E. Palmer (eds) *The Changed Distribution of Well-Being – International Aspects*, Cambridge: Cambridge University Press.

Jenkins, S. P. (1995) 'Accounting for Inequality Trends: Decomposition Analyses for the UK, 1971–86', *Economica* 62: 29–63.

Jensen, P. H. (1996) *Komparative velfærdssystemer*, Copenhagen: Nyt fra Samfundsvidenskaberne.

Johannesson, J. (1995) 'Microeconomic Evaluations of Labour Market Policy Measures in Sweden', in J. Johannesson and E. Wadensjö (eds) *Labour Market Policy at the Crossroads*, Stockholm: EFA, The Ministry of Labour.

Johansson, S. (1979) *Mot en teori för social rapportering* (Towards a Theory of Social Reporting), Stockholm: Swedish Institute for Social Research.

Joppke, C. (1987) 'The Crisis of the Welfare State, Collective Consumption and the Rise of New Social Actors', *Berkeley Journal of Sociology* 32: 237–60.

Julkunen, I. (1996) 'Youth Unemployment and Processes of Marginalisation in the Nordic Countries,' paper presented at the 27th ICSW International Conference, 29 July–3 August 1996.

Kampmann, P. and von Nordheim Nielsen, F. (1995) *Tal om børn*, Copenhagen: Det Tværministerielle Børneudvalg.

Kangas, O. (1994) 'The Merging of Welfare State Models? Past and Present Trends in Finnish and Swedish Social Policy', *Journal of European Social Policy*, 4 (2): 79–94.

Kangas, O. and Ritakallio, V.-M. (1996) Eri menetelmät – eri tulokset? Köyhyyden monimuotoisuus (Different Methods, Different Results? The Many Shapes of Poverty) in O. Kangas and V.-M. Ritakallio (eds) *Kuka on köyhä? Köyhyys 1990–luvun puolivälin Suomessa* (Who is Poor? Poverty in the mid-1990s in Finland). Turun yliopisto, sosiaalipolitiikan laitos. Stakes, Tutkimuksia (Research reports) 65.

Karvonen, L. and Selle, P. (eds) (1995) *Women in Nordic Politics: Closing the Gap*, Aldershot: Dartmouth.

Kautto, M. (ed.) (1997) *European Social Services – Policies and Priorities to the Year 2000*. A report from a European expert meeting on social care services: policies and priorities to the year 2000. Stakes, Ministry of social affairs and health, Finland, Saarijärvi: Gummerus.

Kjoeller, M., Rasmussen, N. K., Keiding, L., Petersen, H. C. and Nielsen, G. A. (1995) *Sundhed og Sygelighed i Danmark 1994 – og udviklingen siden*

1987 (Health and Morbidity in Denmark 1994 – and the Development since 1987), Copenhagen: The Danish Institute for Clinical Epidemiology.

Klavus, J. and Häkkinen, U. (1995) *Terveyspalvelujen käyttö, rahoitus ja tulonjako.* Stakes, raportteja 175, Jyväskylä.

Klein, R. (1993) 'O'Goffe's Tale, or What Can We Learn from the Success of the Capitalist Welfare States?', in C. Jones (ed.) *New Perspectives on the Welfare State in Europe,* London: Routledge.

Klevmarken, A. and Olovsson, P. (1994) *Direct and Behavioral Effects of Income Tax Changes – Simulations with the Swedish Model MICROHUS,* Uppsala University, Department of Economics, Working Papers Series, 1994: 20.

Kolberg, J. E. (ed.) (1991) *The Welfare State as Employer,* Armonk: M. E. Sharpe.

Kolberg, J. E. (ed.) (1992a) *The Study of Welfare State Regimes,* Armonk: M. E. Sharpe.

Kolberg, J. E. (ed.) (1992b) *Between Work and Social Citizenship,* Armonk: M.E. Sharpe.

Kolberg, J. E. and Pettersen, P. A. (1981) 'Om velferdsstatens politiske basis', *Tidsskrift for samfunnsforskning,* 22: 193–222.

Korpi, W. (1983) *The Democratic Class Struggle,* London: Routledge.

Korpi, W. (1985) 'Economic Growth and the Welfare State – Leaky Bucket or Irrigation System?', *European Sociological Review* 1 (2): 97–112.

Korpi, W. (1988) 'Makt, politik och statsautonomi i det social medborgarskapets framväxt', *Sociologisk Forskning* 25 (4): 3–34.

Korpi, W. (1996) 'Eurosclerosis and the Sclerosis of Objectivity: On the Role of Values among Economic Policy Experts', *The Economic Journal* 106 (November), 1727–46.

Korpi, W. and Palme, J. (forthcoming) 'The Paradox of Redistribution and Strategies of Equality: Welfare State Institutions, Inequality and Poverty in the Western Countries', *American Sociological Review.*

Koskinen, S. (1997) *Written Comments to M. Vaarama and M. Kautto (1998): Social Protection for the Elderly in Finland,* Stakes reports at the seminar on 'The state of the debate on social protection for dependency in old age in the 15 EU member states and Norway', arranged at Leuven, Belgium, 27–28 January 1997.

Koslowski, P. (1997) 'Restructuring the Welfare State: Introduction', in P. Koslowski and A. Føllesdal (eds) *Restructuring the Welfare State: Theory and Reform of Social Policy,* Berlin-Heidelberg: Springer.

Koslowski, P. and Føllesdal, A. (eds) (1997) *Restructuring the Welfare State: Theory and Reform of Social Policy,* Berlin-Heidelberg: Springer.

Kosonen, P. (1994a) *European Integration: A Welfare State Perspective,* Helsinki: University of Helsinki, Sociology of Law Series No. 8.

Kosonen, P. (1994b) 'National Welfare States and Economic Integration in Europe', in P. Kosonen and P. Konsghöj Madsen (eds) *Convergence or*

Divergence? Welfare States Facing the European Integration, Brussels: European Commission.

Kosunen, V. (1997) 'The Recession and Changes in Social Security in the 1990s', in M. Heikkilä and H. Uusitalo (eds) *The Cost of Cuts: Studies on Cutbacks in Social Security and their Effects in the Finland of the 1990s*, Helsinki: STAKES report 208.

Kruse, A. (1995) 'An Ageing Population, Public Expenditure and the Pension System in Sweden', in C. Lundh (ed.) *Demography, Economy and Welfare. Scandinavian Population Studies, Vol. 10*, Lund Studies in Economic History 1, Lund: Lund University Press.

Kuhnle, S. (1996) 'Political Reconstruction of the European Welfare State', paper presented at the International Symposium on 'The Welfare State Reconsidered', Tokyo (unpublished).

Labour Market Studies Sweden (1997) *Employment and Social Affairs*, Brussels: European Commission.

Lafferty, W. (1988) 'Offentlig-sektorklassen', in H. Bogen and O. Lageland (eds) *Offentlig eller privat?*, Oslo: FAFO.

Lahelma, E., Manderbacka, K., Rahkonen, O. and Sihvonen, A.P. (1993) *Ill-health and its Social Patterning in Finland, Norway and Sweden*, STAKES, Jyväskylä.

Lahelma, E., Rahkonen, O. and Huuhka, M. (1997) 'Changes in the Social Patterning of Health? The Case of Finland 1986–1994', *Social Science & Medicine* 44: 789–800.

Lane, J-E., Martikainen, T., Svensson, P., Vogt, G. and Valen, H. (1993) 'Scandinavian Exceptionalism Reconsidered', *Journal of Theoretical Politics* 5 (2): 195–230.

Layard, R., Nickell, S. J. and Jackman, R. (1991) *Unemployment*, Oxford: Oxford University Press.

Layard, R., Nickell, S. J. and Jackman, R. (1994) *The Unemployment Crisis*, Oxford: Oxford University Press.

Lazar, H. and Stoyko, P. (1997) *Perspectives on the Future of Developed Social Security Systems*, Geneva: International Social Security Association.

le Grand, C. (1994) 'Löneskillnaderna i Sverige' in J. Fritzell and O. Lundberg (eds) *Vardagens villkor. Levnadsförhållanden i Sverige under tre decennier*, Stockholm: Brombergs.

Lehto, J. (1995) 'Adaptation or a New Strategy? Finnish Local Welfare State in the 1990s', in *Finnish Local Government in Transition*, The Finnish Association of Local Government Studies, No. 4.

Lehto, J. (1997) 'Rahoituksen ja rakenteen muutoksia sosiaali- ja terveyspalveluissa' (Changes in Financing and Structures of the Social and Health Care Services), in H. Uusitalo and M. Staff (eds) *Sosiaali- ja terveydenhuollon palvelukatsaus 1997* (Survey of Social and Health Care Services in Finland in 1997), Stakes, raportteja 214, Jyväskylä.

Lehto, J., Aalto, A.-R., Päivärinta, E. and Järvinen, A. (1997) *Mistä apu ikääntyneille?* (Where to Get Help for the Elderly?), Stakes, aiheita 19, Helsinki.

Leibfried, S. (1992) 'Towards a European Welfare State? On Integrating Poverty Regimes into the European Community', in Z. Ferge and J. E. Kolberg (eds) *Social Policy in a Changing Europe*, European Centre for Social Welfare Policy and Research, Campus/westview, Frankfurt Am Main/Boulder, Colorado.

Leira, A. (1993) 'Mothers, Markets and the State: A Scandinavian Model?', *Journal of Social Policy* 22: 3.

Lindbeck, A., Molander, P., Persson, M., Peterson, O., Sandmo, A., Swedenborg, B. and Thygesen, N. (1995) *Turning Sweden Around*, Cambridge, MA: MIT Press.

Lindqvist, R. and Marklund, S. (1995) 'Forced to Work and Liberated from Work. Historical Perspective on Work and Welfare in Sweden', *Scandinavian Journal of Social Welfare* 4: 224–37.

Lødemel, I. (1994) 'Recent Trends in Cash Benefits: Norway', in N. Ploug and J. Kvist (eds) *Recent Trends in Cash Benefits in Europe*, Copenhagen: The Danish National Institute of Social Research.

Lundberg, O. (1990) *Den Ojämliga Ohälsan – Om Klass- och Könsskillnader i Sjuklighet*, Stockholm: Almquist & Wiksell International.

Lundberg, O. and Manderbacka, K. (1996) 'Assessing Reliability of a Measure of Self-Rated Health', *Scandinavian Journal of Social Medicine* 24: 218–24.

Lunt, N. and Thornton, P. (1993) *Employment Policies for Disabled People: A Review of Legislation and Services in Fifteen Countries*, University of York/London: Social Policy Research Unit/Employment Department.

Maaseide, P. (1990) 'Health and Social Inequity in Norway', *Social Science and Medicine* 31: 331–42.

Mac Cárthaigh, Seosamh (1994) *Resources, Deprivation and Poverty*, Working Paper, Department of Social Policy and Social Work, Dublin: University College, Dublin.

Madsen, M., Folmer Andersen, T., Roestorff, C., Jörgensen, S., Keskimäki, I., Johnsson, M., Paulson, E. and Bay Nielsen, H. (1994) *Rates of Surgery in the Nordic Countries*, Copenhagen: Danish Institute for Clinical Epidemiology.

Mannila, S. (1995) 'Subsidised Employment for Finnish Disabled Jobseekers?', in S. Bengtsson (ed.) *Employment of Persons with Disabilities*, Copenhagen: Socialforskningsinstituttet.

Marklund, S. (1988) *Paradise Lost? The Nordic Welfare States and the Recession 1975–1985*, Lund: Arkiv.

Marklund, S. and Svallfors, S. (1987) *Dual Welfare – Segmentation and Work Enforcement in the Swedish Welfare System*, Department of Sociology, University of Umeå, Research Reports No. 94.

Martikainen, P. T. and Valkonen, T. (1996) 'Excess Mortality of Unemployed

Men and Women during a Period of Rapidly Increasing Unemployment', *Lancet* 348: 909–12.

Matheson, G. (1993) 'The Decommodified in a Commodified World', unpublished PhD Thesis, University of New England, Armidale.

Meisaari-Polsa, T. and Söderström, L. (1995) 'Recent Swedish Fertility Changes in Perspective', in C. Lundh (ed.) *Demography, Economy and Welfare. Scandinavian Population Studies, Vol. 10*, Lund Studies in Economic History 1, Lund: Lund University Press.

Melkas, J. (1993) 'Changing Patterns of Social Relations', in E. J. Hansen, S. Ringen, H. Uusitalo and R. Erikson (eds) *Welfare Trends in the Scandinavian Countries. Part III: Income and Poverty, Part IV: Social Trends, International Journal of Sociology* Summer–Fall 1993, 23 (2–3).

Midre, G. (1995) *Bot, bedring eller brød?* Oslo: Universitetsforlaget.

Miettinen, A. (1997) *Work and Family*, Finnish Institute for Population Research, Working paper E2/1997.

Millar, J. and Warman, A. (1996) *Family Obligations in Europe*, Family and Parenthood, Policy and Practice. Family Policy Studies Centre, November 1996, London.

Ministry of Finance, Sweden (1996) *Fördelningspolitisk redogörelse* (Report on redistributional policies), Prop. 1996/97: 1, Bilaga 1 (Bill to the Parliament), Stockholm.

Ministry of Labour and Ministry of Finance, Denmark (1996) *Labour Market Policy in Transition*, May 1996.

Ministry of Labour, Denmark (1996) *The Danish Labour Market Model and Developments in the Labour Market Policy*, Arbejdsministeriet, June 1996.

Ministry of Labour, Finland (1995) *Operational Programme for the Community Initiative Employment in Finland 1995–1999*. 17 September 1995.

Ministry of Social Affairs, Denmark (1990) *Der er brug for alle. Nye veje til nye muligheder*, Copenhagen: Socialministeriet, 3 April 1990.

Ministry of Social Affairs, Denmark (1995) *Our Common Concern – An Initiative to Promote the Business Sector's Social Commitment*, Copenhagen: Socialministeriet, February 1995.

Narud, H. M. (1995) 'Coalition Termination in Norway: Model and Cases', *Scandinavian Political Studies* 18: 1–24.

Nikander, T. (1997) 'Katsaus viime vuosien perheellistymiseen Suomessa' (A look at families during recent years in Finland), *Hyvinvointikatsaus* 2/1997.

Nolan, B. (1986) 'Unemployment and the Size Distribution of Income', *Economica* 53: 421–45.

Nolan, B. and Whelan, C. T. (1996) *Resources, Deprivation and the Measurement of Poverty*, Oxford: Oxford University Press.

NOMESCO (36: 1991) *Health Statistics in the Nordic Countries 1966–1991*, Nordic Medico Statistical Committee, Copenhagen: Nordic Council of Ministers.

NOMESCO (38: 1992) *Health Statistics in the Nordic Countries 1990*, Nordic Medico Statistical Committee, Copenhagen: Nordic Council of Ministers.

NOMESCO (1996) *Health Statistics in the Nordic Countries 1994*, Nordic Medico Statistical Committee, Copenhagen: Nordic Council of Ministers.

NOMESCO (49: 1997) *Health Statistics in the Nordic Countries 1995*, Nordic Medico Statistical Committee, Copenhagen: Nordic Council of Ministers.

Nord (1986: 5) *Yearbook of Nordic Statistics 1986*, Vol. 25, edited by the Nordic Statistical Secretariat, Stockholm: Nordic Council of Ministers 1987.

Nord (1987: 73) *Yearbook of Nordic Statistics 1987*, Vol. 26, edited by the Nordic Statistical Secretariat, Stockholm: Nordic Council of Ministers 1988.

Nord (1991: 1) *Yearbook of Nordic Statistics 1991*, Vol. 29, edited by the Nordic Statistical Secretariat, Stockholm: Nordic Council of Ministers.

Nord (1992: 1) *Yearbook of Nordic Statistics 1992*, Vol. 30, edited by the Nordic Statistical Secretariat, Stockholm: Nordic Council of Ministers.

Nord (1993: 1) *Yearbook of Nordic Statistics 1993*, Vol. 31, edited by the Nordic Statistical Secretariat, Århus: Nordic Council of Ministers.

Nord (1994: 3) *Women and Men in the Nordic Countries. Facts and Figures 1994*, Copenhagen: Nordic Council of Ministers.

Nord (1995: 1) *Yearbook of Nordic Statistics 1995*, Vol. 33, edited by the Nordic Statistical Secretariat, Århus: Nordic Council of Ministers.

Nord (1996: 1) *Yearbook of Nordic Statistics 1996*, Vol. 34, edited by the Nordic Statistical Secretariat, Århus: Nordic Council of Ministers.

Nordic Statistical Secretariat (1984) *Social Security in the Nordic Countries*, Copenhagen.

Nordic Statistical Secretariat (1987) *Social Security in the Nordic Countries*, Helsinki.

Nordic Statistics on CD-ROM (1996) Danmarks Statistik, Tilastokeskus Suomi, Hagstova Foroya, Gronlands Statistik, Hagstofa Íslands, Statistisk sentralbyrå, Norge, Statistiska centralbyrån, Sverige, Nordiska statistiska sekretariet.

Nordisk Ministerråd (1997) *Budgetkonsolidering i de nordiska länderna*, Köpenhamn: Nordisk Ministerråd.

Nordlund, A. (1997) 'Attitudes towards the Welfare State in the Scandinavian countries', *Scandinavian Journal of Social Welfare* 6: 233–46.

NOSOSCO (1993) *Social Security in the Nordic Countries. Scope, Expenditure and Financing 1990*, Nordic Social-Statistical Committee, Statistical reports of the Nordic Countries 59, Nordic Council of Ministers.

NOSOSCO (2: 1995) *Social Security in the Nordic Countries. Scope, Expenditure and Financing 1993*, Nordic Social-Statistical Committee, Nordic Council of Ministers.

NOSOSCO (6: 1997) *Social tryghed i de nordiske lande 1995* (Social Security in the Nordic Countries), Nordic Social-Statistical Committee, Copenhagen: Nordic Council of Ministers.

NOU (1993) *Levekår i Norge, Er graset grønt for alle?*, Norges offentlige utredninger 1993: 17. Oslo.

NOU (1994): Fra arbeid til pensjon, NOU 1994: 2, Oslo, appendix to St.meld.nr.35.

NOU (1996) *Offentlige overføringer til barnefamilier*, Norges offentlige utredninger, Oslo.

Nyfigen (1997) *Ökonomiske styringsredskaber i sygehusväsenet i Danmark*. Vol. 8, June.

O'Connor, J. (1973) *The Fiscal Crisis of the Welfare State*, New York: St. James Press.

OECD (1990a) *Labour Market Policies for the 1990s*, Paris: OECD.

OECD (1990b) *Lone-Parent Families. The Economic Challenge*, Social Policy Studies No. 8, Paris: OECD.

OECD (1993) 'Active Labour Market Policies: Assessing Macroeconomic and Microeconomic Effects', *Employment Outlook*, Paris: OECD.

OECD (1994a) *Employment Outlook*, July 1994, Paris: OECD.

OECD (1994b) *New Orientations for Social Policy*, Social Policy Studies No. 12, Paris: OECD.

OECD (1995a) *The OECD Jobs Study: Implementing the Strategy*, Paris: OECD.

OECD (1995b) *Labour Force Statistics 1973–1993*, Paris: OECD.

OECD (1996a) *Employment Outlook*, July 1996, Paris: OECD.

OECD (1996b) *OECD Economic Outlook 59*, June 1996, Paris: OECD.

OECD (1996c) *Social Expenditure Statistics of OECD Member Countries, Provisional Version*, Labour Market and Social Policy Occasional Papers No. 17, Paris: OECD.

OECD (1996d) *OECD Economic Surveys. Denmark.* Paris: OECD.

OECD (1996e) *Labour Force Statistics 1974–1994.* Paris: OECD, Statistics Directorate.

OECD (1997) *OECD Statistics CD ROM*, November 1997, Paris: OECD.

OECD (1997a) *OECD Employment Outlook 60,* July 1997, Paris: OECD.

OECD (1997b) *OECD Economic Surveys. Finland.* Paris: OECD.

OECD (1997f) *Health Data.* Paris: OECD.

Østby, L. (1993) 'Main Demographic Trends', in E.J. Hansen, S. Ringen, H. Uusitalo and R. Erikson (eds) *Welfare Trends in the Scandinavian Countries. Part III: Income and Poverty, Part IV: Social Trends, International Journal of Sociology* Summer–Fall 1993, 23 (2–3).

Øverbye, E. (1995) 'The New Zealand Pension System in an International Context, with Special Reference to the Scandinavian Cases', paper presented at NOPSA Conference, Helsinki, 15–17 August 1996, Oslo: INAS.

Øverbye, E. (1997) *Preretirement in the Nordic countries in a European Context,* NOVA Skriftserie 3/97, Norsk institutt for forskning on oppvekst, velferd og aldring.

Offe, C. (1984) *The Contradictions of the Welfare State*, London: Hutchinson.

Orloff, A. S. (1993) 'Gender and the Social Rights of Citizenship. The Comparative Analysis of Gender Relations and Welfare States', *American Sociological Review* 58: 303–28.

Page, B. I. and Shapiro, R. Y. (1984) 'Effects of Public Opinion on Policy', *American Political Science Review* 77: 175–190.

Palme, J. (1994) 'Recent Developments in Income Transfer Systems in Sweden', in N. Ploug and J. Kvist (eds) *Recent Trends in Cash Benefits in Europe*, Copenhagen: The Danish National Institute of Social Research.

Palme, J. and Wennemo, I. (1997) *Swedish Social Security in the 1990s: Reform and Retrenchment*, CWR Working Paper 9, Centre for Welfare State Research, Copenhagen: The Danish National Institute of Social Research.

Pedersen, P. J. and Smith, N. (1995) *Trends in the Danish Income Distribution, 1976–90*, Mimeo, Centre for Labour Market and Social Research, University of Aarhus.

Petersen, E. *et al.* (1987) *Danskernes tilværelse under krisen, I-II*. Aarhus: Aarhus University Press.

Petersen, E. *et al.* (1996) *Danskernes trivsel, holdninger og selvansvarlighed under 'opsvinget'. Træk af den politisk-psykologiske udvikling 1982-86-88-90-94*. Århus: Psykologisk Institut, Aarhus Universitet, i komm. hos Aarhus Universitetsforlag.

Petersson, O. (1995) *Nordisk Politik*, Stockholm: Fritzes Förlag AB.

Pettersen, P. A. (1995) 'The Welfare State: The Security Dimension', in O. Borre and E. Scarbrough (eds) *The Scope of Government*, Oxford: Oxford University Press.

Pettersen, P. A. (1997) *Welfare State Legitimacy: Ranking-Rating-Paying: the Popularity and Support for Norwegian Welfare Programs*, Dragvoll: Department of Sociology and Political Science, Norwegian University of Science and Technology.

Pfaller, A. and Gough, I. (1991) 'The Competitiveness of Industrial Welfare States: A Cross-Country Survey', in A. Pfaller, I. Gough and G. Therborn (eds) *Can the Welfare State Compete? A Comparative Study of Five Advanced Capitalist Countries*, Basingstoke: Macmillan.

Pfaller, A., Gough, I. and Therborn, G. (eds) (1991) *Can the Welfare State Compete? A Comparative Study of Five Advanced Capitalist Countries*, Basingstoke: Macmillan.

Pierson, C. (1991) *Beyond the Welfare State: A New Political Economy of Welfare*, Oxford: Polity Press.

Pierson, P. (1994) *Dismantling the Welfare State: Reagan, Thatcher and the Politics of Retrenchment*, Cambridge: Cambridge University Press.

Pierson, P. (1996) 'The New Politics of the Welfare State', *World Politics* 48: 143-79.

Piven, F. F. (1985) 'Women and the State: Ideology, Power, and the Welfare State', in A. S. Rossi (ed.) *Gender and the Life Course*, New York: Aldine.

Ploug, N. and Kvist, J. (1997) *Overførselsindkomster i Europa. Systemerne i tal*. Social tryghed i Europa 3, Copenhagen: Socialforskningsinstituttet.

Plovsing, J. (1994) 'Social Security in Denmark – Renewal of the Welfare State', in N. Ploug and J. Kvist (eds) *Recent Trends in Cash Benefits in*

Europe. Social Security in Europe 4, Copenhagen: The Danish Institute of Social Research.

Pöntinen, S. and Uusitalo, H. (1986) *The Legitimacy of the Welfare State: Social Security Opinions in Finland 1975–1985,* The Finnish Suomen Gallup Inc Report. No. 15.

Puide, A. (1996) *Den nordiska fattigdomens utveckling och struktur,* (The Development and Structure of Poverty in the Nordic Countries) Köpenhamn: Nordiska ministerrådet, TemaNord 1996: 583.

Ramm, J. (1997) 'God helse, flere sykdommer', *Samfunnsspeilet* 11: 4–9.

Rauhala, P-L. with Andersson, M., Eydal, G., Ketola, O. and Warming Nielsen, H. (1997) 'Why are Social Care Services a Gender Issue?', in J. Sipilä (ed.) *Social Care Services: The Key to the Scandinavian Welfare Model,* Aldershot: Avebury.

Recent Demographic Developments in Europe (1996), Council of Europe. Strasbourg: Council of Europe Publishing.

Recent Demographic Developments in Europe (1997), Council of Europe. Strasbourg: Council of Europe Publishing.

Report to Parliament (1996) *Norwegian Labour Market Policy 1997,* Summary of report No. 1 to the Norwegian Parliament (1996/1997), Oslo.

Rhodes, M. (1996) 'Globalization and West European Welfare States: A Critical Review of Recent Debates', *Journal of European Social Policy* 6 (4): 305–27.

Rikstrygdeverket (1991–94) *Trygdestatistisk årbok,* Oslo: Rikstrygdeverket.

Ringen, S. (1987) *The Possibility of Politics: A Study in the Political Economy of the Welfare State,* Oxford: Clarendon Press.

Ringen, S. (1991) 'Households, Standards of Living, and Inequality', *Review of Income and Wealth* 37: 1–13.

Ringen, S. and Uusitalo, H. (1992) 'Income Distribution in the Nordic Welfare States', in J. E. Kolberg (ed.) *The Study of Welfare State Regimes,* Armonk: M. E. Sharpe.

Rogoff Ramsøy, N. (1987) 'From Necessity to Choice: Social Change in Norway 1930–1980', in R. Erikson, E. J. Hansen, S. Ringen and H. Uusitalo (eds) *The Scandinavian Model: Welfare States and Welfare Research,* Armonk: M. E. Sharpe.

Room, G. (1995) *Beyond the Threshold: The Measurement and Analysis of Social Exclusion,* Bristol: The Policy Press.

Rose, R. (1989) *Ordinary People in Public Policy: A Behavioural Analysis,* London: Sage.

Rostgaard, T. (1996) 'Social Services – A Challenge to the Nordic Welfare Model?' paper presented at ISA Research Committee 19 in Canberra, 19–23 August 1996.

Saltman, R. and von Otter, C. (1992) *Planned Markets and Public Competition,* Buckingham: Open University Press.

Scarpetta, S. (1996) 'Assessing the Role of Labour Market Policies and

Institutional Settings on Unemployment: A Cross-country Study', *OECD Economic Studies* 26(1): 43–98.

Schulte, B. (1996) 'Social Protection for Dependence in Old Age: The Case of Germany', in R. Eisen and F. A. Sloan (eds) *Developments in Health Economics and Public Policy, Volume 5. Long-Term Care: Economic Issues and Policy Solutions,* Dordrecht: Kluwer Academic Publishers.

Schwanse, P. (1997) 'Activating the Unemployed', *The OECD Observer* 209: 10–12.

Schwarz, B. and Gustafsson, B. (1991) 'Income Redistribution Effects of Tax Reforms in Sweden', *Journal of Policy Modelling* 13: 551–70.

Scott, M. B. and Lyman, S. M. (1968) 'Accounts', *American Sociological Review* 33: 46–62.

Sihvo, T. (1997) 'The Consumption Patterns of Low-Income Groups in 1990–1994', in M. Heikkilä and H. Uusitalo (eds) *The Cost of Cuts. Studies on Cutbacks in Social Security and their Effects in the Finland of the 1990s,* Helsinki: Stakes.

Sihvo, T. and Uusitalo, H. (1995) 'Attitudes towards the Welfare State have Several Dimensions. Evidence from Finland', *Scandinavian Journal of Social Welfare* 4: 215–23.

Silver, H. (1994) 'Social Exclusion and Social Solidarity: Three Paradigms', *International Labour Review* 133 (5–6): 531–78.

Sipilä, J. (ed.) (1997) *Social Care Services: The Key to the Scandinavian Welfare Model,* Aldershot: Avebury.

Smart, C. (1997) 'Wishful Thinking and Harmful Tinkering? Sociological Reflections on Family Policy', *Journal of Social Policy* 26 (3).

Social Portrait of Europe (1996), Eurostat, Office for Official Publications of the European Communities, Luxemburg.

Social Security in the Nordic Countries (1996), Copenhagen: Nordiska Ministerrådet.

Socialstatistik (1996) *Den sociale resourceopgørelse 18 januar 1995,* Copenhagen: Danmarks Statistik.

Socialstyrelsen (1996a) *Social service, vård och omsorg i Sverige 1996,* Stockholm.

Socialstyrelsen (1996b) *Barnomsorg 1995,* Stockholm.

Söderström, L. (1988) *Inkomstfördelning och fördelningspolitik* (Income Distribution and Distributional Policy) Kristianstad: Studieförbundet Näringsliv och Samhälle.

SOTKA Database (1997) Electronic Database on Social and Health Care, Stakes, Helsinki.

SOU (1995: 39) *Some Reflections on Swedish Labour Market Policy,* Stockholm: Blanchflower, Jackman and Saint-Paul.

SOU (1997: 40) *Unga och arbete,* Stockholm: Delbetänkande från ungdomspolitiska kommitt[…].

SOU (1997: 64) *Samhall. En arbetsmarknadspolitisk åtgard,* Stockholm: Slutbetankande av LOSAM-utredningen.

Spånt, R. (1981) 'The Distribution of Income in Sweden, 1920–76', in A. Klevmarken, and J. Lybeck (eds) *The Statics and Dynamics of Income*, Clavedon: Tieto.

SSB (1995) *Barnhager og tilbud til 6–åringer in skolen 1994*, Oslo: Statistisk Sentralbyrå.

SSB (1996) *Barnhager og tilbud til 6–åringer in skolen 1995*, Oslo: Statistisk Sentralbyrå.

STAKES (1996) *Facts about Finnish Social Welfare and Health Care*, Helsinki.

STAKES (1997a) Private social welfare providers in Finland by provinces, private correspondence.

STAKES (1997b) *Facts about Finnish Social Welfare and Health Care*, Helsinki.

Statistics Norway (1996) *Levekårsundersøkelsen 1995*. NOS C301. Oslo: SSB.

Statistics Sweden (1991) *Teknisk rapport avseende 1984–95 års, 1986–87 års och 1988–89 års undersökningar av levnadsförhållanden, Serie Levnadsförhållanden Appendix 13*. Stockholm: SCB.

Statistics Sweden (1996) *The Swedish Survey of Living Conditions, Design and Methods, Series Living Conditions Appendix 16*. Stockholm: Statistics Sweden.

Statistics Sweden (1997a) *Inkomstfördelningsundersökningen 1995* (The Household Income Distribution Survey) Stockholm: Statistiska meddelanden, Be 21 SM 9701.

Statistics Sweden (1997b) *Välfärd och ojämlikhet i 20-årsperspektiv 1975– 1995*, Levnadsförhållanden rapport 91, Stockholm.

Stephens, J. (1979) *The Transition from Capitalism to Socialism*, Basingstoke: Macmillan.

Stephens, J. (1996) 'The Scandinavian Welfare States: Achievements, Crisis and Prospects', in G. Esping-Andersen (ed.) *Welfare States in Transition: National Adaptations in Global Economies*, London: Sage.

STM (1994: 9) *Sosiaalimenotoimikunnan mietintö* (Report of the committee on social expenditure), Ministry of Social Affairs and Health, Publications 1994: 9, Helsinki.

STM (1996) *Terveydenhuollon suuntaviivat*, Helsinki.

STM (1997) *Regeringens proposition til Riksdagen med forslag till en reform av lagstiftningen om stöd för vård av små barn*, Helsinki.

St.meld.nr.4 (1992–93) *Langtidsprogrammet 1994–1997* (Report No. 4 to the Storting (1992–93) Long-Term Programme 1994–1997) Oslo.

St.meld.nr.4 (1996–97) *Langtidsprogrammet 1998–2001*, Oslo 1997.

St.meld.nr.35 (1994) *Velferdsmeldingen* (The White paper on welfare), with two expert committee reports as appendices: NOU 1994: 2 Fra arbeid til pensjon (From Work to Pension) and NOU 1994: 6 Private pensjoner (Private pensions).

Stortinget (1997) *Foreløpig innstilling fra finanskomiteen om Langtidsprogrammet 1998–2001*, Innst.S.nr.211 (1996–97), Oslo.

Ström, S., Wennemo, T. and Aaberge, R. (1993) 'Income Inequality in Norway 1973–1990' (original in Norwegian), Rapporter 93/17, Statistics Norway.

Sundberg, J. (1996) 'Finland', *European Journal of Political Research* 30: 321–30.

Svallfors, S. (1991) 'The Politics of Welfare Policy in Sweden: Structural Determinants and Attitudinal Cleavages', *British Journal of Sociology* 42: 609–34.

Svallfors, S. (1995) 'The End of Class Politics? Structural Cleavages and Attitudes to Swedish Welfare Policies', *Acta Sociologica* 38: 53–74.

Svallfors, S. (1996) *Välfärdsstatens moraliska ekonomi. Välfärdsopinionen i 90-talets Sverige,* Umeå: Boréa.

Svenska Kommunförbundet (1995) *Kommunerna fram till 2020*, Stockholm.

Tåhlin, M. (1990) 'Politics, Dynamics and Individualism', *Social Indicators Research*, 22: 155–80.

Taylor-Gooby, P. (1989) 'The Role of the State', in R.R. Jowell, S. Witherspoon and L. Brook (eds) *British Social Attitudes: Special International Report*, Aldershot: Gower.

Teigum, H. (1992) *Levekårsundersøkelsene 1980, 1983, 1987 og 1991*. Bergen: NSD.

Tham, H. (1994) 'Ökar marginaliseringen i Sverige?', in J. Fritzell and O. Lundberg (eds) *Vardagens villkor*, Stockholm: Brombergs.

Therborn, G. (1995) *European Modernity and Beyond: The Trajectory of European Societies, 1945–2000*, London: Sage.

Thomson, D. (1996) *Selfish Generations? How Welfare States Grow Old*, London: The White Horse Press.

Thornton, P. and Lunt, N. (1997) *Employment Policies for Disabled People in Eighteen Countries: A Review*, University of York: Social Policy Research Unit.

Thornton, P., Sainsbury, R. and Barnes, H. (1997) *Helping Disabled People to Work: A Cross-national Study of Social Security and Employment Provisions*, London: SSAC Research Paper No. 8.

Titmuss, R. (1974) *Social Policy*. London: Allen and Unwin.

Townsend, P. (1979) *Poverty in the United Kingdom*, Harmondsworth: Penguin Books Ltd.

Tsakloglou, P. (1997) 'Changes in Inequality in Greece in the 1970s and the 1980s', in P. Gottschalk, B. Gustafsson and E. Palmer (eds) *The Changed Distribution of Well-Being – International Aspects*, Cambridge: Cambridge University Press.

Unemployment Benefits and Social Assistance in Seven European Countries. A Comparative Study (1995) No. 10. Ministerie van Sociale Zaken en Werkgelegenheid.

Uusitalo, H. (1989) *Income Distribution in Finland. The Effects of the Welfare State and the Structural Changes in Society on Income Distribution in Fin-*

land in 1966–1985, Helsinki: Central Statistical Office of Finland, Studies No. 148.

Uusitalo, H. (1997) 'Four Years of Recession: What Happened to Income Distribution?', in M. Heikkilä and H. Uusitalo (eds) *The Cost of Cuts. Studies on Cutbacks in Social Security and their Effects in the Finland of the 1990s*, Helsinki: Stakes.

Valen, H. (1986) 'The Storting Election of September 1985: The Welfare State under Pressure', *Scandinavian Political Studies* 9: 177–88.

Valen, H. (1990) 'The Storting Election of 1989: Polarisation and Protest', *Scandinavian Political Studies* 13: 277–90.

Valen, H. and Aardal, B. O. (1983) *Et valg i perspectiv – en studie av Stortingsvalget 1981*. Samfunnsøkonomiske studier, 54, Oslo: Statistisk sentralbyrå.

Van Parijs, P. (1987) 'A Revolution in Class Theory', *Politics and Society* 15: 453–82.

Vogel, J. (1990) *Leva i Norden*. Statistical Reports of the Nordic Countries 54, Copenhagen: Nordic Statistical Secretariat.

Vogel, J. (1991) *Social Report for the Nordic Countries. Living Conditions and Inequality in the Late 1980s*, Statistical reports of the Nordic Countries 55, Copenhagen: Nordic Statistical Secretariat.

Vogel, J. (1997) *Living Conditions and Inequality in the European Union 1997*, Eurostat Working Papers E/1997/3, Luxembourg.

Waerness, K. (1987) 'On the Rationality of Caring', in A.S. Sassoon (ed.) *Women and the State*, London: Hutchinson.

Walker, A. and Maltby, T. (1997) *Ageing Europe*, Rethinking Ageing Series. Buckingham: Open University Press.

Walker, R. (1995) 'The Dynamics of Poverty and Social Exclusion', in G. Room (ed.) *Beyond the Threshold: The Measurement and Analysis of Social Exclusion*, Bristol: The Policy Press.

WHO (1996) *European Health Care Reforms: Analysis of Current Strategies*, World Health Organization, Copenhagen: Regional Office for Europe.

Wilensky, H. (1975) *The Welfare State and Equality: Structural and Ideological Roots of Public Expenditures*, Berkeley: University of Califonia Press.

Zamanian, M. (1993) *Jämförande nordisk inkomstfördelningsstatistik (II)*, København: Nordisk statistisk sekreteriat, Tekniska rapporter 58.

Zetterberg, H. (1985) *An Electorate in the Grips of the Welfare State*, Stockholm: Swedish Institute for Opinion Polls.

INDEX